"Dr. Robert Cooper has produced a masterpiece. It is a superb resource for all those interested in the highest level of mental and physical well-being. I recommend it highly."
— **Charles A. Garfield, Ph.D.,** clinical faculty member, University of California Medical School at San Francisco, and author of *Peak Performers: The New Heroes of American Business*

"Based on solid scientific and medical fact. . . . The seven-step *Health & Fitness Excellence* plan enables readers to concentrate on the areas that most interest them."
— *American Journal of Health Promotion*

"That's the key: Make an effort to improve your health, but remember to balance what you do. In his new book, *Health & Fitness Excellence*, Dr. Robert K. Cooper calls it a 'golden circle' made up of exercise, nutrition, fat control, good posture, sensitivity to your environment, and control of stress."
— **Miami Herald**

"At last, a book that looks at the wholeness of the human being while effectively dealing with the fitness of each of the parts. . . . *Health & Fitness Excellence* is a drink of pure water in the polluted desert of health fadism, poor science, and dishonest hucksters."
— **Emmett E. Miller, M.D.,** president, Source Learning Systems, and author of *Letting Go of Stress* and *Optimal Performance*

"This book is all-encompassing . . . every page is a call to action."— *Los Angeles Reader*

"*Health & Fitness Excellence* is . . . for anyone looking to begin, enhance, or complete a wellness plan."
— **Mark J. Tager, M.D.,** president, Great Performance, Inc., and coauthor of *Working Well: Managing for Health and High Performance*

"An excellent new book!"— *Women's Sports & Fitness*

"Nothing's more complete than *Health & Fitness Excellence*. . . . Twenty years in the making, this book shows you how you can adjust your lifestyle for optimal health by utilizing the most forward-looking medical and behavioral advice available."
— *Men's Fitness*

"What makes Dr. Cooper's book different from all the other health and fitness publications flooding the market is his reliance on well-documented studies."
— *Rocky Mountain News*

"Dr. Robert K. Cooper explodes myths and fallacies concerning health and fitness, offering a seven-step approach designed for no-nonsense people with no time to waste."
— *Lincoln Park News-Herald*

"*Health & Fitness Excellence* is vital reading for every health-concerned person."
— **Tom Ferguson, M.D.,** award-winning medical writer and contributing editor to *Prevention*

HEALTH & FITNESS EXCELLENCE

THE Comprehensive Action Plan

Robert K. Cooper, Ph.D.

FOREWORD BY Tom Ferguson, M.D.
PREFACE BY Harold H. Bloomfield, M.D.

HOUGHTON MIFFLIN COMPANY
BOSTON

This book is not intended as a substitute for the medical recommendations of physicians. The author does not directly or indirectly dispense medical advice or prescribe treatment of any kind for illness or disease. The intent is to offer information to help you, the reader, cooperate with your physician and other health professionals in your mutual quest for optimum well-being.

Copyright © 1989 by Robert K. Cooper

For information about permission to reproduce selections from this book, write to Permissions, Houghton Mifflin Company, 2 Park Street, Boston, Massachusetts 02108.

Library of Congress Cataloging-in-Publication Data

Cooper, Robert K.
  Health & fitness excellence: the comprehensive action plan / by Robert K. Cooper; foreword by Tom Ferguson; preface by Harold H. Bloomfield.
    p.   cm.
  Bibliography: p.
  Includes index.
  ISBN 0-395-47589-9
  ISBN 0-395-54453-X (pbk.)
    1. Health. 2. Fitness. I. Title. II. Title: Health and fitness excellence.
RA776.C82 1989   88-25790
613—dc19   CIP

Printed in the United States of America

WAK 10 9 8 7 6 5 4 3 2

Quotations from Joan Borysenko's *Minding the Body, Mending the Mind* are used by permission. Copyright © 1987 Addison-Wesley Publishing Company, Inc., Reading, Massachusetts.

Illustrations by Richard Golueke
Text design by Joyce C. Weston

This book is dedicated
to all those who are aware of the gap
between human potential and human performance
and are willing to act to close it.

Acknowledgments

I am deeply grateful for the insights, inspiration, and/or personal support from the following people who helped my dream of *Health & Fitness Excellence* become a reality:

- My wife, Leslie, for her radiant love and deepest friendship
- My son, Christopher, for his courage and joy and for strengthening my commitment to a brighter future for *all* children
- My father, Dr. Hugh Cooper, who taught me the values of science, common sense, and hard work
- My mother, Margaret D. Cooper, who nurtured my idealism and love for humanity
- My sister, Mary, and brother, David, who stood by me at times when I needed it most
- Tom Ferguson, M.D., for his friendship and leadership in the self-care field and for encouraging my first steps as an author
- Harold H. Bloomfield, M.D., for his friendship, unconditional support, and message to let go of limits and keep seeing the world not just as it *is* but as it *could be*
- Ruth K. Hapgood, my Houghton Mifflin editor, for her exceptional wisdom, enthusiasm, and vision
- Others at Houghton Mifflin — Austin Olney, Jonathan Latimer, Nancy Grant, Steven Lewers, Leslie Breed, Marly Rusoff, Becky Saikia-Wilson, and Barbara Flanagan — for their straightforward advice and support
- Karl H. Pribram, M.D., National Institutes of Health Professor of Neuroscience and Professor of Psychology and Psychiatry at Stanford University, for his friendship and for first inspiring me more than twenty years ago to view human potentials through an integrated scientific perspective
- Emmett E. Miller, M.D., for his friendship, global view of wellness, and the quality and warmth in his cassette publications
- William A. McGarey, M.D., and Gladys T. McGarey, M.D., for their friendship and tireless efforts for holistic medicine and a better world
- Anees A. Sheikh, Ph.D., chairman of the Department of Psychology at Marquette University, for his friendship and leadership role in the scientific validation of mental imagery and its uses to enhance life

▶ Kenneth H. Cooper, M.D., M.P.H., for taking the time to share his latest research findings with me and for bringing health and fitness to a far greater level of public understanding

▶ Mauricio Padilla, M.S., for his friendship and scientific perspectives on nutritional biochemistry

▶ Steve Farrell, M.S., exercise physiologist at the Institute for Aerobics Research, for his suggestions as professional reader of the exercise chapters of this book

▶ Trish Ratto, R.D., of the University of California at Berkeley School of Public Health, for her suggestions as professional reader of the nutrition and body fat control chapters of this book

▶ Michael F. Jacobson, Ph.D., and the staff at the Center for Science in the Public Interest, for putting together so many on-the-mark reports

▶ Sheldon Saul Hendler, M.D., Ph.D., of the University of California at San Diego School of Medicine, for helping chart a sensible, scientific path for nutritional wellness

▶ Herbert Benson, M.D., and Joan Borysenko, Ph.D., of Harvard Medical School, for pioneering mind/body programs that benefit thousands of us every day

▶ Charles Garfield, Ph.D., for uncovering the essence of peak performance

▶ Norman Cousins, for so vividly envisioning a more humanistic system of health care and acting to make it a reality

▶ Kenneth R. Pelletier, Ph.D., for his pioneering insights on stress management, mind-body integration, and wellness

▶ William Hettler, M.D., for being instrumental in creating the National Wellness Institute and National Wellness Association

▶ Judith J. Wurtman, Ph.D., and Richard J. Wurtman, Ph.D., both of MIT, for translating discoveries in neuroendocrinology and nutrition into practical guidelines for all

▶ Michael Yessis, Ph.D., for his views on optimum physical fitness

▶ My initial freelance editors, Harvey L. Cohen and Le Trombetta, who helped shape this book in the preliminary stages of writing

▶ My illustrator, Richard Golueke

I am also especially grateful for encouragement and support from Michael Q. Patton, Ph.D., Sherry Eve Penn, Ph.D., Harold V. McAbee, Ed.D., and Fontaine Maury Belford, Ph.D., all of the Union Graduate School; Steven and LaVerne Ross of the World Research Foundation; Grant M. Christopher, M.D., Bernard Jensen, Ph.D., Bill Pearl, Keith W. Sehnert, M.D., Jean Rosenbaum, M.D., Neil Nathan, M.D., Lee Joseph, M.S., Shari Lieberman, M.A., R.D., Richard L. Crews, M.D., and Les Carr, Ph.D.; and for the research insights and inspiration I have received from other leaders, including Oliver Alabsater, M.D., Robert A.

Anderson, M.D., Robert B. Arnot, M.D., Kenneth Blanchard, Ph.D., Marjorie Blanchard, Ph.D., David Bohm, Ph.D., Nathaniel Branden, Ph.D., Jane E. Brody, Barbara B. Brown, Ph.D., Kelly D. Brownell, Ph.D., David D. Burns, M.D., Leo F. Buscaglia, Ph.D., Rene Cailliet, M.D., Michael Castleman, Dolores Curran, Irving Dardik, M.D., Martha Davis, Ph.D., Edward de Bono, Wayne Dyer, Ed.D., Dean Edell, M.D., Gary Emery, Ph.D., Marilyn Ferguson, Viktor E. Frankl, M.D., Sonya Friedman, Ph.D., Bob Goldman, D.O., Daniel Goleman, Ph.D., Joan Dye Gussow, Ed.D., Frederick Hatfield, Ph.D., Dennis T. Jaffe, Ph.D., Gerald Jampolsky, M.D., Susan Jeffers, Ph.D., Spencer Johnson, M.D., Timothy Johnson, M.D., Blair Justice, Ph.D., Ronald M. Lawrence, M.D., Ph.D., Steven Locke, M.D., James J. Lynch, Ph.D., Salvatore R. Maddi, Ph.D., William A. McArdle, Ph.D., Matthew McKay, Ph.D., Roger C. Mills, Ph.D., Gabe Mirkin, M.D., Rochelle Myers, Joyce D. Nash, Ph.D., David C. Nieman, D.H.Sc., M.P.H., Esther M. Orioli, M.S., Jordan Paul, Ph.D., Margaret Paul, Ph.D., Paul Pearsall, Ph.D., Tom Peters, Lynne Pirie, D.O., Michael Ray, Mike Samuels, M.D., Virginia Satir, Cynthia D. Scott, Ph.D., M.P.H., Bernie S. Siegel, M.D., Charles F. Stroebel, M.D., Ph.D., Rick Suarez, Ph.D., Richard M. Suinn, Ph.D., Mark Tager, M.D., Art Ulene, M.D., Denis Waitley, Ph.D., Roy L. Walford, M.D., Robert Waterman, Jr., Andrew Weil, M.D., Hendrie D. Weisinger, Ph.D., Roger Williams, Ph.D., Larry Wilson, Arthur Winter, M.D., Ruth Winter, Georgia Witkin, Ph.D., and Bernie Zilbergeld, Ph.D.

Finally, I want to thank the thousands of dedicated researchers throughout the world who, with little recognition, regularly bring forth vital revelations; my seminar participants over the past two decades who have believed in my message and never wavered in their support of my work; my martial arts instructors, who helped me draw forth the courage to conquer the challenges in my own life and then reach out to help others; and God and the powers of light and love — may our future as a planet be filled with enlightenment, wellness, cooperation, and peace.

Contents

Foreword

The information age is bringing with it many fundamental changes in the way we think about health and fitness. The old model, in which the professional did everything and the client or patient did nothing, will no longer do.

The new health care system of the 1990s and beyond will accept the fact that the major determinants of health, fitness, and longevity are the personal choices made by each individual. *Health & Fitness Excellence* is about those choices.

Health power is moving out of our doctors' offices, clinics, and hospitals. It is moving into our homes, our schools, and the places in which we work. To keep pace with this important shift in responsibility, each of us needs to master important new health skills. We need to keep ourselves up to date on the latest discoveries about fitness, diet, stress, and other self-care priorities. And when we choose to work with health professionals, we must do so as health-active consumers, not as passive patients.

Robert Cooper's *Health & Fitness Excellence* is an important part of this self-care revolution. Robert is an experienced health professional and teacher, a tireless researcher, and a world-class athlete. He combines enthusiasm with open-mindedness and blends the wisdom of ancient traditions with the best of modern science. In his work over the past twenty years, Robert has gathered and refined dozens of effective self-care ideas from hundreds of scientists, physicians, psychologists, educators, and other experts throughout the world. Rather than instructing the reader on how to "do it my way," *Health & Fitness Excellence* provides information, alternatives, options, and resources. You can begin with whatever interests you most. For Robert knows that the best path for you is the one that takes into account your own special background and interests.

Health & Fitness Excellence is important reading for every health-concerned person:

Out-of-condition "couch potatoes" who have decided, once and for all, to get themselves into shape

Adults of every age who'd like to lose body fat and improve their health and appearance

Health-conscious individuals who'd like to be presented with hundreds
of new ideas, perspectives, and options

Committed, fitness-oriented athletes who'd like to deepen and broaden
their training

Achievement-oriented executives in search of maximum performance

Parents and grandparents who'd like to learn all they can about the health
and fitness factors that affect their children and grandchildren

Business leaders in search of increased productivity — for themselves and
their employees

Educators who acknowledge the wide range of factors that affect learning
and performance

All those ready to build new vitality in their lives by designing a balanced, integrated, up-to-date program

This book is also for all those who realize that the steps to *Health &
Fitness Excellence* — exercise, nutrition, stress management, body fat control, posture, living environments design, and mental development — are
more than just a way to health, happiness, and best performance. They
are also a Way.

Tom Ferguson, M.D., graduate of Yale
University School of Medicine, editor-in-
chief of *Medical Self-Care* magazine, and
contributing editor to *Prevention* magazine

Preface

Health & Fitness Excellence is the very best book on the subject I have ever read, a superb integration of the best scientific evidence with practical ancient wisdom. It is must reading for anyone who wants to live on that most delightful edge of more health, fitness, joy, and success. Robert K. Cooper, Ph.D., has harmonized theory and practice in a well-written, clear, and imaginative way. He dispels myths and introduces state-of-the-art options, alternatives, and possibilities to produce immediate and lasting benefits for the reader.

Dr. Cooper describes the latest scientific and medical evidence that the health of the average individual can be vastly improved. It appears that only a small fraction of the population currently enjoys anywhere near its full capacity for health. Furthermore, the failure of people to make use of this capacity seems to be the single most important cause of much of today's illness.

To put it plainly, research is showing that by not achieving your full, natural measure of vigor and vitality, you invite not only unnecessary minor illness and unnecessary rapid aging but also heart attack, lung disease, and cancer, the most serious diseases of our era. One in five men will have a heart attack before age sixty; half of all smokers will have serious lung disease by that age, and the incidence of some cancers is still rapidly rising. These alarming facts underline the importance of reconsidering your full capacity for health and fitness and taking Dr. Cooper's steps to begin making use of it.

This book will show you how to achieve a state of fitness and well-being that will afford improved resistance to disease and provide a physical-emotional springboard for greater enjoyment of living. You will learn how to slow the aging process. You will learn how to look better and feel better and with each succeeding year look forward to further rewards from living, not to illness, incapacity, or isolation.

Clearly health and fitness isn't just a matter of finding the "right technique" and adjusting the body to run smoothly. Something more is required, and this book provides it: *a new vision of the fully functioning person, a new model of health and fitness.*

This program will show you how to tap your deepest capacities for vitality, performance, and well-being. Medical investigators have evolved a new concept of health, called "positive wellness." It does not denote a state of exceptional physical health or ability such as that attained by a champion athlete; rather it refers to a level of fitness and physical-emotional-mental harmony that affords maximum resistance to disease and supports a sustained joy of living. People enjoying positive wellness are

Trim and physically fit; full of energy and vigor; rarely tired
Free from destructive lifestyle habits
Free from minor complaints, such as indigestion, constipation, headaches, or insomnia
Aware and alert; able to concentrate and think with great effectiveness
Radiant in appearance, with clear skin, glossy hair, and sparkling eyes
Able to relax easily, free from worry and anxiety
Self-assured, confident, optimistic, active, and creative
Satisfied with work and the direction of their lives
Fulfilled and at peace with themselves

You can achieve positive wellness by following Dr. Cooper's integrated, medically sound program for better living. Contrary to popular belief, the average person need not remain at the mercy of many of today's most ravaging illnesses. Disease is not just a matter of chance, destiny, or fate. An overwhelming body of scientific evidence indicates that most of today's illnesses, whether major or minor, have their roots in inactivity, poor lifestyle habits, and failure to develop and follow a complete, balanced health and fitness program.

In short, *you,* not your doctor, determine whether you will achieve positive wellness or whether you will face high medical bills and meet premature aging and death. You can, and should, take matters into your own hands. This program will show you how.

Health & Fitness Excellence will bring you positive wellness and deep personal satisfaction, but it also leads to something more. It changes your perception of yourself and your relationship to your world. As you become more cognizant of your personal power, you develop a new appreciation of your interdependence with every other human being and with the whole living, evolving biosphere that we call earth. You become committed to the well-being of each and every person on this planet.

Follow *Health & Fitness Excellence* and join millions of others in this great, much-needed adventure.

Harold H. Bloomfield, M.D., graduate of Yale University School of Medicine, adjunct professor at the Union Graduate School, and best-selling author of *The Holistic Way to Health and Happiness, Inner Joy, The Achilles Syndrome: Turning Your Weaknesses into Strengths,* and *Lifemates: The Love Fitness Program for a Lasting Relationship*

Health: The positive condition of being sound in body, emotions, mind, and spirit, especially with freedom from pain and disease.

Fitness: The self-directed development of awareness, competence, and adaptability — on physical, emotional, mental, and social levels — that promotes optimal performance within the environment.

Excellence: The state or condition of excelling, demonstrating highest-level vision, values, mission, knowledge, integrity, commitment, and actions.

1 Invitation

Human capacities have never been measured; nor are we to judge of what we can do by any precedents, so little has been tried.

— *HENRY DAVID THOREAU*

Myths or Facts: Which Are You Choosing?

At this moment, how many popular myths are taking their toll on your health and performance and that of your family, your business? Here's a sample, with more to come, of the common misconceptions that may be limiting you right now:

MYTH: To lose weight, you must diet.

FACT: Researchers have proven that fad diets fail. Any pounds lost are usually water or muscle tissue, not fat. Just as serious, many diets damage health and make it easier for you to *gain* — not lose — more body fat in the future. You can cut through the myths of diet with a five-part scientific formula that helps eliminate excess body fat once and for all. (*See Chapter 29.*)

MYTH: There's no way to take time out to relax or calm down when you're hit with problem after problem all day, forced to meet deadlines, prevent mistakes, and keep performing at your best.

FACT: You can learn a five-step "instant calming sequence" (ICS) that requires *less than one second* to neutralize stress and help keep you in command of your thoughts, energy, and emotions whenever you're under pressure. (*See Chapter 7.*)

MYTH: "Positive thinking" is simply a matter of filling your mind with "good" thoughts and blocking out the "bad."

FACT: Surprising new research reveals that much so-called positive thinking is really negative. Whether or not we consciously notice the many thoughts that flash through our minds, we *feel* their effect because our thoughts create or influence our emotions. You can learn two key elements in positive thinking and five steps for forming mental images to help you relax, boost your body's immune power, and achieve your goals. You will discover how to tap into your vast mental potentials and let go of whatever self-defeating thoughts and attitudes are holding you back. (*See Chapter 44.*)

MYTH: By doing lots of sit-ups or leg-lifts you can melt fat from your stomach.

FACT: Not a chance. First of all, spot reduction doesn't work. Fat is metabolized ("burned") during aerobic exercise; it is not *melted*. And traditional sit-ups and leg-lifts are ineffective — in fact, they often contribute to lower back pain, protruding abdomen, and poor posture. To have a slim, strong waist, you must exercise five key abdominal muscles including the little-known transversalis and pyramidalis. (*See Chapter 14.*)

MYTH: As long as you eat "good" foods, you've taken care of your nutritional health.

FACT: While choosing healthful foods is very important, scientists have discovered that an extraordinarily varied diet and five or six carefully planned meals and snacks per day are also crucial to nutritional health. In addition, there is compelling new evidence about a mind-mood-food connection. You can learn how *your* best food choices may give you greater control of your emotions, energy, mental sharpness, and performance. (*See Chapters 21 and 27.*)

MYTH: It's all but impossible to pay much attention to health and fitness on work breaks, especially on hectic days when you're lucky to find more than a free minute or two here and there.

FACT: Thirty seconds is all it takes for a rejuvenation-in-motion routine. You can release tension and balance your posture; send a "wave of relaxation" through your body; lift your mood; clear and focus your mind; and help replenish nutrients and fluid. It's a new secret weapon against stress and fatigue. (*See Chapter 10.*)

MYTH: Most of us use only about 10 percent of our brain power.

FACT: Neuroscientists now estimate that we use only about *one-hundredth of one percent* of our potential brain power! And the brain can steadily deteriorate, becoming flabby as unused muscles do. Another discovery: Senility is *not* a normal part of aging. With the right mental exercises and environment, the size, number, and function of many types of brain cells may be increased at any age. Your mind can keep developing and be as sharp — or *sharper* — at age ninety as at twenty. (*See Chapter 43.*)

Worldwide Discoveries: The Whole Picture

One of the biggest challenges we all face is finding the facts we need to know for best health and performance and getting rid of the myths and fads that seem to be everywhere. We all want a personal program that takes the least amount of time but doesn't miss anything crucial.

That's why *Health & Fitness Excellence* was developed. It's the first program that replaces myths with facts and gives fast new ways to master stress, lose body fat, become fit, and unlock peak achievement.

Health & Fitness Excellence is also the first scientific action plan that doesn't go off on a tangent — as "exercise only" or "diet only" programs do. Instead, it's based on the whole picture, bringing together the latest recommendations of leading experts in seven key areas:

1 Stress strategies
2 Exercise options
3 Nutritional wellness
4 Body fat control
5 Postural vitality
6 Rejuvenation and living environments design
7 Unlimited mind and life unity

This book began twenty-five years ago when, as a young teenager, I survived street gang terrorism by learning martial arts. That's when I first started to understand the capabilities of the body and mind. I also watched both of my grandfathers — heroes in my life — die years before they should have. One, a humanitarian medical doctor, died from cancer. The other, an educator, died from his fifth heart attack. Those crises motivated me to begin learning everything I could about the sciences of health and fitness. And I have continued ever since.

Over the years I have studied and taught martial arts, competed in sports as an All-American athlete, and served in organizations dealing with health and human relations. I earned my first doctoral degree in health education (combining health sciences and human services), and at the time of this writing I am completing a second Ph.D. in health education and psychology at the Union Graduate School in Cincinnati. I have been certified as a Health and Fitness Instructor by the American College of Sports Medicine and as a Fitness Specialist by the Institute for Aerobics Research (Kenneth H. Cooper, M.D., M.P.H., president).

I have taken graduate work in biomedical journalism, conducted computer database searches of the world's scientific and medical literature, and learned from physicians, psychologists, educators, and research scientists in the United States and Europe. Rather than emphasizing traditional health education, I have focused on health and fitness enhancement and promotion — developing a comprehensive model for high-level wellness. I have checked, rechecked, and updated findings, incorporating valuable feedback from professionals who have attended lectures and seminars I have presented since 1975. You hold the results in your hands: *Health & Fitness Excellence* is an integration of scientific discoveries by experts around the world.

Choosing a Health and Fitness Program

Chances are that your busy lifestyle leaves you little time for exercise. Daily pressures drain your energy. Eating on the run is a frequent necessity. These and other challenges in our fast-paced world make it harder and harder to get into your best possible shape — in body, emotions, mind, and spirit — and stay that way.

Millions of health-conscious Americans are trying to follow some kind of regular program. Perhaps, like many of them, you've been investing hundreds, even thousands, of dollars trying diet after diet, attending health lectures, buying home fitness equipment and videotapes, traveling to health clubs and spas, untangling contradictory advice — in short, trying to piece together a plan that doesn't overlook anything essential *or* tie up too much of your time. It's a huge task.

Are You Staying Up to Date?

Adding to the pressure is the realization that staying up to date is getting harder all the time. Many valuable discoveries have remained locked away in research journals around the world, and some aren't even translated into English.

According to the *Annals of Internal Medicine,* health professionals who want to keep up with discoveries in the biomedical world now have to read more than thirty-nine thousand articles every week.[1] And then there are hundreds of books and popular magazines to contend with.

Public confusion is growing as fast as this tidal wave of news flashes and data. It has become a major challenge *to eliminate misinformation and pinpoint priorities*. That's where *Health & Fitness Excellence* comes in.

There is strong new evidence that what many Americans have come to accept as "good health" falls far short of what it could — and should — be. According to Dr. William H. Foege, assistant U.S. Surgeon General and special assistant for policy development of the Centers for Disease Control in Atlanta, about two-thirds of the deaths in the United States are *premature* "given our present knowledge," and about two-thirds of the years of life lost before age sixty-five are "theoretically preventable given our current capabilities."[2] It has become evident that our behavior — our lifestyle — is of tremendous significance to health, fitness, and longevity. But disease prevention and health enhancement research is still allocated less than 5 percent of overall health funding in the United States. It's time for that to change.

Science and Synergy

"We are at the beginning of *the age of public participation in science,*" says Maurice Goldsmith, director of the International Science Policy Foundation in London. "This has occurred as it has become clearer that science is not a private game, but is for everybody; that it has a function in society; and that if used in a planned way could improve our condition immeasurably."[3]

Health & Fitness Excellence is founded on *science* — on the recommendations of top researchers, educators, and clinicians around the world. It's also based on *synergy* — the concept that a comprehensive, balanced program can give far greater results than the mathematical sum of the individual parts of the program.

Science has brought us answers in bits and pieces, but fragmented expert advice — an isolated little section of the puzzle — no matter how good it is, just isn't enough. *Health & Fitness Excellence* is the first program designed to put all the pieces together in a coherent picture within easy reach.

"In an ideal whole," says medical researcher Andrew Weil, "the components are not only all there, they are there in an arrangement of harmonious integration and balance."[4]

Why One Book Instead of Seven?

Several professional readers who reviewed the manuscript for this book suggested that it might be divided into seven different publications, one for each step. I said no — *Health & Fitness Excellence* depends on an integrated program. My goal is to provide you, the reader, with a complete action plan right now, not doled out in pieces.

I agree with John Morrison, president of Anderson College, when he said, "Knowledge comes by taking things apart, by analysis; wisdom comes by putting things together."

Results Begin Right Now

Unlike so many other programs, *Health & Fitness Excellence* isn't a faraway goal or endpoint. Some of the recommendations in this book give immediate results — such as the ICS (instant calming sequence), 30-second rejuvenation-in-motion routines, posture techniques, breathing changes, insights on the mind-mood-food connection, and why much so-called positive thinking is really negative — and how to change that. Many other suggestions — all recommended by experts — produce benefits in just a few short weeks.

You may be wondering, Do I really need to learn and do *everything* in this book? My answer: Absolutely not. You can begin anywhere in this program and proceed, step by step, at your own pace, with whatever first interests you. Other programs are often loaded with contradictions, but in *Health & Fitness Excellence* the seven steps complement each other. This book offers advanced strategies for closing the gap between human potential and human performance.

It's time to get rid of the myths and fads. We are all entitled to know the scientific facts we need to achieve our best possible health and performance in today's pressure-filled world. But here's the key question: Are you ready to *act* on those facts? If yes, then I have written *Health & Fitness Excellence* for you.

2 The Seven Steps to Health & Fitness Excellence

Designing Your Personal Program

As you read this book, keep a notebook close at hand. Label a section of the notebook for each of the seven steps in *Health & Fitness Excellence*. Note the facts and recommendations that seem most important to *you*. You can devise a "daily/weekly checklist" to organize and schedule your priorities. Every new idea, each choice you make, adds momentum to success in all areas.

The "Golden Circle"

Scientists around the world have identified a "golden circle" of seven key steps to *Health & Fitness Excellence*. And each of us needs them all. You can't eat a good diet but skip exercise; or exercise regularly but forget to manage stress; or learn how to relax but overlook good posture; or sit up straight but fill your mind with negative thoughts; or try to lose body fat by just changing your diet; and so on.

There are also golden circles within each of the seven steps. To be balanced and complete, every step must build its own foundation. Here are highlights of what you will learn:

Step 1: Stress Strategies

▶ How to use the instant calming sequence (ICS) to neutralize negative stress *in less than one second* and keep you in command of your thoughts, energy, and emotions whenever you're under pressure

▶ How to improve relationships and expand and strengthen your support network of friends and co-workers

▶ How to enhance the quality of your nightly rest — sleeping more deeply and healthfully, in fewer hours, than you do now

▶ Ten ways to speak with greater clarity and insight, turning resistance into support and avoiding communication pitfalls that sabotage personal and business relationships

▶ How to turn work breaks into health-and-energy breaks using 30- second rejuvenation-in-motion routines, which release tight muscles and balance your posture; send a "wave of relaxation" through your body; replace nutrients and replenish fluids; revitalize your vision; lift your mood; and clear and refocus your mind

Step 2: Exercise Options

▶ How to increase mental and physical stamina on even the most hectic days

▶ How to use the latest scientific strategies for exercising smarter to accomplish the best results in the shortest amount of time

▶ How to flatten and tone your waist using simple, scientifically advanced exercises to strengthen five abdominal muscles, including the little-known transversalis and pyramidalis

▶ Seven key guidelines for aerobic exercise; if you don't know them, there's a good chance you're wasting time, missing benefits, or risking needless injuries

▶ A European method for developing full-body flexibility quickly and safely

▶ The fastest ways to build strong, toned muscles

▶ Balance and agility exercises to develop the body and mind in ways that no other exercises can — all in as little as six minutes a week

Step 3: Nutritional Wellness

▶ The latest discoveries in nutritional science

▶ Eight key principles of optimal nutrition that will help you design a superior diet that will cost no more — in time or money — than a mediocre one

▶ Why eating five or six times a day (three light meals and the right kind of between-meal snacks) helps your body burn excess fat and function at its best

▶ How to best ensure that your food is fresh and not contaminated with pesticides, antibiotics, hormones, bacteria, molds, or additives

▶ Compelling new evidence on the mind-mood-food connection: how certain meals and snacks may promote faster thinking, greater energy, increased attention to detail, and quicker reaction speed while other foods may help produce a calm, focused state of mind and relaxed emotions

▶ Tips for planning and preparing fast, delicious recipes based on the principles of *Health & Fitness Excellence*

▶ How to continue enjoying restaurant meals without counting calories or gaining weight

▶ Why vitamin and mineral supplements can be valuable but are widely overrated as factors for top health and performance

Step 4: Body Fat Control

▶ Why fad diets fail and make it easier to *gain* — not lose — body fat

▶ Which exercises to select (and, just as important, which *not* to select) for fast, safe weight loss

▶ Why skipping meals and struggling to resist feelings of hunger push you toward overeating binges — and how to solve this problem

▶ Why drinking water will *not* cause bloating or puffiness and why not drinking enough water can slow down fat loss

▶ Why spot reducing — trying to lose weight in isolated areas of the body — doesn't work; you will learn the fastest ways to become fit, lean, and toned in *every* part of your body and stay that way

Step 5: Postural Vitality

▶ Why most of us tense dozens — sometimes *hundreds* — of the wrong muscles when we sit, stand, and move and then suffer from fatigue, muscular pain, headaches, eyestrain, decreased blood and oxygen to the brain, and diminished productivity

▶ The fastest, easiest ways to create buoyant, balanced posture when you sit, stand, walk, work, drive a vehicle, or participate in sports

Step 6: Rejuvenation and Living Environments Design

▶ How to more fully develop your senses (sight, hearing, touch, etc.) and how this increased sensitivity can build brain power and slow or reverse many effects of aging

▶ Eight of the most serious indoor pollution problems and the simplest means to solve them (the Environmental Protection Agency has reported that indoor pollution levels are up to one hundred times greater than outdoor pollution levels)

▶ Ways to improve oral hygiene and dental health, including new recommendations on frequent toothbrush replacement and not using mouthwash

▶ How to give an easy 10-minute seated massage to release muscular tension, increase circulation, and relieve pain

▶ Ways to improve intimate relationships and the latest research discoveries on how to solve many male and female sexual problems

Step 7: Unlimited Mind and Life Unity

▶ Why we rarely ever find solutions to emotional distress by dwelling on shortcomings or repeatedly getting negative feelings "out in the open"

▶ The latest scientific techniques for switching negative moods into positive ones and how to let go of self-defeating thoughts and attitudes that are holding you back

▶ The straight truth about why so much "positive" thinking is really negative — and what to do about it

▶ New ways to sharpen concentration and creativity

▶ Mental exercises to help build your brain power at any age, increasing the size, number, and function of many types of brain cells

▶ Five key steps for forming mental images that help you relax, boost your body's immune power, and achieve your goals

Medical Advice for Illness

A mutually trusting relationship with a family physician provides each of us with accesss to medical information and services. *Health & Fitness Excellence* doesn't replace medical resources or advice. Consult your personal physician with all questions about illness and disease. A good medical assessment is an important part of responsible self-care. If you have any symptom or illness that seems serious or is recurrent or persistent, see your doctor for a diagnosis and for treatment recommendations. Medicine is an immense, rapidly changing field. Consequently, we can't expect every medical doctor to be up to date on all nonmedical aspects of the sciences of health, fitness, and performance.

High-Level Wellness

Rather than focusing on the depth and span of illness, *Health & Fitness Excellence* is directed toward the height and breadth of wellness. It offers a new model for health promotion and fitness enhancement.

"I would argue that [medicine and nursing] have their hands full staying abreast of the knowledge explosion in biomedical sciences," writes Dr. Lawrence W. Green, director of the Center for Health Promotion Research and Development at the University of Texas Health Science Center at Houston. "A revolution would be necessary in the curriculum of medical schools and, to a lesser extent, in nursing schools for either of these professions to assume a primary role in health promotion. We have seen little evidence that medical schools are prepared to reorient the education of physicians to include a primary emphasis on disease prevention, much less health promotion."[5]

"Even so-called preventive programs and health maintenance organizations are primarily designed to keep people from sinking into illness rather than to help them rise higher into wellness," adds Dr. Calvin W. Taylor of the University of Utah.[6]

"A true wellness program goes far beyond traditional health education and preventive medicine. It involves learning about yourself and why you tend to make the choices you do," says Dr. Grant M. Christopher, a graduate of Mayo Medical School and the University of Minnesota School of Medicine and author of *Well Now!* "It involves reviewing a complete set of options — physical, emotional, mental, social, and spiritual — and then taking personal steps to improve your *total* well-being."[7]

Health & Fitness Excellence is designed to complement modern medicine and provide the greatest benefits beginning where traditional health care leaves off — at the point where you have no symptoms of illness or disease but are still thinking, feeling, and performing far below your unlimited best.

Step 1

STRESS STRATEGIES

3 Introduction

MYTH: All stress is bad.

FACT: Life is filled with changes, and stress seems to be everywhere. But that pressure can be good or bad depending on how you *perceive* it and *react* to it. Researchers have discovered fast new ways to manage stress so that it can be used to *improve,* rather than break down, your health and productivity.

MYTH: You're stuck with stress when you're achievement-oriented. Headaches, stomachaches, and backaches are a small price to pay for success.

FACT: That's ridiculous. Nagging tension and health complaints don't promote success, they *block* it. You can learn how to get them out of your way. (*See Chapters 4, 7, and 10.*)

MYTH: When bad things happen, it's normal to get depressed for a while — some days are just a pain in the neck.

FACT: You can do a lot about feeling anxious when bad things happen in your life, and stress shouldn't give anyone a pain in the neck. To a surprising extent, the way you think about bad experiences — and how you explain them to yourself and others — determines your stress load. (*See Chapter 6.*)

MYTH: Relaxing is easy if you have the time for it. You just listen to music, watch TV, read a book, or something like that.

FACT: While those activities may be good choices for a change of pace, they aren't deeply relaxing. You can learn to do a step-by-step "tension scan" and produce a "wave of relaxation" to revitalize your body and mind. (*See Chapter 4.*)

MYTH: The best way to deal with anger is to vent it — to yell, rant, and rave and immediately get your feelings out in the open.

FACT: That's wrong. Recent studies report that suppressing anger *and* explosively venting it are both linked to a death rate (from all causes) that is over two times greater than that related to "reflective coping." (*See Chapter 6.*)

MYTH: It's all but impossible to talk to some people. When you say what you mean, they misunderstand it, which leads to arguments and bad feelings. No matter how hard you try, there's just nothing you can do about it.

FACT: *How* we say things can be even more important than *what* we say. Differences in conversational style cause many conflicts. You say what you mean, but the other person hears what he or she *thinks* you mean, which may not be what you meant. In many relationships communication mix-ups are a major stress, but you can correct them by using precise language and developing better listening skills. (*See Chapter 9.*)

MYTH: There's no time to relax or calm down when you're racing to meet deadlines and being pounded by stress all day.

FACT: Now you can learn fast, powerful techniques to manage stress, including the 1-second instant calming sequence (*Chapter 7*) and 30-second rejuvenation-in-motion routines (*Chapter 10*).

Demystifying Stress

Stress is the subject of more and more headlines nationwide — in newspapers, magazines, health journals, business reports, educational reviews, and on television and radio. It has emerged as one of the biggest obstacles to optimum health and performance. In fact, mismanaged stress costs American businesses more than $200 billion a year[1] and is linked to 65 to 90 percent of all illnesses.[2]

Pressure is the name of the game today — our world is unpredictable, competitive, and swirling with change. In less than half a century the industrial age has vaulted into the atomic age, space age, and computer age. We've landed right in the middle of unprecedented opportunity — and anxiety. This stress turbulence reaches deep into every nation, business, and family. Our options? We can blow up, freeze, burn out, or break down. *Or* break through . . . with *Health & Fitness Excellence.*

"We are warned every day about the potential dangers of stress," says Georgia Witkin, professor of psychology at Mount Sinai Medical College. "We are told that stress can be held responsible for high blood pressure and low blood pressure; for overeating and loss of appetite; for fatigue and for hyperactivity; for talkativeness and withdrawal; for hot flashes and cold chills. We are advised that under stress we are more susceptible to infection, depression, accidents, viruses, colds, heart attacks, and even cancer. We worry about the aging effects of stress and then worry about the effects of worrying! We are stress-conscious and stress-concerned. We are not, however, sufficiently stress-educated."[3]

Stress originates from the Old French word *estrece*, meaning narrowness. Some authorities say that stress is the everyday wear and tear on our bodies and minds as we respond to the people, places, and events in our lives.[4] "*Stress is the nonspecific response of the body to any demand made upon it*," wrote Dr. Hans Selye, a pioneer in stress research for more than fifty years. "The stress-producing factors — technically called *stressors* — are [varied and] different, yet they all elicit essentially the same biological stress response. . . . From the point of view of its stress-producing or stressor activity, *it is immaterial whether the agent or situation we face is pleasant or unpleasant;* all that counts is the intensity of the demand for readjustment or adaptation. . . . *Stress is not merely nervous tension . . . [or] something to be avoided.*"[5]

Good Stress, Bad Stress

New evidence reveals that the amount of stress we feel and whether it is good stress or bad stress depend not on the situations we face in life but on how we *perceive* and *react to* those situations.

Positive stress generally occurs when you view a demand as a challenge rather than a threat. You feel a sense of commitment, an attitude of curiosity and involvement in what is happening. You also feel in control and believe that you can influence events in your life and are willing to take action.

Negative stress generally occurs when you view a demand as a threat. You feel a sense of alienation, of frustration, or of helplessness. You perceive yourself as the victim of circumstances, powerless to influence the events in your life. Repeated or prolonged negative stress leads to an exhaustion of mental and physical energies and increased susceptibility to disease. Stressors trigger a complex response that involves more than fourteen hundred physiochemical reactions in the brain and body, channeled through the autonomic nervous system and neuroendocrine system.

Destructive Effects of Negative Stress

Scientists continue to unravel the mystery of the ways in which stress affects the body, emotions, and mind. In a landmark Harvard study, people who coped poorly with stress became ill four times more often than those with good coping styles.[6]

Negative stress affects the immune system, heart function, hormone levels, the nervous system, memory and thinking, physical coordination, and metabolic rate; raises blood cholesterol, blood pressure, and uric acid levels; and it increases the risk of many diseases, including heart disease, cancer, immunodeficiency diseases, and even the common cold.[7]

Beyond that, negative stress can kill brain cells and appears to prematurely age the adult brain.[8] A continuous bombardment of stress hormones on the brain seems to destroy cerebral hormone receptors and weaken the brain areas that control emotions.[9] Then adrenal stress hormones — glucocorticoids — can block the entry of glucose into brain cells, killing them.[10] We all need ways to break the grip of negative stress.

"Clearly, the magnitude of stress-related disorders in terms of cost to society, as well as human suffering, is enormous," write Drs. Kenneth R. Pelletier and Robert Lutz of the University of California School of Medicine at San Francisco. "The tragedy, or promise, depending on your perspective, is that many stress-related health problems are preventable."[11]

Little Daily Hassles Take a Big Toll

The chronic, unavoidable stresses of everyday life may accelerate aging, according to new research at Bowman-Gray School of Medicine in North

Carolina.[12] How we respond to the irritations of everyday life — such as anger, rejection, interruptions, broken appointments, the inescapable telephone, financial anxieties, bad weather, traffic jams, and deadlines — is often a more powerful predictor of psychological and physical health than is our reaction to major life crises.[13]

It's not just the big pressures — final exams, marriage, parenting, divorce, job changes, deaths of friends and relatives — that overload us with stress; it's the lives of quiet desperation that millions lead. Which smaller stresses are most annoying? They vary from person to person, but the evidence is clear: daily hassles — and the way we respond to them — shouldn't be ignored.

Differing Female and Male Stress Syndromes

When under prolonged stress, both males and females are at increased risk of conditions such as ulcers, hypertension, indigestion, tight muscles, and chronic fatigue. But because of their differing physiology and conditioning, men and women experience some different stress symptoms.

Women under negative stress are threatened with stress-related disorders such as premenstrual syndrome, infertility, and anxiety neurosis, conditions that are unique to women or are reported more often by women than men.[14]

In contrast, men under prolonged negative stress face added risk of persistent physical conditions such as muscle aches and headaches (which are often overlooked as simply fatigue or flu) and psychological symptoms such as decision-making difficulties and chronic distraction.[15]

Stress Thresholds: How Do You Respond?

As individuals, we each have a "stress threshold" — a tolerance level for certain situations — beyond which we begin to experience physical or psychological damage.

Even when we're unaware of stress, we may be reacting negatively. Some people are "muscle responders," holding tension in the jaw, tongue, shoulders, face, chest, abdomen, or back. Others are "autonomic responders," displaying heightened nervous system activity evidenced by cold hands or feet, increased heart rate, mental distractions, and changes in breathing. By ruminating about past mistakes or upcoming events, people can provoke anxiety, headaches, "butterflies" in the stomach, tight muscles, irritability, or fatigue.

Precisely how do *you* respond to the pressures of different daily circumstances? To best manage stress it's essential to first become fully aware of it. Different kinds of stress require different responses.

Your Stress List

Make a list of the main negative stresses in your life right now — the things that bother you today, this week. They can be inner conflicts, relationship problems, sexual distress, illnesses, work pressures, unanswered mail, unpaid bills, the stock market, world affairs — anything. Next, pull out your time planner and divide the list into three categories.

First category: stresses that need to be clarified. Many work and relationship problems come from poor communication and false assumptions. Clarify these stresses on your list and plan to resolve them by listening, observing, and questioning.

Second category: stresses that require action. Identify all those situations that can be resolved or helped through action and then write down precise times on your schedule to take those actions. If you know that you are handling these specific issues or will soon handle them, they won't haunt you as much right now.

Third category: stresses that can't be avoided. The remainder of the list consists of stresses that you're stuck with, at least for a while — downturns in the economy or world affairs, traffic, the weather, deadlines at work, ailments of friends, and so on. These stresses can best be handled philosophically, through changes in mental focus (using meditation, imagery, or releasing), compensatory self-improvements (such as an exercise program, relaxation sessions, or educational seminars), or spiritual insights.

Be alert for those quick symptoms that signal that stress may be starting to overload you:[16] Your pulse gets unusually rapid; you notice unnecessary muscle tension anywhere in your body; your breathing gets shallow, rapid, or interrupted; you perspire from nervousness; or the temperature in your hands drops (indicated by your hands feeling cool if you place them on your neck just above your collar). When you notice any of these symptoms, it's time to take some immediate action to identify and manage whatever has caused the stress.

A stress list lets you get a better grasp on current pressures in your life. If you'd like to complete a detailed stress measurement and self-assessment, I recommend *StressMap* by Esther Orioli, M.S., Dennis Jaffe, Ph.D., and Cynthia Scott, Ph.D., M.P.H. (Newmarket Press, 1987; available from Essi Systems, Inc., 126 S. Park, San Francisco, CA 94107; 415-541-4911).

What Is Your "Type"?

A pessimist is someone who, when confronted with two unpleasant alternatives, chooses both.

— ROBERT S. ELIOT, M.D.[17]

In the 1960s and 1970s, cardiologists linked type A behavior — "a sense of time urgency, aggressiveness and excessive achievement striving"[18] — to high blood pressure, heart attacks, and other health disorders. While predominantly a male trait, type A behavior is also found in women and children.[19]

At first, type A individuals were advised to switch to type B behavior, a lethargic state in which zest for work was viewed with suspicion. Type B people seemed better suited for life in Tahiti than in the Western world. But new research has helped clear things up.[20]

The MR FIT study, conducted by the National Heart, Lung, and Blood Institute with twelve thousand subjects, failed to find any link between type A behavior and heart disease. At the same time, relying on mortality data from long-term studies, researchers at Duke University Medical Center pinpointed the deadly personality trait: a cynical, mistrusting, pessimistic attitude.[21]

Now you can take steps to minimize the destructive characteristics of type A behavior (such as overcompetitiveness, impatience, cynicism) while preserving the positive traits (such as dedication, enthusiasm, and persistence).

What Is Your Coping Style?

Why do some stress-loaded people exhibit very little illness and maintain happy, satisfying lives, while many others with matching stress burdens cope poorly and get sick often? The answer is *hardiness*.

Scientists have discovered that people with a hardy, resilient personality have a variety of stress buffers that keep them from being debilitated by stressful life events.[22]

One of the most effective ways to diffuse stress is known as *transformational coping*. "Committed people who believe they are in control and expect situations to be challenging are likely to react to stressful events by *increasing* their interaction with them — exploring, controlling, and learning from them," says Joan Borysenko, director of the Mind/Body Clinic at Harvard Medical School. "This attitude transforms the event into something less stressful by placing it in a broader frame of reference that revolves around continued personal growth and understanding."[23]

In contrast is *regressive coping* — thinking about stressful events pessimistically and avoiding interactions with them. Regressive copers feel alienated from activities, powerless to influence the events in their lives, and threatened by change. And they're most likely to become ill when pressures rise.

Stress as an Opportunity

Stress management programs of all kinds are being offered in the United States these days — various collections of risk profiles, relaxation exercises, biofeedback, and related activities. Most have what is known as a "lack of transference" or surprisingly poor "carry-through." Once you leave the clinic or peaceful seminar setting the techniques are not easy to apply to the real world, to the *stress-filled everyday situations where you really need them.* It's hard to find the time for a formal relaxation or meditation session when you're in rush-hour traffic or hit with one problem after another all day.

Health & Fitness Excellence gives fast, simple ways to take charge of the stresses in your life. You can prime your mind and body to clear a path of least resistance to your goals. And you can learn to catch the first signs of negative stress, neutralize them, and transform mental confusion into clear thinking, tension into calmness, and anxieties into personal power.

The stress strategies in *Health & Fitness Excellence* are divided into seven areas, which are presented in detail in Chapters 4–10:

1 Present-moment awareness and relaxation
2 Time competency
3 Positive support system: self, others, and environment
4 ICS: "instant calming sequence"
5 Optimum sleep
6 Listening and communication skills
7 30-second rejuvenation-in-motion routines

The "Golden Circle"

How you manage or mismanage stress affects and is affected by the other six major steps to *Health & Fitness Excellence.* By neutralizing negative stress, you alleviate the tensions that sap energy, stall digestion, and choke off blood to the brain and muscles. And you can stop overproducing stress hormones that can ignite negative emotions and confuse the mind.

To be fully successful, stress management depends on all seven areas of *Health & Fitness Excellence.* For example, a lack of regular exercise is linked to anxiety states and related psychological disorders.[24] Aerobic exercise promotes positive attitudes and relaxation and helps the body metabolize stress hormones before they cause damage. Frequent small meals and snacks change brain chemistry, giving you greater control over your mind and mood. Good posture keeps blood flowing throughout the body, preventing or unraveling the muscle knots that create tension and pain. Positive-on-positive thoughts can reverse the negative thinking that causes so much emotional turmoil and fatigue.

It's the golden circle of *Health & Fitness Excellence*. Every choice you make in one area supports and accelerates improvements in other areas. Take a few minutes to scan the next seven chapters containing strategies for stress management. Pick whatever area interests you most right now, and begin there.

4 Present-Moment Awareness and Relaxation

Present-Moment Awareness

One of the first steps to managing stress is becoming aware of your stress-producing thoughts, feelings, and habits. Most of us live in a state of chronic distraction — a chaotic mixture of excitement, goals, guilt, impatience, and worry.

Distraction is defined as a state in which attention is easily diverted. Chronic distraction is an early warning sign that your stress burden is nearing the maximal level.

"We all get distracted from time to time, but when we enter a state of chronic distraction, life becomes an endless cycle of frustrations," says Kenneth R. Pelletier, assistant clinical professor at the University of California School of Medicine at San Francisco. "It feels as though we never get anything accomplished. Our days seem like unbroken strings of interruptions."[25]

A major part of the problem is conditional happiness. "How many times has your mind told you that you could be happy *if* you lost ten pounds? made more money?" asks Joan Borysenko, director of the Mind/Body Clinic at Harvard Medical School. "Then, even if these things come to pass, you just move on to the next set of conditions for happiness. The conditions are like the proverbial carrot that dangles in front of the donkey. You never reach them. . . . Deferring happiness until any condition is met — a new job, a new relationship, a new possession — leads to suffering."[26]

Calm, attentive, *present-moment awareness* is a dynamic, productive state. It's the opposite of distraction. Your mind is alert, your body relaxed and efficient. You can unknot tension patterns and change negative thoughts because you're aware enough to notice them. When you feel yourself becoming distracted from an important task, you can clear your mind to focus on the subject at hand without concern about what's coming up later or what happened before.

The Japanese word *muga* describes present-moment awareness. Abraham Maslow wrote: "The [*muga*] is the state in which you are doing whatever you are doing with a total wholeheartedness, without thinking of anything else, without any hesitation, without any criticism or doubt or inhibition of any kind whatsoever. It is pure and perfect and total spontaneous acting without any blocks of any kind."[27]

Developing present-centered awareness takes regular practice using techniques such as breathing, sensory openness, and meditation.

Breathing

Your stress response hinges on your breath. Neuroscientists have discovered what martial arts masters, yogis, spiritual teachers, and advanced thinkers have realized for centuries: Proper breathing enhances blood flow to the brain and helps quell destructive emotions such as anxiety, anger, envy, jealousy, fear, frustration, and even shyness.[28]

By changing the way you breathe, you can change the way you think and feel. When you notice stress signals — tense muscles, cold hands, irregular breathing, rapid pulse, nervous sweating — use smooth, deep breathing to regain control.

"Your breath should be light, even, and flowing, like a thin stream of water running through the sand," advises Zen master Thich Nhat Hanh. "Your breath should be very quiet, so quiet that a person sitting next to you cannot hear it. Your breathing should flow gracefully, like a river . . . not like a chain of rugged mountains or the gallop of a horse. To master our breath is to be in control of our bodies and minds."[29]

Take some time to listen to your breathing, to *feel* it. Smoothly, slowly, draw each breath into the lower lungs, expanding your ribs out to the sides. Feel greater relaxation each time you exhale. Chapter 12 presents a variety of breathing enhancement exercises.

Sensory Openness

Many of us live out of touch with our senses. We're so busy, so tense, that we have drifted away from the landscape of sights, sounds, smells, tastes, and touches around us. And stress wins. Without sharp awareness, we can't catch — and neutralize — negative pressures.

One way to open your senses is with a *body tension scan*. This technique helps you become alert to your muscles and relax them more easily.

Scanning uses your inner awareness, rather than your eyes, to check for tight muscles. With practice, this technique can be used quickly — even instantly — to help you find and release tension.

To learn scanning, choose an environment that's free from distractions. Set aside about 10 minutes. Sit comfortably in a chair or lie on your back on a padded surface. Spread your legs slightly and relax your body. Close your eyes and begin taking smooth, deep breaths.

After 30 seconds or so, mentally scan a muscle area as you inhale. As you breathe out, imagine the tension releasing as that muscle becomes more comfortably relaxed. After several breaths, shift your attention to another area. Systematically search the entire body: Begin at the scalp and work down through the face, eyes, ears, jaw, tongue, neck, shoulders, upper arms, forearms, wrists, hands, fingers, chest, upper back, abdomen, lower back, pelvis, thighs, lower legs, ankles, feet, and toes.

Scan for tight areas on each inhalation and then visualize the tension melting away as you exhale. Don't be alarmed if your mind wanders. Just bring your attention back and continue scanning.

Once you've finished, remain completely relaxed for half a minute more. Notice the warm sense of ease in your body, especially in those places — perhaps the face, neck, jaw, tongue, shoulders, abdomen, or back — where you tend to hold tension.

There are many other ways to increase your sensory awareness. Can you feel your breath as it comes in and goes out? The slightest breeze on your cheeks or hands? The surface beneath your feet, legs, or back? Which arm or leg is more relaxed right now? The more senses you involve — sight, touch, sound, smell, and taste — the greater your gains in awareness. (See Chapters 36 and 37 for more ideas and recommendations.)

Meditation

Within you there is a stillness and a sanctuary to which you can retreat at any time and be yourself.

— *HERMANN HESSE,*
SIDDHARTHA

Meditation is any activity that keeps your attention pleasantly drawn to the present moment. It has been practiced since the beginning of civilization, and various methods are found in all cultures, from Judeo-Christian to Oriental.

"The primary goal of meditation is not relaxation — it is awareness," writes Joan Borysenko. "This is what eventually leads to getting the mind back under control. . . . The state of meditation occurs . . . whenever we are fully engaged in what we are doing. . . . For once, the mind is not reading its list of things that must happen before we can be happy. It's not reciting the list of awful things that could happen to steal our happiness. It has taken a back seat to just *being*. This is the meditative state that elicits the relaxation response. It is peace."[30]

There are two paths in developing stress hardiness: *taking action* whenever required and *letting go* when no further action is advisable or possible. Meditation is a great means of letting go — enjoying the moment, surrendering any feelings of worry and guilt, quickly rejuvenating the body and mind. Researchers suggest that regular meditation may also improve learning, provide a buffer against stress, and even slow the aging process.[31]

Basic meditation is a simple process of paying attention to the reality of the moment. Many traditional forms of meditation teach focusing your awareness on the breath — coming in, going out. To further anchor the mind, a word or phrase may be repeated silently with each breathing cycle. In research at Harvard, Dr. Herbert Benson found that repeating the word *one* on each exhalation of breath worked well.[32] In Oriental meditation, sounds with *mmm* and *nnn* are traditionally used because they evoke a release of tension and an enjoyment of the moment. Other people prefer prayers or phrases with heartfelt meaning — *love, calmness, letting go, peace,* and so on.

The particular object or technique doesn't matter. What's important is keeping the mind focused; if it wanders — and it often does — gently bring it back without judgment. Meditation takes effort, but it's not a battle. It's more like a friendly way of getting in touch with yourself.

Meditation opens the door to all kinds of self-improvement, reports Dr. Benson after more than two decades of medical studies. "We've found that the Relaxation Response [meditation] also acts, in a rather extraordinary fashion, as a kind of door to a renewed mind and changed life. It can enable you to change even the most deeply ingrained bad habits. It can enable you to develop new, beneficial disciplines, and enhance your health in ways which you had always felt were beyond your grasp."[33]

Here is a basic meditation process:

1 *Select a quiet place where you will not be disturbed*. Schedule 10 to 20 minutes. Once you've learned to meditate on a more advanced level and draw inward, environmental distractions will disturb you much less.

2 *Sit in a comfortable position,* with good posture and no unnecessary muscle tension. Close your eyes to make concentration easier. Put a half smile on your face — this increases blood flow to the brain and promotes positive thoughts and emotions (see Chapter 7 for more details).

3 *Relax all your muscles* systematically, from scalp to fingertips and toes, using one of the techniques suggested in the next section, letting go of tension with each breath out.

4 *Become aware of your breathing* in an easy, effortless way, without forcing it.

5 *Repeat your silent focus word or phrase on each breath out.* Or, if you have a two-part phrase like the old Sanskrit mantra *Ham* ("I am") *Sah* ("that"), imagine that the first word is spoken silently on the breath in, the second on the breath out.

6 *Don't judge how you are doing.* If you begin to wonder how you are doing or why your mind keeps dancing off on other thoughts, you'll become anxious. Don't be concerned about your performance or try to stop your mind from wandering. Practice gently bringing it back into focus.

7 *Practice 10 to 20 minutes a day.* Meditation takes practice. An ultimate goal is to apply your meditation skills — such as calm, attentive awareness — to all kinds of daily activities.

Present-moment awareness is an inner thread of *Health & Fitness Excellence*. "What would it be like if we lived each day, each breath, as a work of art in progress?" asks Tom Crum, cofounder of Windstar Foundation. "Imagine that we are a masterpiece unfolding, which means that every minute, every second of the day we are a masterpiece now and now and now and now. We are art-forming and masterpiecing with each breath. What would it be like if we lived life like that? [A] major component of making your life a work of art . . . is a heightened sense of awareness, a heightened sense of clarity, of sensory acuity of everything that is going on at that moment."[34]

Relaxation Skills: Creating "Islands of Peace"

Learning how to relax — quickly, deeply, thoroughly — is a major health asset, according to decades of scientific and medical research. Relaxation is a prerequisite to exceptional thinking. It also sets the stage for guided imagery techniques that have proven effective in sports, education, and healing. However, it's easy to miss out on benefits by not learning how to *apply* relaxation skills in the real world of day-to-day stress. That's why the following chapters in this section focus on ways to use a *calm body and alert mind* to meet the challenges of everyday life.

There are many effective relaxation techniques. No matter which you choose, it's important to take several minutes a day — every day — to systematically and completely release muscle tension in your body. For some people, the best time is early evening, when the day's work is over and the start of a good night's rest is only hours away.

We can all benefit from scheduling daily "islands of peace" — Dr. Kenneth Pelletier's term for "relaxed, no-hassle periods in which no stressful messages are coming either from inside or outside. . . . Modern society does have its chronic stresses. But there's usually a way to break that frantic cycle and build some islands of peace and tranquility into our lives."[35]

While deep relaxation sessions are valuable, don't mistakenly assume that relaxation or meditation practice will automatically protect your body and mind against stressful events and let you break out of anxiety cycles. Fast, practical techniques are important, too — such as the instant calming sequence (ICS) presented in Chapter 7 and the 30-second rejuvenation-in-motion routines in Chapter 10. The following are some basic techniques for achieving deep relaxation.

Relaxation Tapes

Listening to audiotapes is a helpful way to learn relaxation skills. You can write out your own script and have a friend read it to you or record a tape to use during relaxation sessions. Be certain the voice is calm, interested, and pleasing. Or you may find it easier to purchase a prerecorded tape (a list is included under "Resources" at the end of the chapter).

Specific Relaxation Sequences

1 *Select a quiet place and a comfortable position*. Take a moment to loosen all constricting clothing.
2 *Give yourself full permission to relax*. Missing this simple step is one reason many relaxation plans don't succeed. This is a critical first step, explains Dr. Emmett E. Miller in his book *Self-Imagery: Creating Your Own Good Health*. "Allow yourself to rest in a comfortable position, choose some object in the distance to look at and keep your eyes fixed upon it as you repeat silently to yourself 'There's no place I have to go right now, nothing I have to do and no problem I have to solve. . . . I give myself permission to relax.'"[36] Repeat several times.
3 *Focus on your breathing as you begin to release tension*. "After repeating these words [above] several times," says Dr. Miller, "and really hearing their meaning, let your eyelids close and take a deep breath in, filling your abdomen, your middle chest and your upper chest. Hold this breath for a moment without closing off your throat, then let it go, imagining that as you breathe out, you're breathing all unnecessary tension out of your body. As you breathe out repeat to yourself the words, 'Letting go . . . and relaxing.'" Repeat several times.
4 *Have a strategy for dealing with unnecessary thoughts*. You may discover that as your body relaxes and your emotions calm, unnecessary thoughts continue to parade through your mind. It's important not to fight or resist those thoughts — that only makes their distraction more powerful. "Imagine," Dr. Miller suggests, "that your nostrils are like

two tiny exhaust pipes that go up into your mind and that with each breath out you are breathing out unnecessary thoughts. Imagine that with each breath in, fresh clean air is being breathed in through your nostrils and is cleansing your mind of unnecessary thoughts."

5 *Relax by letting go.* You can't force yourself to relax — it doesn't work. Relaxation is basically a letting-go process and there's simply no need to *try* to become relaxed. Just let it happen.

6 *Select a specific relaxation technique — either the progressive relaxation method or the autogenic approach.* Try both methods to find which works best for you. Then you may want to record your own relaxation audiotape and listen to it while you follow the step-by-step sequence. Write your script to include whatever suggestions make it most meaningful and effective for you.

Add the following areas, one at a time, using either relaxation method: (a) right leg, foot, and toes; (b) left leg, foot, and toes; (c) hips and buttocks; (d) abdomen; (e) chest; (f) back; (g) shoulders; (h) right arm, hand, and fingers; (i) left arm, hand, and fingers; (j) neck; (k) jaw; (l) tongue; (m) eyelids; (n) face and scalp.

Progressive Relaxation

Progressive relaxation was developed by Dr. Edmund Jacobson, whose research on stress and relaxation began in 1908 at Harvard University. Also known as the "tense-relax" method, progressive relaxation systematically tightens and releases every major muscle group of the body. Dr. Jacobson discovered that people can relax a muscle to a much greater degree after first tensing it.

Progressive relaxation employs the body tension scan principle discussed earlier and boosts your ability to detect — and eliminate — unnecessary tension. For an in-depth study of Dr. Jacobson's program, see *You Must Relax* in "Resources" at the end of this chapter.

Instructions: Repeat for each body area in sequence from (a) through (n) as listed above: "I am becoming fully aware of my ———— and any sensations I feel there. Next, I am tightening *all* the muscles in that area, taking several seconds to become completely aware of holding tension there. What does it feel like? Now, after taking a smooth, deep breath and holding it for a moment, I'm exhaling as I tell those muscles to *relax and let go,* fully releasing *all* tension and feeling a wave of deep relaxation spreading into that area."

Autogenic Relaxation

Autogenic ("self-regulation") relaxation was developed by Dr. Johannes H. Schultz and Dr. Wolfgang Luthe in Germany. More than fifty years of medical documentation verify its effectiveness. Autogenic relaxation uses mental imagery and verbal cues to regulate breathing, heart rate, blood pressure, and muscle tension. The autogenic method emphasizes calm, rhythmic breathing, a slow heartbeat, and muscular sensations of heaviness (relaxation) and warmth (increased circulation). For an in-depth study, see *Autogenic Methods* in "Resources."

Instructions: Repeat for each body area in sequence from (a) through (n) as listed above: "Warmth and heaviness are flowing into my ———. Warmth and heaviness fill my ——— and it feels relaxed, comfortable, heavy, and warm. I feel my whole body relaxing ever more deeply as the heaviness and warmth fill my ———. I am letting go of all my tensions and worries. I feel peaceful and calm."

Once you have completed a relaxation sequence, take a few extra moments to remain quiet and relaxed, enjoying the calmness. Then return slowly to the active world; count from 1 to 10, completing a breath cycle with each number and becoming ever more alert while maintaining your sense of peacefulness. Now slowly move and stretch your body before returning to your daily activities.

Fight, Flee, or Flow?

It takes wisdom to effectively manage stress. Even with the best strategies and skills, some situations remain beyond our control. To neutralize anxiety in those cases, the best advice may be that given by Dr. Robert Eliot: "If you can't fight and you can't flee, flow."[37]

RESOURCES

Meditation

▶ *Meditation: An Instructional Cassette* by Daniel Goleman, Ph.D. (Psychology Today Tapes, Box 059073, Brooklyn, NY 10025; 800-345-8112). An audiotape that explains basic meditation, its Eastern origins, and common problems faced by beginners.

▶ *Meditation in Action* by Chogyam Trungpa (Shambhala, P.O. Box 308, Boston, MA 02117; 1969). A direct, nonmystical book by a modern Tibetan master who teaches meditation "concerned with seeing what *is*."

▶ *Minding the Body, Mending the Mind* by Joan Borysenko, Ph.D. (Addison-Wesley, 1987). A warm, practical book on meditation, mental imagery, and the mind-body connection.

▶ *The Miracle of Mindfulness! A Manual on Meditation* by Thich N. Hanh (Beacon Press, 1976; available from Parallax Press, P.O. Box 7355, Berkeley, CA 94707). Introductory book by a poet and Zen master nominated for the Nobel Peace Prize by Dr. Martin Luther King, Jr.

▶ *The Relaxation Response* by Herbert Benson, M.D. (Avon, 1975). Simple, straightforward book backed by solid medical documentation.

▶ *Zen Mind, Beginner's Mind* by Shunryu Suzuki (Weatherhill, 1970). An all-time classic on Zen meditation.

Relaxation

▶ *Autogenic Methods* by Johannes H. Schultz, M.D., and Wolfgang Luthe, M.D. (Grune and Stratton, 1969).
▶ *Letting Go of Stress* and *Ten Minute Stress Manager,* two popular relaxation skills audiocassettes by Emmett E. Miller, M.D. (Source Cassette Learning Systems, P.O. Box W, Stanford, CA 94309; 415-328-7171). A videotape called *StressBreak* is also available, combining Dr. Miller's warm, encouraging message with beautiful nature scenes.
▶ *Mind Power Exercises,* audiotapes by Bernie Zilbergeld, Ph.D. (Mind-Power Project, 2847 Shattuck Ave., Berkeley, CA 94705; 415-839-4200). Good instruction in basic relaxation and imagery.
▶ *Stress Talk/Stress Release; Relax . . . Let Go . . . Relax;* and *Daydreams,* audiotapes by Donald Tubesing, Ph.D. (Whole Person Associates, Inc., P.O. Box 3151, Duluth, MN 55803; 218-728-6807). Good relaxation instruction and quick, pleasant imagery "vacations."
▶ *You Must Relax,* 5th edition, by Edmund Jacobson, M.D. (McGraw-Hill, 1978).

5 Time Competency

Planning is bringing the future into the present so that you can do something about it now.

— *ALAN LAKEIN*

The number of minutes and hours available each day is the one resource we all have in common. Time consciousness has reached a predominant place in the American mind. Time urgency and time mismanagement are major stress factors for people in all walks of life. Time competency — using time wisely — is a prerequisite to success in health and fitness programs.[38]

Time frustrations generate and intensify other stresses and undermine self-confidence. Feelings are held inside or are vented prematurely. Conflicts mount. When a couple lacks adequate time together, communication suffers. And when communication is hurt, couples deal less capably with issues like children's behavior and financial concerns.

Another problem is that being *busy* often creates the illusion of being *productive* — and the two aren't the same. You can be maximally efficient — in motion every moment of the day, accomplishing long lists of tasks — and get nowhere in terms of your long-term goals and mission or purpose in life.

Time competency empowers us because (1) it increases the amount of functional time available to take care of high-priority activities because we can identify and reduce sources of wasted time, delegate certain time-consuming activities to others, and fit our long-range goals step by step into our daily schedules, and (2) it reduces the perception of time-urgent conditions that leads to anxiety.

Don't Overdo It

Time-competency goals include reducing stress and making the best use of time in ways that help us achieve our highest objectives. But it's important not to *over*manage time — imploding so much impatience and clock-watching tension that you actually lose time each day. Time effectiveness is the goal, not time warfare.

Beware of "the Time Nuts," says Alan Lakein, author of *How to Get Control of Your Time and Your Life*. These compulsive clock watchers fall into three undesirable categories:[39]

First, the *overorganized person,* who "is always making lists, updating lists, losing lists. . . . He's so intent on being well-organized that he's often blind to changes, new opportunities, and the needs of others."

Second, the *overdoer,* who "is so busy doing things that he has no time to assess their true value. . . . He lacks spontaneity and flexibility. He's terribly efficient, but as often as not is eagerly clambering up the wrong tree. With every moment of his time, both at home and at work, filled with activity, he never has a moment to relax."

Finally, the *time nut,* who "is overwhelmingly preoccupied with time. He makes himself and everyone else nervous with his concern about never wasting a minute. He's always rushing around to meet an impossible schedule."

Choosing the Right Level of Organization for You

"Once you wholeheartedly accept that being better organized really is in your best interest," says Dr. Tom Ferguson, editor-in-chief of *Medical Self-Care* magazine, "there are tools and resources available to help you attain the level of organization that feels right for you."[40]

Here are ten ways to boost time competency:

1. Controlling Your Time

Time is a precious resource but, unlike many resources, it can't be borrowed, bought, saved, or changed. It can only be spent. Beyond increasing your personal effectiveness, don't expend energy trying to save time; instead, improve the ways you *spend* it.

There's *always* time for the most important things in your life. "People these days are so busy with the things that are *urgent,*" says stress researcher Dr. Emmett Miller, "they haven't time for those things that are *important*. . . . I wish I had a nickel for every time I've heard people say: 'I can't *afford* to take the time' and [then a crisis occurs] — and PRESTO! — they suddenly *do* have the time for the things and people they really care about. . . . It's all a matter of priorities."[41]

The challenge is identifying the most important uses of your time — personal, family, work, social, and other — and then scheduling your time so you keep track of priorities. State your objectives precisely, using detail-rich descriptions, and be certain they are attainable within a measured period of time. Post your goals in a conspicuous place where you can't easily overlook them from day to day.

It's also important to reduce your sense of time urgency. Unexpected delays are a poor excuse for tying yourself up in stress knots. Instead of fuming about bad weather, scheduling difficulties, traffic jams, delayed airline flights, and countless other inevitable events, plan for them. First, stop getting upset about situations that are beyond your control. Learn the ICS (instant calming sequence) in Chapter 7. Expand your willingness to accept change and try new strategies for handling difficulties.

Next, keep some emergency resources in your purse, backpack, or briefcase — a low-fat, high-carbohydrate snack to help calm your mind and emotions (see Chapter 27), a notebook for new ideas, a book or periodical you're looking forward to reading, a musical or educational audiotape, and so on. Start filling unavoidable time-delay periods with positive actions. What used to seem like a catastrophe can become an unexpected bonus in the midst of your busy schedule.

Time competency combines calm, attentive awareness to whatever task is at hand with periodic time checks — keeping track of planning, scheduling, and completing your priorities. Lakein suggests that throughout the day you use the question "What is the best use of my time right now?" By frequent mental check-ins, you can lose less time to nonproductive, nonfulfilling activities.

2. Meaningful Directions, Achievable Goals

You can't make time. You can only make *choices*. All the planning in the world won't get you anywhere without action. Whether your dreams are big or small, whether you're reaching for optimal performance or simply a better way to handle day-to-day living, identifying the specific steps to achieve your objectives really pays off.

"It's not goals, it's *directions*," says neuroscientist Dr. Karl H. Pribram from Stanford University. "We need to get away from endpoints, closed systems, zero sums. We feel energized, involved, and motivated when we choose a *direction;* life becomes coherent. Goals are just signposts along the paths of our lives."[42]

Remember, it's easy to get lost in *setting* goals, not appreciating what we're *becoming* on the way to achieving them. And in nearly every case what we become means far more than where we arrive or what we get. It's also important to stop putting off happiness — getting so tangled up in *wants* that we start thinking we can't be happy without satisfying them. As the Zen saying reminds us, There is no way to happiness; happiness *is* the way.

Big dreams are fine, of course, but make step-by-step goals reachable. Don't forget to savor the small wins, the one-at-a-time choices and changes you make, the day-in-day-out efforts and accomplishments.

Goals can be divided into short-term and long-term categories. *Long-term goals* include your chosen mission and lifetime goals. Use a planning notebook and divide these goals into a manageable series of steps. How are you going to bring them to life each day and each week of this coming year?

"Think about what a perfect day would be — five years from today," suggests Dr. Ferguson. "Describe where and how you'll be living. Make it a day that you would find fully satisfying in terms of work and play, friends and family, health and environment. Then list your lifetime goals as that day reveals them."[43]

State your goals in positive terms, describing what you want, not what you don't want. Make sure your goals deal with things you can change directly rather than depending on other people to make changes that affect you. Be as specific as possible and define your goals in sensory-rich ways. The more you can see, touch, hear, smell, or taste your goals, the more powerful they become.

3. Clear Priorities, Specific Plans

There's never enough time to accomplish everything you'd like to do. When you create a daily "to do" list (see number 4 about scheduling), rate each proposed activity on the basis of whether it is (a) essential, (b) important, or (c) trivial.

Focus on the essentials first, followed by the important concerns. Delete or delegate the trivial tasks, except — and this is a vital exception — those seemingly minor choices that warm your heart, ground your feet, or lift your spirit. You know the kind I mean: puttering in the garden; sitting out on the lawn watching the stars or seeing the sun come up or go down; reading a novel or tackling a crossword puzzle; taking time out to play with the kids, cuddle with your pet, or smell the flowers along a park path; seeing a special movie or TV show; raking the leaves, polishing the car, knitting a sweater, baking an exotic loaf of bread, playing a board game . . . whatever gives your psyche a boost. But try to get rid of most trivial tasks you don't enjoy.

Rate your planned daily activities with a priority code. Make it a habit to evaluate every urgent-looking activity you are faced with. Is it really important or urgent? In what way(s) will it help you achieve your objectives? Can it wait until later? Does it require *your* attention or can you delegate it?

Block out time for family activities. Make these times sacred and commit to them in indelible ink — a full year in advance whenever possible. If you and your family don't plan for time together, you'll rarely get around to it and will be plagued by feelings of guilt over neglecting important relationships.

Drifting, dreaming, drowning, *or* deciding: time competency takes regular planning and organizing the specific activities necessary to accomplish your objectives. For those of us who are compulsive note keepers, a planning notebook provides space for recording goals and plans. Review your entries in this journal during daily and weekly planning sessions. A small spiral notebook can serve as your planning record, or you may want to purchase a special planning notebook (see "Resources" at the end of the chapter).

Once your plan is in hand, it's time to schedule your priorities.

4. Effective Scheduling

Scheduling brings your plans to life, setting up precisely when to complete each step or activity.

Daily to-do list. For many of us, a daily to-do list is the main secret of getting more accomplished. Start a rough draft of tomorrow's to-do list today. Tomorrow morning, quickly review the list, prioritize the activities, and focus your attention on the most vital commitments, making deletions and delegating whenever appropriate. Then check off your accomplishments throughout the day as they occur.

Activity calendars. The families that are most in control of their time, say researchers, are likely to keep a family calendar and individual calendars, even for young children.[44] These calendars are reviewed each week in a family meeting, during which members focus on the amount of time they will have to eat together and see one another during the upcoming week. If the schedule looks overloaded with stress, they work together to find ways to reschedule or eliminate some of the proposed activities.

One more tip: Keep some "safety valve" time slots in your schedule for dealing with emergencies and wrapping up unfinished projects.

5. Conquering Procrastination

A lot of people — including bright, successful people — live with a tremendous sense of anxiety because they can't conquer procrastination, the practice of doing low-priority tasks while delaying more important ones. It's a habit that can lead to negativism and self-doubt.

Perfectionism can also contribute to procrastination, causing you to delay moving on to new, important activities because you are never quite satisfied with current activities. Try to avoid perfectionism by doing your very best, accepting the results, and moving forward.

For persistent overloads, try the "done, delegated, or ditched" philosophy expounded by one of my favorite time-management authorities, Edwin C. Bliss, author of *Doing It Now.* His philosophy sounds a bit harsh, but it's a good way to cut excess baggage from your stress caravan.

Delete trivial time wasters from your to-do list, and either delegate unpleasant tasks to someone else or perform them first, at the beginning of the day. Divide difficult duties into small, manageable steps.

What about the odds and ends that you *know* won't be accomplished today? Bliss recommends setting aside a separate tray or drawer for them called a "back burner." Some people call it a "Friday afternoon file." Whatever the name, it should be limited to low-priority items that, about half the time, seem to take care of themselves. Sift through that file every week, discarding those tasks that simply won't get done.

One final recommendation: Don't get dragged into the mindset of focusing entirely on *problems,* which seem urgent, and missing out on taking advantage of *opportunities,* which usually aren't urgent. "Beginning immediately," suggests Bliss, "make it an ironclad rule to schedule a block of time every day for something that does not have to be done that day — but that is important in the long run. (Usually it will turn out to be something relating to one of your long-range goals.) Make it a substantial block of time, perhaps an hour. And guard it jealously: whatever urgent tasks you have to do surely can be accomplished sometime during the remaining twenty-three hours. This one habit can help you to overcome the most pernicious variety of procrastination, which is the postponing of those important (but not urgent) tasks that would move you toward your major goals."[45]

"But how do I get *motivated?*" ask many people ready to start a new program. If you find yourself waiting until everything is perfect before you move toward your goals, stop waiting. "Motivation always follows behavior; it does not precede it," says psychologist Paul Pearsall, founder and director of the Problems of Daily Living Clinic at Mount Sinai Hospital in Detroit. "You must change your behavior first; do not wait for the 'mood to strike.'"[46]

6. Dealing with Interruptions and Paperwork

"Interruptions are *people* — people who want to shift your attention from what you're doing to something else," say Merrill Douglass and Larry Baker in *The New Time Management.* "While people are important, many of the issues they call or walk through your door with are *not* important. Learning to separate people from issues and then dealing with the issues makes it easier to cope with interruptions. Be gracious with people, but be serious about time."[47] When faced with frequent interruptions, act decisively to prevent, screen, consolidate, or delegate them.

To avoid the ocean-of-paperwork syndrome, learn to sort your papers and mail using a priority system. First, deal immediately with paperwork requiring action of some kind — responding right away or at least scheduling the response on your calendar or to-do list. Dr. Tom Ferguson recommends not opening mail until you're ready to respond to it — each piece of paper should be handled only once if possible.[48]

Sort materials you want to read, send to others, or file. *All* other paperwork and mail should be thrown out immediately and with finality; avoid cluttering your environment with mountains of junk mail and unread miscellaneous items — they become sources of unfinished business and needless anxiety.

7. Organizing a Work Space That Fits Your Needs

Set up a private work space in your home or office where your personal planning and scheduling can take place with minimum distractions. Good lighting, proper ventilation, easy access to materials, and pleasant pictures and posters will contribute to the right atmosphere. It's amazing how good it feels to have an uncluttered spot where you can organize your time.

8. Speed Learning, Memory, and Communication Skills

By increasing your reading speed and improving your memory, you can accomplish more in each time slot on your schedule. Research shows that most of us can at least double our reading speed and memory power in six to eight weeks by following simple recommendations (see "Resources" at the end of this chapter). Another important time consideration is how well you listen to and communicate with others (see Chapter 9). The more clearly you express yourself and the better you handle conflicts, the less time and energy you waste coping with recurring interpersonal problems.

9. Controlling Time in Group Situations

With some practice, you can learn to humanely but firmly say no to requests for unnecessary or unpleasant uses of your time.

"To say no is difficult," says Leo Buscaglia. "But so is accepting no for an answer. Why is it that 'no' always seems to infer a rejection or imply rudeness? We seem obliged all too often to say 'yes' when we should be saying 'no.' . . . We forget that we have the right to say no to anything that concerns our own person or time. It seldom occurs to us that a no answer can be the most considerate and positive one we can give. Saying yes from a sense of obligation, fear of rejection or guilt makes no sense. It's degrading to us and unfair to others. . . . It's apparent that saying no can, in many cases, become an act of loving. . . . 'No' at the right time can help others to better understand us and our special needs. It's something we have a right to expect from one another."[49]

"When faced with the prospect of a new task, ask yourself, 'Would anything terrible happen if I didn't do this?'" suggests Dr. Tom Ferguson. "If the answer is no, consider not doing it. . . . When reviewing your problem lists, look for tasks that could just as well remain undone — then cross them off. . . . If you find it difficult to say no to a request, say you'd like some time to think about it and say no later."[50]

10. Making Time for Self, Family, Friends, and Recreation

It isn't easy to schedule and protect times for yourself, your family, your friends, and recreation. But it's certainly important from a health and fitness perspective.

Couples and families who manage stress well devote quality time to each other every day. They also allocate personal time for each family member. And they check in with each other at key points in the day. "In one quiet minute with myself, I can first *become aware* of what I am doing and then I can *choose* to see a better way," writes Dr. Spencer Johnson in *One Minute for Myself.* "I invite you to take one minute to stop and gently ask *yourself* the . . . quiet question: *Is there a way, right now, for me to take better care of myself? . . . Am I asking another person or our relationship to do the impossible — to take good care of me — or are we each taking better care of ourselves and thus enjoying an even better relationship together?* . . . In one minute I can change my attitude and in that minute I can change my entire day."[51]

Finally, don't forget to take time for play. Families that play together are consistently healthier than those that don't.[52] Post the activities your family finds most fun-filled and look for new options, checking in each week with the question How much fun have we had together lately?

Delegating

Delegation is the practice of appointing someone else to perform a task. It's *not* the carefree abandonment of responsibility. *Effective* delegation requires awareness and follow-through. If the task is essential and you can't ensure the outcome, don't delegate it. If you can maintain control and select the right person to complete the activity, then delegate.

RESOURCES

Planning and Scheduling Notebooks

▶ Day-Timers, Inc. (Allentown, PA 18001; 215-398-1223).
▶ Memogenda (Norwood Products, Inc., 1000 S. Thompson Lane, Nashville, TN 37211).
▶ Personal Planning System (R. Webster Systems International, Inc., Suite 260, 500 W. Wilson Bridge Rd., Columbus, OH 43085; 614-436-5300; or Higher Education Management Institute, 924 Talus Dr., Yellow Springs, OH 45387).
▶ Time/Design (11835 W. Olympic Blvd., Suite 450, Los Angeles, CA 90064; 800-637-9942).

Time Management and Speed Learning

▶ *Creativity in Business* by Michael Ray and Rochelle Myers (Doubleday, 1986). Gives innovative, practical ideas for making decisions and managing time, based on the Stanford University course taught by Ray and Myers.

▶ *Doing It Now* by Edwin C. Bliss (Bantam, 1984). Banishes the top forty cop-outs and gives a straightforward 12-point plan.

▶ *Don't Forget: Easy Exercises for Better Memory at Any Age* by Danielle C. Lapp (McGraw-Hill, 1986). Excellent book by a Stanford University memory skills instructor.

▶ *Evelyn Wood Reading Dynamics* (Nightingale-Conant Corp., 7300 N. Lehigh Ave., Chicago, IL 60648; 1987). A top-rated speed-reading course presented in an audiotape collection with study guide.

▶ *Getting Organized* by Stephanie Winston (Warner Books, 1978; Warner Audio, 1985). Focuses on getting all aspects of daily life in order — from the basics of managing time through setting up a desk/work area, dealing with paperwork and money arranging your kitchen and other rooms of the house, and educating children about time and organization.

▶ *Harry Lorayne's Page-a-Minute Memory Book* by Harry Lorayne (Ballantine, 1985). A concise memory skills book.

▶ *How to Get Control of Your Time and Your Life* by Alan Lakein (Signet, 1973). A classic step-by-step orientation to time management.

▶ *The Insight System for Planning Your Time and Your Life* by Charles R. Hobbs (Nightingale-Conant Corp., 7300 N. Lehigh Ave., Chicago, IL 60648; 1986). An audiotape collection offering a comprehensive approach to time management that is simple to apply.

▶ *Make the Most of Your Mind* by Tony Buzan (Linden Press, 1984; Simon and Schuster Sound Ideas, 1986). Introduction to memory enhancement, speed reading, numerical skill, creativity, observation, logic, and analysis.

▶ *Putting the One Minute Manager to Work* by Kenneth Blanchard, Ph.D. and Robert Lorder, Ph.D. (Berkley, 1984). Fast, practical techniques that support effective delegation, including "One Minute Goal Setting," "One Minute Praisings," and "One Minute Reprimands."

▶ *Total Recall* by Joan Minninger, Ph.D. (Pocket Books, 1984). A thorough book on memory improvement.

6 Positive Support Systems

Positive Self-Support

The more I take good care of myself, the less resentment and anger I feel and the more loving I become toward myself and others.

— *SPENCER JOHNSON,*
ONE MINUTE FOR MYSELF

Your wellspring of confidence comes from within. If you support yourself poorly — with criticism, pessimism, fear, anger, guilt, or worry — it's easy to end up plodding through life in a cloud of negativity. Positive self-support is a cornerstone of *Health & Fitness Excellence*. Here are several areas to consider.

Your Thoughts and Mental Images

Men are disturbed not by things, but by the view which they take of them.
— *EPICTETUS*

Your thoughts and mental images can contribute to one of the biggest stress knots of all. Thoughts create emotions, and emotions shape our thinking. It's a continuous cycle.

Your brain uses neurochemicals, electrical impulses, and trillions of special receptors to spread the influence of your thoughts to every cell in your body. These chemicals change in response to the way we each perceive ourselves and interact with the people and events in our lives. Every pressure triggers a host of questions: Can I handle this? What happens if I can't? What are my options?

One way the mind affects health is through *explanatory style* — the way we describe our experiences to ourselves and others. Evidence shows that when we consistently make certain assumptions about the cause of bad things that happen to us, we increase our risk of disease and undercut our performance.[53]

According to the results of more than one hundred experiments involving nearly fifteen thousand subjects, people with negative explanatory style tend to explain the bad things that happen to them in terms that are internal ("It's all my fault"), stable ("It's going to last forever"), and global ("It's going to spoil everything I do"). These individuals are at the greatest risk for depression, repeated mistakes, and illness.

Some researchers call this phenomenon *cognitive distortion* — distorted thinking — the automatic negative thoughts that lead to distress and conflict. Distorted thoughts include *filtering* (magnifying the negative details of your experiences and filtering out the positive); *all-or-nothing thinking* (life is either good or bad; if you're not perfect, you're a failure); *overpersonalizing* (seeing yourself as the cause of all the bad things in your life); *overgeneralizing* (viewing single setbacks as a never-ending treadmill of defeat); *catastrophizing* (considering every mistake and bad situation as the end of the world); and *jumping to conclusions* (concluding the worst without evidence).[54] Each negative thought encourages and amplifies others. It's easy to end up trapped in a labyrinth of pessimism, and it takes dedication to break out.

Chapter 44 reviews the most common types of distorted thinking and presents advice from the experts on how to stop it. For right now, begin with awareness — pay closer attention to the way you explain mistakes and unpleasant situations to yourself and others — and start catching distorted thoughts. Replace them with constructive attributions. Be specific, honest, and positive. And be gentle to yourself. Life is challenging enough without letting your mind stack the odds against you.

Letting Go of Guilt

How much time do you spend shackled to the past? Each of us has made mistakes, suffered injustices, been criticized, envied, and rejected by others, and failed to reach certain goals. We can — on an instant's notice — clobber ourselves with negative memories and end up paralyzed in the present.

Shedding self-blame is crucial to best health and fitness. "If unchecked, our natural tendency to blame ourselves for our suffering becomes . . . unreasonable and immobilizing," writes psychologist Julius Segal in *Winning Life's Toughest Battles: Roots of Human Resilience.* "The danger is especially great because our readiness to indict ourselves is often reinforced by the attitudes of people around us. . . . The capacity to nurture an optimistic attitude is obliterated by self-blame. So, too, is the capacity to turn our thoughts outward, toward others. Self-blame means wallowing in private ruminations, cutting ourselves off emotionally from [other people]."[55]

"The fact is that *the past is over,* and, whatever may have happened 'then,' it will never come again, and you can never get it back," adds Wayne Dyer, author of *The Sky's the Limit.* "Any time you find yourself using up your present moments being immobilized because of something that occurred in the past, you are victimizing yourself unnecessarily. The first step in transcending your past is to *surrender* the attitudes toward it that immobilize you now. . . . 'Surrendering' does not mean giving up your memories, or that you should forget anything you have learned that can make you more happy and effective in the present. . . . I am talking about ridding yourself *immediately* of those learned attitudes which inhibit you from functioning effectively and happily today."[56]

That's easy to say but harder to achieve, you're probably thinking. But with a commitment and some work, the past *can* be released. Here are some suggestions.

First, increase your awareness. Begin to identify the circumstances, attitudes, viewpoints, feelings, or physical tensions you want to release. Some of them spring from hidden beliefs and life decisions based on painful experiences that happened long ago.

Experts recommend a number of ways to release the past, including meditation, which draws your attention away from guilt or worry and into the present moment; changing distorted thinking patterns by changing your mood (see Chapter 44); using mental imagery to rewrite past scripts in a more positive way (see Chapters 44 and 45) and to imagine that things had been different (which doesn't erase the facts but substitutes more positive thoughts and feelings so that you're unimpaired right now); practicing an instant calming sequence (see Chapter 7) in which you can begin catching and neutralizing the first signs of anxiety, remaining calm and productive; or writing a letter expressing your hurt or anger and then (without mailing it or letting anyone else know about its existence) destroying it.

When you feel you must change what you can't change — something about yourself, others, or the world — you get caught in an emotional bind. One of the fastest ways to fuel feelings of guilt is to keep hitting yourself with "should" statements. Cognitive therapist Dr. David D. Burns, author of *Feeling Good: The New Mood Therapy,* recommends finding a variety of ways to catch and stop irrational "should haves" or "shoulds," replacing them with something less upsetting like "It would have been (or would be) nice if ———" or "I wish I could have done (or could do) ———."[57]

Stop letting other people make you feel inferior. One of the biggest disadvantages of being guilt-prone is that others can and will use your feelings of guilt to manipulate you. Whiners, complainers, belittlers, and blamers show up in most families and businesses. Don't let their doubts and worries become yours.

Use precise language (see Chapter 9) to cut through generalizations, "should" statements, and other communication pitfalls. Be clear and specific about how much your goals and feelings mean to you, and experiment with different strategies to eliminate pessimistic whining and nagging.

According to Dr. Burns, a typical pattern works like this: "The whiner complains to you about something or someone. You feel the sincere desire to be helpful, so you make a suggestion. The person immediately squashes your suggestion and complains again. You feel tense and inadequate, so you try harder and make another suggestion. You get the same response. Anytime you try to break loose from the conversation, the other person implies he or she is being abandoned, and you are flooded with guilt."[58]

One effective technique, say cognitive therapists, involves finding some way to agree with nags, complainers, and whiners rather than trying to help them. That's because these people are usually feeling irritated and insecure. When you make an effort to help them, it sounds to them like criticism implying that they aren't handling things properly. On the other hand, if you find some way to agree with them and add a compliment, they feel endorsed and usually relax and quiet down.

Moving Beyond Fear

Fear is a question. What are you afraid of, and why? Our fears are a treasure-house of self-knowledge if we explore them.

— *MARILYN FERGUSON,*
EDITOR OF BRAIN/MIND BULLETIN

For millions of Americans, the idea of "risk" is frightening. "It is surprising how little most people know about taking risks," says psychiatrist David Viscott in *Risking.* "Often they become inhibited by fear at the very moment they must commit themselves to action. At the first sign of a reversal they hesitate and, fearing that the situation is about to fall apart, retreat untested, convinced that they were in over their heads, thankful just to escape."[59]

Not risking destroys lives. People who don't risk never learn who they are, never test their potential, never stretch or reach. They become comfortable with fewer and fewer experiences, living as victim in an increasingly rigid world. The fears that we deny can end up dominating our lives.

"What is stopping you, at this very moment, from being the person you want to be and living your life the way you want to live it?" asks psychologist Susan Jeffers, author of *Feel the Fear . . . and Do It Anyway.* "The answer — beneath all the other answers — is *fear.* Whether it relates to work, relationships, money, or simply life in general, fear can keep you from doing what you really want and need to do in order to grow and achieve a sense of well-being."[60]

Dr. Jeffers divides fear into three categories: (1) surface-level fears (such as of aging, accidents, being alone, retiring, dying, natural disasters, changing careers, making friends, ending or beginning relationships, losing weight, public speaking, or intimacy); (2) inner-state-of-mind fears (such as of rejection, success, failure, vulnerability, envy, or helplessness); and (3) the biggest fear of all — the one that really keeps people stuck — the fear that "I can't handle it!"

Fear leads to conflict — upset feelings, fighting, winners/losers, compromising, rejection, humiliation — and worsening relationships. In *Do I Have to Give Up Me to Be Loved by You?*[61] psychologists Jordan and Margaret Paul cite research showing that, although conflict is an inevitable part of all relationships, it can be an opportunity to learn rather than a calamity. Two possible chain reactions — one positive, one negative — occur every time we have a conflict. We must choose between an *intent to protect* (against threats, real and imagined, of emotional pain) and an *intent to learn* (in which we stop blaming and take responsibility for our own thoughts and feelings). The intent to protect includes control, compliance, and indifference and ranges from violent reactions to total silence. The intent to learn is based on openness — the willingness to discover why each of us is feeling and behaving as we do.

Everyone experiences some fear when going into unfamiliar experiences, explains Dr. Jeffers. As long as you keep learning and growing, that fear won't go away — so you need to accept it. Not only are you going to experience fear when you're venturing into something new, but so is everyone else. The way to get rid of the fear of doing something is to go out and do it. No amount of thinking and talking will get you unstuck — it takes action. In other words, you may have to make the first step while still afraid. Remember, in the long run pushing through fear is less frightening than anxiously living with it.

One final note: If you are afraid of being violently assaulted, consider learning martial arts. If you choose an instructor with care, you'll find new ways to be fit, open your senses, clear your mind, and resolve most conflicts before they occur — without force. Over the past twenty-five years, I have studied and taught a number of martial arts systems. I am partial to those styles that emphasize a peaceful attitude, sharp senses, fluid movements, timing, and positioning. These skills can be developed by people of all ages and sizes.

If, in spite of all precautions, you are forced into a confrontational situation, this training can enable you to remain calm and alert instead of appearing menacing or afraid. The assailant will sense an unexpected lack of resistance or intimidation and may quit the attack. If the assault proceeds, the right martial arts skills can give you an advantage — a state of awareness and relaxation that permit movement in any direction, suddenly and powerfully.

You can learn to make your thoughts and actions simultaneous and neutralize an assailant's aggression not by clashing with it head-on but by merging with the attacking energy and guiding it, diverting it, and neutralizing it. These physical principles are a good metaphor for dealing with *any* embattled situation.

Enhancing Self-Esteem

Nobody can make you feel inferior without your permission.
— *ELEANOR ROOSEVELT*

Esteem is derived from the Latin and means "to value highly." Of all the judgments that we pass in life, none is more important than the one we pass on ourselves. Self-esteem combines self-respect and self-confidence and is based on the belief that an individual is competent and worthy of living. Our self-concept tends to be our destiny. And self-doubt is one of the most debilitating and widespread psychological problems affecting men and women today.

"The greatest barrier to achievement and success," says psychologist Nathaniel Branden in *Honoring the Self: The Psychology of Confidence and Respect,* "is not lack of talent or ability but, rather, the fact that achievement and success, above a certain level, are outside our self-concept, our image of who we are and what is appropriate to us. . . . Self-esteem is an evaluation of my mind, my consciousness, and, in a profound sense, my person. It is not an evaluation of particular successes or failures, nor is it an evaluation of particular knowledge or skills. . . . *Genuine self-esteem is not competitive or comparative.* Neither is genuine self-esteem expressed by self-glorification at the expense of others, or by the quest to make oneself superior to all others or to diminish others so as to elevate oneself. Arrogance, boastfulness, and the overestimation of our abilities reflects inadequate self-esteem rather than, as some people imagine, too high a level of self-esteem. In human beings, joy in the mere fact of existing is a core meaning of healthy self-esteem. It is a state of one who is at war neither with self nor with others."[62]

How can you build self-esteem? There are a number of ways. You may want to approach it indirectly. For example, every lifestyle change you make from this book can lift self-esteem through what researchers call *compensatory self-improvement*.[63]

Then there are direct approaches, such as those already mentioned in this chapter. To build self-esteem, you need to catch negative thoughts and images that buzz around in your head and substitute objective, positive ones. Why? Because the automatic, critical inner voice we each hear is almost always wrong. Most of us have years of practice with put-downs. In fact, the national average of parent-to-child criticisms is 12 to 1 — a dozen criticisms for every single compliment or positive comment. And in the average secondary school classroom, the ratio of criticisms to compliments from teacher to student is 18 to 1.[64]

It's time to begin complimenting yourself often and genuinely. Be specific and detailed. You do lots of things right every day — so make the effort to stop focusing undue attention on mistakes.

Anger

"Now we know that anger is a killer." With these words, CBS News medical correspondent Dr. Robert Arnot recently summarized research on the effects of unresolved anger. When you lose your cool, you lose your performance edge, your health, maybe even your life.

For years, researchers have known that anger contributes to high blood pressure and heart attack risk.[65] A recent fifteen-year controlled study of husbands and wives by the University of Michigan School of Public Health measured the effects of expression of anger, supression, and "cool reflection." The researchers discovered that ineffectively managed anger was linked to 2.5 times greater risk of death from all causes.[66] The findings held true for both sexes and all age groups and education levels, regardless of whether the individuals smoked or had any other common risk factors for heart disease. "The key issue," says Dr. Ernest Harburg, one of the researchers, "is not the amount or degree of your anger, but *how you cope with it*."

Three standard responses to anger are (1) "anger-in" — suppressing your angry feelings altogether; (2) "anger-out" — explosively venting your anger immediately; and (3) "reflective coping" — waiting until tempers have cooled to rationally discuss the conflict with the other person or sort things out on your own. Reflective coping is by far the best choice because, as the research team discovered, it restores a sense of control over the situation and helps resolve it. Those people who kept their cool — who acknowledged their anger but were not openly hostile, physically or verbally — felt better faster and had superior health. While venting anger does relieve tension, it can also contribute to guilt feelings, which become an added source of stress.

What conclusions can we draw from all this? The events of life don't make us angry — our "hot thoughts" do. Anger is usually a defense against loss of self-esteem and comes from frustration and unmet expectations. Most thoughts that generate anger contain distortions (see Chapter 44), and most anger can be quickly defused if you take a moment to see the world through the other person's eyes. Remember, conflicts are rarely caused by only one. Although we all have the *right* to get angry whenever we want, in almost every case it's not to our advantage.

"Reflective anger-coping," says Dr. Mara Julius, who headed the study, "not only promotes better problem solving but better health, and possibly longer life." And it affects our children too. A recent study by researchers at the National Institute of Mental Health reported that young children are especially susceptible to psychological problems from angry exchanges they see or hear in the home.[67] This "background anger" of heated arguments clearly distressed the children studied, causing them to freeze in place, cry, cover their ears or eyes, or run away from the scene. Their reactions suggest that background anger may have a cumulative effect, perhaps even more detrimental than television violence.

Begin using the instant calming sequence (Chapter 7) to help stop surges of anger. Pause for a moment each time you get frustrated to ask, Is my anger useful? Does it support my integrity and help me achieve my goals — or does it just defeat me?

Criticism

Anger is frequently triggered by criticism. Shaming people, assigning blame, giving incomplete or inaccurate feedback, and overemphasizing the negative aspects of a situation all make problems worse.

Criticism is a two-way street; in addition to being given, it's also taken. Stonewalling ("I've always done it this way" or "That's just the way I am") and excuse making are common examples of inappropriate criticism taking.

To give criticism effectively and constructively,[68] tell people beforehand that you're going to honestly let them know how they are performing. Then wait for the appropriate time and place. Focus your comments on the problem behavior, not on the person. Use "I" and "we" statements, not the accusatory "you." Be certain that the behavior you are criticizing *can* be changed and state it as your opinion, not fact, using neutral gestures and voice tones that do not ridicule, accuse, or threaten. And avoid absolutes and generalizations (discussed in Chapter 9).

Make your comments as specific and brief as possible. Tell the person exactly how you *feel* about what went wrong. Then pause for a few seconds of silence to let the person feel how you're feeling.

Finally, demonstrate empathy for the other person's feelings and problems and, if appropriate, offer to help resolve them. Shake hands or touch the other person in a way that genuinely communicates that you are on his or her side, that you value him or her. Reaffirm that you think highly of the person, but not his or her actions in this situation. Then let go. When the criticism is over, it's over.

To learn to take criticism more productively, first use an "instant calming sequence" (Chapter 7) to keep yourself relaxed and under control. Then ask yourself how important the criticism is, how objective the source is, and how emotional the climate is where it arises. And then, if the comments seem the least bit valuable, take the point of view that constructive change can make you a healthier, more productive person — and welcome the ideas.

Cutting Back on Competition

Do people perform better when they're trying to beat others than when they're working *with* them or alone? Instead of taking competition's reputed benefits for granted, research teams have put them to the test. And with astonishing consistency, scientists have discovered that competition — by definition, making one person's success another's failure — *doesn't* support best performance.[69] Seven different studies have been conducted since the late 1970s by psychologist Robert Helmreich at the University of Texas using different groups of subjects — scientists, academic psychologists, businesspeople, elementary school students, college students, airline pilots, and airline reservation agents. Every study showed that competitiveness results in poorer performance.

David and Roger Johnson, professors of education at the University of Minnesota, reviewed 122 studies conducted between 1924 and 1981 — every evaluation of performance or achievement data in competitive, cooperative, or individual educational settings. Sixty-five studies showed that cooperation promoted higher achievement than competition, 8 indicated the opposite, and 36 showed no significant difference. The superiority of cooperation held for all subject areas and all age groups.[70]

"Once we move from such achievement measures as speed of performance, number of problems solved or amount of information recalled and consider the quality of performance, competition does even worse," says Alfie Kohn, author of *No Contest: The Case Against Competition*. "There are two important reasons for competition's failure. First, success often depends on sharing resources efficiently, and this is nearly impossible when people have to work against each other. Cooperation takes advantage of all the skills represented in a group as well as the mysterious process by which that group becomes more than the sum of its parts. . . . Second, competition generally does not promote excellence because trying to do well and trying to beat others simply are two different things."[71]

Success is not the same as victory. Goals can be achieved in three ways: competitively, cooperatively, or independently. Competition, it turns out, is almost always inferior to the other two.

Humor, Laughter,
and Play

Laughter is the shortest distance between two people.

— *VICTOR BORGE*

Very few things so instantly form a bond between people as laughter. It's a universal language. And research suggests that it may enhance the body's immune system.

Scientists theorize that laughter stimulates the production of brain hormones called catecholamines, which affect hormonal levels in the body, some related to feelings of joy, an easing of pain, and strengthened immune response.[72]

In response to the pioneering work of Norman Cousins, author of *Anatomy of an Illness*,[73] a growing number of hospitals have opened "humor rooms" where patients can view comical movies and select books from a humor library. One company (Laughter Therapy, P.O. Box 827, Monterey, CA 93942) will loan one-hour humor tapes free for a month to people suffering from serious health problems.

The healthy family has a great sense of play and humor, reports Dolores Curran in *Traits of the Healthy Family*. "A sense of humor keeps things in perspective and works as an antidote to drudgery, depression, and conflict within the family. . . . In good families humor is used to defuse potentially stressful situations. . . . Healthy families tend to laugh *with* one another while unhealthy families laugh *at* one another."[74]

Of course, humor isn't something you can cultivate in cold blood. You *allow* it to happen naturally — through a sense of relaxation and fun. Begin noticing the absurd, silly, incongruous events that go on all around you. Look for positive humor in your life experiences, and seek out other people you can laugh with. The healthiest laughs may be the all-out, side-splitting variety. One way to defuse anger with friends and relatives is to momentarily change the conversation focus to a time when you laughed together. But avoid telling jokes based on ridicule — they inflict pain. And skip hurtful sarcasm. A good pun that gives you a twist of expectancy can be wonderful. And cosmic humor — an appreciation of life's paradoxes and absurdities — is the most fun of all.

Physical play — the laughter-filled games of youth — should be guaranteed a small block of time every single day of our lives. Group play activities have moved beyond the winner-loser games most of us grew up with. New versions of table games (such as Scrabble and bridge) and outdoor games (such as basketball) have been developed using an exciting non-zero-sum (NZS) approach in which everyone is inspired to perform his or her best *and* cooperate, and nobody loses.[75]

"New Games" are another great development in fun-filled activities, a humanistic way for people to play. In small or large groups, New Games create an exciting, "everybody wins" spirit, offering a safe but challenging array of activities — from running, tagging, hugging, and throwing soft objects in the air through laughter-filled pantomime — all at any intensity level you choose. New Games are easy to learn and require little or no special equipment. And they're for everyone — your sex, age, or size doesn't determine your ability to have fun and improve your fitness. (See *Play* in "Resources" at the end of the chapter.)

Personal Rewards

Nothing succeeds like success. Reward yourself in some way every time you respond successfully to a stress-provoking situation. *Every* time. Doing *anything* more quickly, easily, effectively, or enjoyably than before is cause for personal congratulations, perhaps even a celebration. The same holds true for the times you make others feel better — your family, friends, co-workers, neighbors, or community.

Personal rewards don't have to be edible or cost anything. They can be as simple as spending quiet time in a special place, listening to music, reading a favorite book, playing a game of tennis, treating yourself to a massage, a new plant or flower, or relaxing in a hot bath. And frequent small perks are more effective than one big reward after years of sacrifice.

Positive Support of and from Others

The rise of human loneliness may be one of the most serious sources of disease in the 20th century.

— *JAMES J. LYNCH, PH.D.*

Human connectedness — a positive and supportive social network — helps us resist disease, enjoy life, and live longer.[76] In fact, some medical researchers have even reported that nonsmokers who live alone have shorter life spans than smokers who have a mate or even a pet!

"Researchers have repeatedly demonstrated a vital link between the strength of our social support systems and our emotional and physical resilience under severe stress," says psychologist Julius Segal. In reviewing the evidence to date, Hebrew University psychiatrist Gerald Caplan adds that "when the stress level is high, people without psychological support suffer as much as ten times the incidence of physical and emotional illness experienced by those who enjoy such support."[77]

"Every time I found evidence of disrupted social relationships, I found evidence of some sort of negative health outcome," reports S. Leonard Syme, epidemiologist and professor in the School of Public Health at the University of California at Berkeley. "And the range of disease outcomes is very broad indeed. For example, people with interrupted social ties exhibit more depression, unhappiness, and loss of morale, more complications of pregnancy, higher mortality rates for many diseases, including heart disease and cancer, higher morbidity rates for such illnesses as gastro-intestinal upset, skin problems, arthritis, and headaches."[78]

Improving Your Current Relationships

There is no longer any doubt that the quality of our relationships — intimate, family, neighborhood, business, social, and so on — is closely related to our health, productivity, and well-being.

Good relationships are those that can deal well with differences in values, perceptions, and interests. In contrast, bad relationships are filled with conflict, selfishness, disruption, and emotional trauma.

It's time for all of us who care about our health to take a close look at our relationships (see "Resources" at the end of this chapter for recommendations for further reading). Clear communication (Chapter 9) is critical, as is the instant calming sequence (Chapter 7), positive thinking (Chapter 44), and many other *Health & Fitness Excellence* elements presented throughout this book.

In their book *Getting Together: Building a Relationship That Gets to Yes* (Houghton Mifflin, 1988), Roger Fisher and Scott Brown, leaders of the Harvard Negotiation Project, advise strengthening qualities essential to coping successfully with the inevitable differences found in all relationships.

First, although it takes two or more people to have a relationship, it's important to realize that it takes only one to change the quality of that relationship. Second, try to separate people from problems. Don't entangle substantive issues (money, dates, time, property, terms, conditions) with human aspects (how we deal with each other).

Third, learn to be unconditionally constructive, which means checking partisan perceptions; don't forget how differently we each see things. In a relationship with another person, do whatever is good for the relationship and you — whether or not the other person reciprocates.

The extensive research by Fisher and Brown suggests that the following actions will help strengthen a relationship: Even if the other person is acting emotionally, try to balance emotions with reason. Even if you feel you are being misunderstood, keep trying to understand the other person. Even if you think the other person isn't listening, consult him or her before making decisions on matters that affect you both. Be reliable, whether or not you trust or feel deceived by the other person. Operate beyond coercion; try to persuade the other person and be open to persuasion yourself. Even if you feel that you and your concerns are being rejected, care about others, accept them and their ideas as worthy of your consideration, and be open to learning from them.

Expanding Your Support Network

How can you explore ways to nurture and enlarge your support network? Dr. Tom Ferguson, editor-in-chief of *Medical Self-Care* magazine, offers these suggestions: After taking three pieces of paper, draw a circle in the center of one and, inside this circle, write your name. In circles near yours, write the names of the people with whom you have the strongest, closest bonds. Include those who have been sources of warmth and approval during earlier periods of your life, as well as those who actively support you now.

"List the people you have warm feelings for," advises Dr. Ferguson. "People you are comfortable with. Nurturing people. People you would like to be able to talk with if you were having a hard time. Think of all the people you would feel comfortable hugging — or being hugged by. All the people you would enjoy sharing a meal with. All the people you'd enjoy receiving a letter from. Don't worry about being 'fair' or reasonable or logical — this exercise is for you alone."[79]

As you list the names, you may find yourself wishing you were closer in touch with some of them. If so, list these people on the second sheet of paper. Entries may include old friends you haven't seen in a long time or new friends you'd like to get to know better.

There may be some people for whom you would like to do something special — a hug, a phone call, a letter, or a gift to let them know they're really important to you. If such feelings come to mind, list them with the names of these friends on the third sheet of paper.

When you've finished your social support system diagram, take several minutes to review each name, remembering the kinds of support you've received from and given to that person. Is there anyone you'd like to be in touch with right now? What ongoing use can you make of your lists?

"Most of us take our friendships for granted," says Leo Buscaglia. "We become passive in maintaining them and lose sight of the fact that they need constant effort, care and attention. . . . We forget that even the most secure among us needs reassurance from time to time. . . . The space that so often expands between people is so easily bridged with the right words at the right time."[80]

An added benefit of nurturing friendships is that lending a helping hand to other people may be good for your own vitality — and even for your heart and immune system. New research in this area looks promising, and the benefits of altruism continue to be investigated.[81]

Self-Help Groups in the Computer Age

The computer age has ushered in the era of high-speed networking. Self-help groups are being formed for special needs of all kinds. In fact, there's a support group for virtually every problem and interest these days — physical and psychological health concerns of all descriptions, sports and fitness specialties, learning abilities, communication skills, family needs, education, politics, hobbies, travel, and spiritual growth. Computer databases can put you in instant contact with groups in your community that share your interests or needs. And Self-Help Clearinghouse director Ed Madara says, "If there's not one nearby, we encourage callers to start their own."[82]

To link up with groups in your area, talk to relatives, friends, psychologists, physicians, co-workers, and community service offices. Check the white pages of your phone book under "Volunteer Bureau" or "Volunteer Center." Or send a stamped, self-addressed envelope to VOLUNTEER — The National Center (1111 N. 19th St., Suite 500, Arlington, VA 22209). VOLUNTEER provides groups with information sharing, training, and promotion. You can also obtain a partial list of support groups by sending a stamped, self-addressed envelope to Self-Help Clearinghouse (St. Clares–Riverside Medical Center, Pocomo Road, Denville, NJ 07834; 201-625-9565 or 800-367-6274). Be certain to specify the kind of group you're interested in joining or forming.

RESOURCES

Letting Go of the Past

▶ American Imagery Institute (P.O. Box 13453, Milwaukee, WI 53213). Directed by Dr. Anees Sheikh, chairman of the department of psychology at Marquette University, this institute offers books, tapes, and a journal on mental imagery.

▶ *Good-Bye to Guilt: Releasing Fear Through Forgiveness* by Gerald G. Jampolsky, M.D. (Bantam, 1985). Straightforward philosophical advice.

▶ *Necessary Losses* by Judith Viorst (Simon and Schuster, 1980). A compassionate, scholarly analysis of how to view life's many losses and separations in a constructive way.

▶ *Rapid Relief from Emotional Distress* by Gary Emergy, Ph.D., and James Campbell, M.D. (Fawcett, 1986). A fast, clinically proven method for overcoming emotional problems, using the ACT formula: accept current reality; reaffirm where you choose to go; take action to get there.

▶ *Releasing: The New Behavorial Science Method for Dealing with Pressure Situations* by Patricia Carrington, Ph.D. (William Morrow, 1984; audiotapes available from Pace Educational Systems, Inc., P.O. Box 113, Kendall Park, NJ 08824). Innovative technique for letting go of the desire to change situations that can't be changed now.

▶ *Sanity, Insanity, and Common Sense* by Rick Suarez, Ph.D., Roger C. Mills, Ph.D., and Darlene Stewart, M.S. (Fawcett, 1987). A groundbreaking book on neo–cognitive psychology, or the psychology of mind. Discusses the sources of our perceptions, feelings, thoughts, and behaviors. Audiotapes and research papers are available from the Advanced Human Studies Institute (P.O. Box 140223, Coral Gables, FL 33114).

▶ *Smart Cookies Don't Crumble* by Sonya Friedman, Ph.D. (Pocket, 1986). A close look at what blocks our progress or gives us the courage and persistence to overcome life's disappointments.

▶ *Software for the Mind* by Emmett E. Miller, M.D. (Celestial Arts, 1987). Practical exercises for using visualization to release tension and anxiety and create new habits, attitudes, and experiences in life.

▶ *When Bad Things Happen to Good People* by Harold Kushner (Avon, 1983). The story of a father whose child died and the struggle of a rabbi to understand why we lose those people dearest to us. Universal message.

▶ *Writing Your Own Script* by Emmett E. Miller, M.D. (Source, P.O. Box W, Stanford, CA 94309; 415-328-7171). This warm, supportive audiotape includes "Setting Your Image Goal," "Letting Go of the Past," "Writing Your Own Future Script," and "Applauding Your Progress."

Fear

▶ *Feel the Fear . . . and Do It Anyway* by Susan Jeffers, Ph.D. (Harcourt Brace Jovanovich, 1987). Clear, practical advice.

▶ *Freeing Yourself from Fear* by Emmett E. Miller, M.D. (Source, P.O. Box W, Stanford, CA 94309; 415-328-7171; 1981). An audiotape program for deconditioning fears and phobias and succeeding with future challenges.

▶ *Life Without Fear: Anxiety and Its Cure* by Joseph Wolpe, M.D. (New Harbinger, 1988). Discusses a "systematic desensitization" program.

▶ *Love Is Letting Go of Fear* by Gerald G. Jampolsky, M.D. (Bantam, 1981). A wonderful addition to the self-help field, teaching that by increasing the love in our lives we naturally reduce fear.

Self-Esteem

▶ Advanced Human Studies Institute (P.O. Box 140223, Coral Gables, FL 33114; 305-445-2155). Offers audiotapes and books on neo–cognitive psychology.

▶ L.A. Center for Cognitive Therapy (630 S. Wilton Place, Los Angeles, CA 90005; 213-387-4737). The center, directed by Dr. Gary Emery, coauthor of *Rapid Relief from Emotional Distress* (Fawcett, 1986), offers books, tapes, and a newsletter that deal with self-esteem issues.

▶ *One Minute for Myself* by Spencer Johnson, M.D. (William Morrow,

1985). Encourages each of us to take a minute out several times a day to become fully aware of how we are doing and to find better ways to take care of ourselves while still helping others.

▶ *The Psychology of Self-Esteem* (Bantam, 1971), *Honoring the Self: The Psychology of Confidence and Respect* (Bantam, 1980), and *How to Raise Your Self-Esteem* (Bantam, 1987), all by Nathaniel Branden, Ph.D., are recognized standards in the field.

▶ *The Sky's the Limit* by Wayne Dyer, Ed.D. (Pocket Books, 1980). A fast-paced presentation of techniques for becoming a "no-limit" person.

▶ Denis Waitley, Ph.D. (P.O. Box 1641, Ames, IA 50010). Offers books, audiotapes, and videotapes for building self-esteem in children, teenagers, and adults on individual, family, school, and community levels.

Anger and Criticism

▶ *Anger: The Misunderstood Emotion* by Carol Tavris (Simon and Schuster, 1982). A fresh, well-researched look at understanding anger; exposes common myths.

▶ *Dr. Weisinger's How to Give Criticism and Get Results* (William Morrow, 1986). Audiotape series is also available (Nightingale-Conant Corp., 7300 N. Lehigh Ave., Chicago, IL 60648; 1986).

▶ *The One Minute Manager* by Kenneth Blanchard, Ph.D., and Spencer Johnson, M.D. (Berkley, 1983). Best-selling guidance on quick praisings and reprimands.

Play

▶ *The New Games Book* (1976) and *More New Games* (1981) both by the New Games Foundation, edited by Andrew Fluegelman (Doubleday/Dolphin).

▶ Let's Play (1327 6th St., Boulder, CO 80302) offers training seminars and organizes special events with New Games and more than 100 related activities for public and private groups across America.

Relationships

▶ *The Caring Question: You First or Me — Choosing a Healthy Balance* by Donald A. Tubesing, M.Div., Ph.D., and Nancy Loving Tubesing, Ed.D. (Whole Person Press, P.O. Box 3151, Duluth, MN 55803; 218-728-4077; 1985). Thought-provoking questions inviting readers to develop a life that balances self-care with caring for others.

▶ *Do I Have to Give Up Me to Be Loved By You?* by Jordan Paul, Ph.D., and Margaret Paul, Ph.D. (CompCare, 2415 Annapolis Lane, Minneapolis, MN 55441; 1983). Audiotape program is also available. One of the best books on self-discovery and building intimate relationships.

▶ *Getting Together: Building a Relationship That Gets to Yes* by Roger Fisher and Scott Brown (Houghton Mifflin, 1988). Offers proven guidelines for solving disputes, avoiding cycles of hard feelings, keeping emotions from getting in the way of agreement, and accepting others and being accepted.

▶ *How to Talk So Your Kids Will Listen and Listen So Your Kids Will Talk* by Adele Faber and Elaine Mazlish (Avon, 1980). Based on their parenting workshops, the authors give guidelines for family communication, including helping children deal with their feelings, giving praise, encouraging cooperation and autonomy, and alternatives to punishment.

▶ *Making Peace with Your Parents* by Harold H. Bloomfield, M.D., and Leonard Felder, Ph.D. (Ballantine, 1983). Important reading for all of us — highly recommended.

▶ *The Psychology of Romantic Love* by Nathaniel Branden, Ph.D. (Bantam, 1981). A best seller on creating and nurturing romantic relationships.

▶ *Sanity, Insanity, and Common Sense* by Rick Suarez, Ph.D., Roger C. Mills, Ph.D., and Darlene Stewart, M.S. (Fawcett, 1987). Clear advice on finding happiness in relationships.

▶ *The Secret Life of the Unborn Child* by Thomas Verney, M.D. (Delta, 1981). A bright look at the development of consciousness and feelings.

▶ *Siblings Without Rivalry* by Adele Faber and Elaine Mazlish (Norton, 1987). An eminently helpful book about one of the toughest problems parents must handle.

7 ICS: Instant Calming Sequence

ONE OF THE MOST POWERFUL SECRET weapons against stress is centuries old. It can be quickly learned and then used to neutralize negative stress in *less than one second* — whenever and wherever it occurs.

According to neuroscientists, one of the most effective ways to master pressure-filled situations is to learn to *catch the first stimulus or signal of stress* and *trigger an immediate control response*. Chemical and hormonal changes in the brain and body can tighten muscles and unleash negative emotions so quickly that it's much more difficult and time-consuming to reverse bad stress effects once they've occurred. And yet that's where most programs focus their attention — on unraveling stress knots after they have been securely tied. But now there's a new option — a way to instantly stop the negative effects of stress and stay in control of your thoughts, feelings, and actions whenever you're under pressure.

Science Supports 5-Step ICS Method

Years ago in martial arts training, I learned about a skill which I call an "instant calming sequence" or "instant control sequence" (ICS). This simple 5-step technique gives the user exceptional inner control — of the mind, emotions, and body — whenever peak stress situations occur. The ICS can help each of us avoid anguishing over life's misfortunes and unexpected crises. And it can provide a buffer against worry and guilt while preserving our best physical and mental capabilities in the present moment.

Recent research confirms the benefits of each of the 5 ICS steps. The "instant" and "automatic" stress management concept is verified through successful results with thousands of behavioral medicine patients and seminar/workshop participants and is endorsed by experts in the United States and Europe.[83]

One of the main problems with many stress management programs — including biofeedback, relaxation training, and passive meditation — is "lack of transference."[84] That is, techniques that may work well when you're alone in a quiet meditation room or doctor's office are extremely difficult to apply to situations in the real world. It seems all but impossible to calm down when you're hit with problem after problem all day and you just can't take time out to go relax or meditate. The ICS solves this dilemma.

The need for stress strategies like the ICS has become even greater with recent medical discoveries that "minor, daily mood fluctuations are associated with immune functioning"[85] and that small, persistent, mishandled stresses of daily life may accelerate aging.[86] Roller-coaster emotions and tense, anxious moments pile up. Without a way to neutralize the pressure that accumulates, our health suffers. The ICS offers a practical solution.

Best of all, the technique can be quickly learned. But be forewarned that, like any new skill, *mastering* the ICS takes time. At first the 5 steps have to be practiced consciously, but they soon become automatic.

Applying the ICS in Everyday Stress Situations

No matter what pressures you face — major "out in the open" crises and performance challenges or quiet, nagging self-doubts that worsen each time something or someone reminds you of past mistakes or present weaknesses — the ICS is a powerful skill you can start using right away. Its applications can be grouped in two basic categories.

1 The ICS is ideal for the *very first instant of a crisis,* such as when you are

▶ Receiving unexpected bad news
▶ Forced to make a sudden critical decision and "it's all on the line"
▶ On the verge of plunging into an unnecessary argument or negative self-statements (put-downs)
▶ Caught in a traffic jam or at a red light when you're late for an appointment
▶ Forced into a physical confrontation or self-defense situation
▶ Starting to feel guilty about something in the past or anxious about the future
▶ Facing other problems or emergencies — large or small

2 The ICS also gives you a great edge during the moments *right before important situations,* such as when you are

▶ Making a key phone call
▶ Entering a job interview or sitting for an exam
▶ Communicating what's on your mind — with your boss, employees, loved ones, friends, neighbors, a loan officer at the bank, or the person who just dented your car or cut into line ahead of you
▶ At a key performance point of any kind — on the job, in school, at home, during public speaking, in sports competition, while driving in rush-hour traffic, when negotiating (in business or with a spouse, parent, child, or friend), or when making a critical decision

In short, the ICS is effective whenever you don't want stress clouding your thinking, lowering your mood, or interfering with your actions.

Using the ICS Against All Kinds of Stress

Because an ICS is performed while you are fully alert, with eyes open, the technique may be used unobtrusively in a wide range of circumstances. The ICS is successful whether you're standing, sitting, or moving. You can learn to trigger the following response at the first sign of irritation, tension, or anxiety.

Instant Calming Sequence (ICS)

1 Uninterrupted breathing
2 Positive face
3 Balanced posture
4 Wave of relaxation
5 Mental control

The 5-step sequence is followed by the appropriate response to the stress situation.

ICS Step 1: Uninterrupted Breathing

Be certain that you *continue* breathing without interruption. Most of us halt our breathing for several seconds or more during the first moments of a stressful situation. This catapults us toward feelings of anxiety, panic, anger, frustration, faulty reactions, and a general loss of control.[87]

Whereas some techniques require you to complete an entire new breath cycle to maintain calmness, the ICS command is simple: *continue breathing* — smoothly, deeply, and evenly, no matter where in the inhalation or exhalation you happen to be when the pressure cue first captures your attention.

ICS Step 2: Positive Face

In addition to breathing control, a "positive face" can make a big difference during stressful situations. It has been recommended for thousands of years in martial arts and meditation systems, and new evidence suggests that even the slightest smile may "reset" the nervous system so that it is less reactive to negative stress.[88]

A positive facial expression — no matter what your mental state — increases blood flow to the brain and transmits nerve impulses from the facial muscles to the limbic system, a key emotional center of the brain.

Smiling changes neurochemistry toward favorable emotions, and recent research shows that these changes are powerful and swift. In a twitch of an eyelid, you can learn to flash a slight smile the moment stress strikes. "Smile inwardly with your mouth and eyes, and say to yourself, 'Alert mind, calm body,'" advises Dr. Charles F. Stroebel, professor of psychiatry at the University of Connecticut School of Medicine and author of *QR: The Quieting Reflex*.[89]

ICS Step 3: Balanced Posture

A common self-victimizing response to stress is "somatic retraction," a slouching posture characterized by collapsing the chest, rolling the shoulders forward and down, and tensing the abdomen, back, or neck. It may be obvious (doubling over as if someone hit you in the stomach) or very subtle (a slight shoulder movement and tensing of the neck, jaw, and chest wall). Somatic retraction not only restricts breathing and reduces blood flow and oxygen to the brain and senses, but it adds needless muscle tension, slows reaction time, and magnifies feelings of panic and helplessness.[90]

With balanced posture (see Chapters 33 and 34) you have an exhilarating sense of no effort in action, of moving buoyantly, comfortably in space. Your chest is open and "floats" upward; your head is up — with neck long and chin slightly in; jaw and tongue are relaxed; shoulders are broad and loose; pelvis and hips are level; back is comfortably straight; abdomen is free of tension. An imaginary sky hook is gently lifting your whole spinal column upward from a central point on top of your head.

During an ICS, the key — assuming you have learned to maintain good balanced body positions — is *to keep your posture buoyant and "up"*; don't let it become tense or collapse even slightly.

ICS Step 4: Wave of Relaxation

In this step you perform a "tension check" by scanning all of your muscles in one fast sweep of your mind — from your scalp, jaw, tongue, and face to your fingertips and toes — to locate unnecessary tension. At the same time, you flash a mental "wave of relaxation" through your body, as if you're standing under a waterfall that sweeps away *all unnecessary tension*. Your mind remains fully alert, your body calm. In meditation and martial arts terminology you are centered. The more deeply you learn to relax, the more effective the calming wave. But be careful not to overdo it: relaxing too much may pull down your posture.

To increase your ability to handle a wide range of situations, you can learn to instantly elicit surges of your best energy using a technique called *anchoring*. Anchors call forth positive physical, emotional, and mental states by linking multisensory cues to mental images of competence. See Chapter 45 for details.

ICS Step 5: Mental Control

"Acknowledge reality." That's how Tibetan martial arts instructors suggest focusing the mind for the first response to a sudden challenge. It's similar to what performance psychologists call the "flow state," in which you perform at your absolute best by avoiding the paralysis of analysis. Far too many of us get tangled up bemoaning every challenge we face. "Not *another* problem! Why does this *always* happen to me?" Or "Well, that blows the day! It's just been one disaster after another." Or "Please — not *now!* I need more (time, money, energy, rest, experience . . .) to prepare for this." Or "Oh no! Why couldn't I be somewhere — *anywhere* — else right now?"

By wishing the situation weren't happening, regretting you didn't have more time to prepare, wanting to be somewhere else, or anguishing over life's unfairness, you set off a biochemical avalanche of victimizing thoughts and feelings. Without realizing it, you actually *help* yourself lose control and get loaded up with anxiety and frustration. A single stressful event can disrupt an entire day.

You have to break that pattern if you want the ICS to work. Practice this key thought again and again: *What's happening is real and I'm finding the best possible solution right now.*

The second mental response priority in an ICS is "focus your mind." In large part, what you do with your mind in the initial moment of a challenge determines the outcome. In the first split second of a crisis, the nervous system reacts — and can choose a panic-paralysis or positive-action response.

If you look back at times in your life when you reacted poorly to situations, it's usually obvious that, had you remained calmer and thought more clearly during the first moments of the crisis (big or small), you could have chosen a better response. That's the key to the ICS — learning to insert that calm, clear-mindedness *in precisely the right place* at the very *beginning* of each stress scene.

With practice, you can train your mind to quickly seek solutions instead of getting locked on problems and to focus on what you can control rather than what you can't. This fifth and final ICS step is the place to choose an intent to learn instead of your old reactionary habits; to pause for a moment, to listen with an open mind instead of blindly responding; to resolve, rather than create, conflict; to apply your personal golden rule or spiritual philosophy in place of anxiety or anger; to be skilled enough to protect yourself without harming other people; to think clear, honest thoughts instead of distorted ones; and so on.

The idea in this step is to develop powerful mental "radar" that instantly scans each new situation, magnetically seeking and drawing out all your options for most effectively dealing with it.

Here's an example: Let's say someone is starting to criticize you for something you've done. Let's imagine the scene in slow motion: You catch the first critical remarks coming and fire off the ICS — continue breathing, positive face, balanced posture, "wave of relaxation," acknowledge reality. And when you get to the focus part of this fifth step, pause. Can you see that your past habits are primed to hurl you into the old "Uh-oh, here it comes again" options — getting down on yourself, blurting out excuses, bracing yourself to angrily lash back at the critic, and so on? If you don't learn to substitute a new mental focus right here, you'll probably be stuck repeating these old victimizing responses for the rest of your life.

The alternative — if we keep our example in slow motion and you choose the outcome you really want — paints an entirely different picture: your mind zeroes in on the specifics of the challenge, putting the importance (or unimportance) of the criticism in immediate perspective and looking at *every possible way* you can benefit — or at least learn — from the situation. In short, you're neurologically derailing negative habits and turning a potential blowout into a moment for self-improvement. It takes practice, but it works.

And if this all sounds a bit overoptimistic, note that I'm not suggesting that you have to *pay attention* to criticisms that are irrelevant or that ridicule, accuse, or threaten. If you do opt to stand there while someone is berating you, you might elect to send your mind on a short, pleasant mental vacation and leave your body relaxed, emotions calm. However, you give up this option whenever you've already launched into some kind of victimizing reaction.

The bottom line is that the dozens of little daily bursts of anger, clumps of tension, and bundles of anxiety take a serious toll — little by little they break down the body, mind, and spirit. If you find it especially difficult to keep from overreacting to daily hassles, don't get discouraged. Like millions of us, you've probably had years of practice reacting unproductively.

For a fresh perspective on problems, you might try this tip from cardiologist and stress expert Dr. Robert Eliot: "Ask yourself, 'Is it worth dying for?'"[91] If it isn't, keep practicing the ICS and other *Health & Fitness Excellence* techniques until you can consistently catch and overcome negative reactions.

One final note on this mental control step of the ICS: a number of psychologists and motivational speakers suggest that all you really need is the right mental self-talk to master stressful situations. That's a myth. *All five* ICS steps are critical. I am all for positive thinking (as discussed in Chapter 44), but by itself it just isn't enough. In fact, it's all but impossible to think truly positive thoughts (you can recite empty mental jingles perhaps, but not thoughts with meaning) when you've halted your breathing, frowned, collapsed your posture, tensed your muscles, and opened the floodgates to negative emotions — all about as fast as you can blink your eye. Try it and you'll see what I mean.

The ICS is a simple, logical, scientifically founded skill that enhances every aspect of *Health & Fitness Excellence*.

Appropriate Response   With your senses alert, your breathing steady, your posture erect, your emotions controlled, and your mind clear and looking for solutions, you're far better prepared to constructively meet each new challenge in life's parade; to learn, to adapt to change, to grow; and to respond appropriately.

Taking an Inventory of Your Own ICS Targets

To see where the ICS can best help, check out your own crunch points. What critical performance situations do you face? What problems (thoughts, feelings, attitudes, people, places, circumstances) tend to really upset you? Take a quick inventory. This list may also include persistent day-to-day burdens, guilt-loaded memories from the past, or worries about upcoming events. Think of all areas of your life — self-image, family, work, daily responsibilities, time urgency, ethics, sexual relationship, friendships, finances, health concerns, environmental pressures, communication conflicts, politics, philosophical issues — and note whatever you associate with especially stressful thoughts or emotions.

Select one problem situation in which you would especially like to use the ICS right away. First, vividly imagine the circumstance. Roll the slow-motion mental videotape backward in your mind's eye until you catch *the very first signal* that the problem is starting to distract or hurt you. For each situation on your list, this is the key moment. Write down a short phrase or sentence — a "red flag" — that gives you the first clue that a stress onslaught feels imminent. This is *exactly* the place where you need to begin inserting an ICS.

Using Fluid Intelligence

Instantaneous? How can five separate steps occur in an instant? you may be wondering. Just as the eye blinks faster than you can register what's coming, neuroscientists know that the brain can use "fluid intelligence" pathways — at speeds measured in thousandths and ten-thousandths of a second — to produce complex interactions and sequences in perception, attention, neuromuscular activation, and responsiveness.[92] The brain can recognize the meaning of more than one hundred thousand words or images in less than one second.[93] It takes only one-hundredth of a second for the eye to blink completely. At least six hundred individual muscular actions can occur in a single second, and the number may be much higher, say researchers.[94] Some scientists believe that skilled actions — such as the ICS — may be stored in the nervous system as "chunks of instructions . . . that can be called up and executed by a single command."[95] This may account for the deep relaxation and control — the "flow state" — felt by top musicians and athletes.[96]

With practice, your nervous system can enact the entire ICS in a fraction of a second — at the first instant stress strikes. *All you're learning to do is substitute a powerful, positive self-command reflex in place of an unconscious, habitual response of tension, anger, or anxiety.*

I recently spent several days studying with Dr. Karl H. Pribram, National Institutes of Health Professor of Neuroscience, Professor of Psychology and Psychiatry at Stanford University, and director of Stanford's Neuropsychology Laboratory. He is an expert on perception and reactions and has pioneered the holonomic brain theory. Dr. Pribram's research indicates that the human brain and nervous system can use what he calls "holonomic parallel processing" to function outside many time-space limitations — and instantaneous responses like the ICS can indeed be created with practice.[97]

Practice — Slowly at First

How do you learn to use the ICS? You rehearse it in slow motion, gradually increasing the speed. And you *choose* to use it every day. Notice I didn't say *try* or *hope*. *Choose* means bringing the skill to life right now. Here's how:

First, let's go back to the stressful situation you selected from your inventory list earlier. Sit down, take some time to relax, and vividly imagine — *in extra-slow motion* — that this particular stressful situation is just beginning to happen at this very moment. Stall the stress signal right there. Now picture yourself effortlessly, successfully going through the ICS: (1) continue breathing, (2) positive face, (3) balanced posture, (4) wave of relaxation, and (5) mental control.

Now repeat the process, a little faster. Remember, the ICS is a *natural, flowing sequence*. You unleash it; you don't force it. Practice a number of times a day, using different stress cues, increasing the vividness of the mental images and the speed of your ICS response. If at first you have difficulty with any of the steps, practice them one at a time until they become comfortable. If you get partway into the ICS and feel yourself starting to lose control, back the sequence up and slow things down. Be absolutely certain that you freeze the image of the stress cue at the first instant — *don't* let the stressful image keep rolling to the point at which you become anxious.

You are training to automatically slip the ICS into the situation right behind the first signal of stress. This can make all the difference in the world in the outcome. When rehearsing for especially intense situations, you might try lightening the image of the stress signal (by seeing yourself move farther away from it in your mind or by dulling the vividness of the scene) until you're at ease with using the ICS to handle it.

Developing the ICS as an Automatic Response

You can begin applying the ICS to many everyday situations. How long does it take until you don't have to think about it anymore? In some cases, only a month or so; but it takes an average of four to six months for the ICS to become an automatic part of your response to stress — and then it should last for a lifetime.

Be patient with yourself, especially during the first weeks. The really tough stress challenges often require quite a bit of rehearsing before you can handle them with ease. Remember, most of us have had years of practice strengthening the bad habits the ICS is going to replace. If you try an ICS for a particularly difficult challenge and happen to get impatient and revert to an old victimizing response, don't worry about it. Simply take some time later that day to sit down in a quiet place, relax deeply, and replay the beginning of the scene in slow motion in your mind, clearly seeing the ICS succeeding this time. Each time you use it, the sequence will flow more easily and become more automatic.

Daily Reminders

A number of my seminar participants report fast progress in learning the ICS when they set up a reminder system. One effective plan is using small colored dots (the kind available at an office supply store) and sticking them wherever you'd like a reminder to practice the ICS. Put a colored dot on your telephone. Whenever it rings, go through an ICS before you pick up the receiver. It will help you be more calm and confident in conversations. Put other dots on your watchband, in the corner of your television screen and remote control, on your bathroom mirror, on your car dashboard, in your wallet or checkbook cover, on your alarm clock, in your appointment calendar — in short, anyplace you think an

ICS reminder could be helpful. You might also begin practicing the ICS before you get out of bed each morning and whenever you have to wait in line or stop for a red light. You'll find hundreds of situations for using the ICS in response to daily stress cues — every single time you start to feel annoyed, anxious, tense, guilty, worried, or angry.

One final note: *Keep practicing* — dozens of times a day. It may be the best health and performance investment you ever make.

8 Optimum Sleep

Sleep engenders energy, clarity and optimism and provides the physical and emotional fuel needed to cope well with the day's demands.

— *LYNNE LAMBERG*[98]

How to Get Better Rest from Less Sleep

Most of us sleep poorly, or at least not as deeply and healthfully as we could. Good sleep provides many benefits and is a central thread in the golden circle of *Health & Fitness Excellence*. This chapter examines ways to improve the *quality* of your nightly rest — sleeping better and perhaps in fewer hours than you do right now.

An estimated thirty million Americans have DIMS — "disorders of initiating and maintaining sleep."[99] DIMS include difficulty in falling asleep, staying asleep during the night, or in rising early in the morning. Poor sleep all but guarantees decreased productivity, social irritability, and lowered resistance to disease.

We depend on sleep for healing. The *British Medical Journal* recently published a study from the Royal Edinburgh Hospital in Scotland in which researchers found that the same processes that renew our normal cells during sleep also promote accelerated healing.[100] While you are sleeping, your body secretes hormones that stimulate red blood cell production and bone synthesis and inhibits hormones that destroy cells.

Beyond the health benefits, sleep quality is an important performance factor. Even a single night of poor sleep can cut your physical performance the next day by as much as 30 percent![101]

How Much Sleep Is Enough?

One of the most pervasive myths about sleep is that everybody needs eight hours a night. Although two-thirds of adult Americans sleep seven to eight hours per night, about one-fifth sleep less than six hours.

People who sleep between six and eight hours often have more effective rest than those who sleep more, say scientists.[102] In most cases, those of us who now sleep poorly can easily improve the quality of our nightly rest. And those of us who may be sleeping more hours each night than we actually need can safely, progressively reduce sleep time.[103]

People who naturally sleep six to seven hours a night are reportedly, on average, happier, better adjusted, and more active than longer sleepers, say sleep scientists at the University of Florida and Tufts University School of Medicine in Boston.[104] Researcher Larry Beutler of the University of Arizona agrees, adding that such people seem to "have their whole nervous system wired quite efficiently. They may have more energy, make more social contacts and establish better social-support systems than more sluggish people."[105]

After comparing people sleeping an average of 5.6 hours a night and those averaging 9.7 hours, Dr. Ernest Hartmann, director of the Sleep Laboratory at West-Ros-Park Mental Health Center in Boston, concludes, "The differences that were most clear were in what I call lifestyle. The long sleepers tended to be worriers. They took things seriously in all kinds of ways. Some of them were a bit anxious, but they were all pretty much within the normal range. The short sleepers tended to be nonworriers. Their style was to keep busy, to get a lot done, and they would tend to push away their problems."[106]

Perhaps the reason for the difference is that, compared with non-worriers, people who ruminate about the future or past may accumulate more stress symptoms — increasing their need for longer and deeper rest so they can better recover. Some of us need less sleep when things are going well and more when life seems rough.

The message from these findings is not to put the cart before the horse. Instead of trying to reduce the amount of time you sleep each night, direct your attention toward improving the *quality* of your rest and implement stress management skills, a change of mental outlook, exercise, and other *Health & Fitness Excellence* priorities.

What about going to bed early to be sure we get enough sleep? That's usually a waste of time unless we're ill, say scientists at the Montefiore Sleep-Wake Disorders Unit in New York. Each of us has an internal body clock tuned to our personal metabolism and other health functions that governs when our best sleep should be taken. Trying to force more sleep than we actually need is counterproductive.

But how much sleep do *you* need? The best way to know is to experiment. Can you rest completely in fewer hours than you sleep now? Maybe. First, cut your stress burden and begin a healthier lifestyle. Then, very gradually, reduce your sleep time. If you now sleep eight hours a night, try seven hours and fifty minutes each night for one week, then take off another ten minutes the next week, and so on. Try the following suggestions and stop reducing your sleep time when you notice a sense of weariness after awakening. Over several months, you may still be able to function optimally while sleeping about an hour less every night.[107] Here are some important considerations for best sleep.

Get up at the same time every day. No matter how many hours you sleep, set a regular schedule and get up at the same time every day. No matter how short or poor the night's sleep may have been, by getting up at the same time every morning you reset the body's circadian rhythm and synchronize all other sleep and wake cycles.[108]

Oversleeping or "sleeping in" on the weekends is a sure way to confuse your body clock. You'll not only become less alert after too much sleep, but you reduce the number of waking hours, making it more difficult to fall asleep the next night.[109] And the luxury of sleeping late on Sunday morning leads to "Sunday night insomnia" and "Monday morning blahs," says Lynne Lamberg, author of the *American Medical Association Guide to Better Sleep.*[110] If you *must* sleep in, limit your sleep to not more than an extra hour or so and do it as infrequently as possible.

Exercise regularly. Studies link physical fitness — achieved by regular exercise — with improved sleep quality.[111] Physical and mental inactivity are prime causes of insomnia.

Ensure good nutrition. Your diet can support your body and mind in improving the quality of your sleep. An optimal diet, discussed in detail in Chapters 20–28, includes five or six small meals and light snacks a day, emphasizing recipes that are high in complex carbohydrates and fiber, adequate but not excessive in protein, and low in fat, cholesterol, and salt. Avoid alcohol and caffeine near bedtime; and don't go to bed hungry. A drop in blood sugar in the middle of the night can interfere with sleep. A carefully planned, moderate-sized evening meal is important. A very small midevening snack that is low in fat and protein and high in complex carbohydrates also helps many people have a smoother transition into deep, restful sleep (see Chapter 27).

Keep business out of the bedroom. If you want the best sleep, and especially if you suffer from insomnia, reserve your bed for sleeping and for a warm, positive sexual relationship. Nothing else. Keep heated discussions and intense brainstorming sessions out of your bedroom. Schedule a time each evening to write down concerns and challenges, planning how you will take steps to solve them *tomorrow,* and then release your personal and business concerns before falling asleep.

Establish a relaxing bedtime ritual. The most common causes of sleep difficulties are related to stress.[112] If you don't let go of accumulated tension each evening, you prevent yourself from getting the best possible sleep. Choose a favorite relaxation technique (see Chapter 4) and use it regularly *before* falling asleep. Release tight muscles throughout your body: from the face, scalp, jaw, neck, and tongue down to your back and abdomen and out to your fingertips and toes.

Let go of emotional baggage you may be carrying from the day's events. Positive music helps some people unwind; for others, sleep researchers at Northwestern University have found that the static "white noise" at the end of the FM radio dial is even more calming than music.[113] Relaxation and guided mental imagery tapes have helped many people fall deeply asleep. *Easing into Sleep* by Dr. Emmett E. Miller (Source, P.O. Box W, Stanford, CA 94309; 415-328-7171) features two good listening options: "Put the day to rest," and "Escape from insomnia."

And don't forget to bring your spiritual beliefs to light each evening — bedtime prayers and positive affirmations help create a state of mind conducive to deep, revitalizing rest.

Design an optimal sleeping environment. Although the room where you sleep is one of the most valuable spaces in your home, bedrooms usually receive the least design attention. Considerations include the following.

Fresh air, cool temperatures. Fresh, circulating air boosts sleep quality. Temperature is important, too. Many people find the range between 65 and 70°F to be ideal.[114] If you are too cold, you must fumble for covers; if you're too hot, you become restless in sleep.

Proper bed. Good beds can be expensive, but they're worth the investment. Firm beds are preferable to soft ones, but some extra-hard mattresses contribute to back pains rather than relieving them. Experts recommend a bed that is level, with no sags, and just firm enough to fully support the lower back. Top-quality waterbeds are also worth considering. With a thermostatically controlled heater and natural fiber bed linens, "flotation sleep systems" provide many people with excellent back support and great rest all year round.

Woolen mattress cover. According to Australian medical studies, a fleecy woolen pad placed between the mattress and bottom sheet improves sleep quality.[115] People sleeping on the wool pad tossed and turned less and felt better each morning than those who slept on a conventional mattress pad. This is apparently due to wool's ability to cushion the body and let the skin "breathe" — helping to keep you comfortably cool in summer and warm in winter.

Natural fiber bed linens. Natural fiber sheets and pillowcases — usually made from cotton — help sleep quality by reducing potential skin irritation from synthetic fabrics. Blankets and quilts of all-natural fabrics (cotton, wool, linen, flax, down) are a good choice for most of us, although less expensive quilts filled with lightweight sleeping bag insulation materials are also fine.

If you have difficulty finding all-cotton bed linens and wool- or down-filled mattress covers in your area, contact Garnet Hill (Main St., Franconia, NH 03580; 800-622-6216) or the Company Store (500 Company Store Rd., LaCrosse, WI 54601; 800-356-9367). *Nontoxic & Natural* by Debra Lynn Dadd (J. P. Tarcher, 1984) lists many other mail order sources.

Quiet, dark sleeping room. Most people sleep most deeply when their bedroom is dark. New curtains or window blinds may be in order if outside light filters into your room from a street lamp or the moon. Even dim light causes unnecessary eye movements that can sabotage your sleep.

Noise control is also important for deepest rest. Soundproofing your bedroom and educating family members and neighbors about peace and quiet at night are good steps to take. You might also consider earplugs or, as a last alternative, "white noise" generating devices that produce oceanlike sounds to mask outside clamor. Even ticking clocks in the bedroom can create sleep problems for some people!

Best sleeping position. While there are many sleep postures, the one most frequently recommended by experts is the semi-fetal position.[116] "Sleeping in the semi-fetal position, lying on the side with the knees drawn partway up, has the physical advantage of conserving heat without closing off the circulation of air around the body," says Dr. Samuel Dunkell in *Sleep Positions.* "Also, the center of the body is protected, especially its psychological center, the heart. The semi-fetal position allows greater maneuverability in the course of the night than any of the other most common positions. . . . The semi-fetal position thus makes good 'common sense' in terms of physical comfort and functioning. The personalities of those who choose this position show a parallel degree of sensible adjustment to the world. Such individuals are usually fairly well-balanced and secure."[117]

For most people, the semi-fetal position minimizes tossing and turning during the night. This is important because deep rest is very difficult amid excessive movement. Cramped positions and beds that sag or are too firm cut off circulation and can trigger hundreds of position changes during the night.

Your pillow matters too. For best sleep, your head and neck must be well supported in a variety of sleep postures since most of us change position during the night. Special neck-support pillows may be fine when you are sleeping on your back or side, but when you change positions they can add more pressure to your shoulders, neck, or back than traditional pillows.

Choosing the right personal pillow takes some experimentation, but it pays off with better sleep. To help keep your head in a neutral, relaxed position when on your side, pull the side or corner of your pillow down between the top of your lowermost shoulder (the one resting directly on the bed) and the side of your chin.

Be certain to consciously release tension spots before falling asleep. Areas of particular concern include your hands, wrists, elbows, neck, shoulders, lower back, abdomen, jaw, and tongue. If the semi-fetal position is uncomfortable for you, try placing a soft pillow beneath the knee of your upper leg. This generally reduces strain on the hip and back. You might also try a soft pillow between your upper arm and chest wall; this helps keep your upper shoulder from collapsing downward and straining muscles of the back and neck.

A gentle awakening. How you wake up has a lot to do with your physical and emotional tone all day. Awakening forces your body to go through a dramatic shifting of gears. Leaping out of bed to shut off an alarm clock is an abrupt jolt to your entire being — triggering racing heartbeat, muscle tension, and other stress "emergency" symptoms. In fact, as you merely *step* out of bed, two pints of blood go into your legs, your blood pressure shifts and then shoots up by 30 points, and a cascade of hormones enters your system.[118]

If possible, wake up at least several minutes early to lie in bed and allow your body to slowly shift into being wide awake. Positive music — set to come on with a timer and with the volume just loud enough that you'll pay attention — is a far better choice for most people than a traditional alarm clock.

9 Listening and Communication Skills

I see communication as a huge umbrella that covers and affects all that goes on between human beings. Once a human being has arrived on this earth, communication is the largest single factor determining what kinds of relationships he makes with others and what happens to him in the world about him.

— *VIRGINIA SATIR*[119]

Communication is a subject that is little recognized as a health factor. Communicating is perhaps the profoundest way to change brain chemistry, according to Steven Paul, chief of clinical neuroscience at the National Institute of Mental Health.[120] Good communication means expressing yourself clearly through verbal and nonverbal language, and — even more important for most of us — it means actively *listening* so that you understand what other people are saying.

Simple human dialogue — the process of talking and listening — dramatically affects the heart and blood vessels, say researchers, and, in turn, every aspect of our health and well-being.[121] As people begin to speak, their blood pressure goes up, and microscopic blood vessel changes are detectable at far distant points in the body. Conversely, when people listen attentively or tune in to the external environment in a relaxed manner, their blood pressure usually falls and heart rate slows, often slightly below normal resting levels.

"Study after study reveals that human dialogue not only affects our hearts significantly but can even alter the biochemistry of individual tissues at the furthest extremities of the body," reports James J. Lynch, codirector of the Psychophysiological Clinic and Laboratories at the University of Maryland School of Medicine and author of *The Language of the Heart: The Body's Response to Human Dialogue*. "Since blood flows through every human tissue, the entire body is influenced by human dialogue. Thus, it is true that when we speak we do so with every fiber of our being. The 'language of the heart' is integral to the health and emotional life of every one of us."[122]

Moreover, communication is our lifeline for survival. During periods of great stress, communicating with others can pull us through, renewing our inner strength, lifting our vision, and reaffirming the meaning in our lives.

As researchers have discovered, the *rise* in blood pressure experienced when we speak should be balanced by the *lowering* of pressure that occurs when we listen in a relaxed manner. This talk-listen combination helps keep blood pressure evenly regulated. Unfortunately, most of us have learned to listen defensively and talk too much.

In addition, our "inner communicator" — often called self-talk — shapes attitudes, moods, and performance (see Chapter 44). For couples and families, it can make or break nurturing relationships. To a great extent, the quality of our lives is determined by our communication.

Listening Skills

"It can be stated with practically no qualification that people in general do not know how to listen," says Dr. Ralph G. Nichols, who developed classes on listening at the University of Minnesota. "They have ears that hear very well, but seldom have they acquired the necessary . . . skills which would allow those ears to be used effectively for what is called *listening*."[123]

Listening Is More Than Hearing

Here are some key components of effective listening:

Attending skills. Attending consists of giving your physical attention to another person, demonstrating that you are truly interested in what is being said. Nonattending, on the other hand, dramatically thwarts the speaker's expression.

Listening posture. Good listeners communicate attentiveness through the relaxed alertness of their bodies. They face the other person squarely and incline slightly, with arms and legs uncrossed, leaning toward the speaker.

Eye contact. Eye contact improves communication by permitting speakers to determine the listeners' receptiveness to them and their message.

Nondistracting environment. Removing physical barriers such as desks and minimizing interference from television, music, and noise can help people let go of tension and open up communication.

Active listening. Listening is an active process that requires your full participation — not just sitting there like a statue. In *Messages: The Communication Book,* Matthew McKay, Martha Davis, and Patrick Fanning offer several guidelines for active listening:[124]

Paraphrasing. This means stating in your own words what you think someone said. It keeps you focused on understanding what the other person means. Paraphrasing lead-ins include "In other words . . ."; "What I hear you saying is . . ."; "So essentially what happened (or how you felt) was . . ."; and so forth. Paraphrasing helps avoid miscommunication and breaks down false assumptions, errors, and misrepresentations. It also helps you to remember what was said and to avoid comparing, judging, derailing, advising, and sparring.

Clarifying and feedback. Clarifying, which often accompanies paraphrasing, means asking more questions until you clearly understand the issue. After observing the speaker's tone of voice, facial expressions, gestures, and body language, you can check the congruency of the message (do the words say one thing and the eyes and body language another?). You verify your perceptions by creating a tentative description: "I want to understand your feelings (or this situation); is this (give your own description of the message you've received) the way you feel (or what really happened)?" You are not approving or disapproving, you're simply checking to be certain your interpretation is correct.

Listening with empathy and openness. Listening with empathy puts you on a heart-to-heart level with the speaker. It is difficult to listen when you're judging another person or finding fault. You need to hear the *whole* statement, the entire communiqué. You can compare what is being said — without judgment — to your own knowledge of life, people, history, and similar events. As Tom Crum, cofounder of Windstar Foundation, puts it:

To let go of our old images, of the way we think people are, and to see, hear and touch them anew, like a precious being or flower that we've come across for the first time — this is the joy we get from listening. We all know how truly empowering it is to have a person truly listen to us, without judgement or answers, as an interested and attentive partner, a true friend. Let us explore the power and blessings that result when we are able to give this gift freely in our daily lives and receive its rewards.[125]

Communicating What You Really Mean

When it comes to communication skills, small things make a big difference. Most of us operate on the premise that everyone else understands what we *mean* to communicate whenever we speak. Yet there are countless ways that our messages get mixed up and, in spite of our best efforts, we fail to communicate clearly. You say what you mean — but the other person hears what he or she *thinks* you mean, which wasn't what you meant.

The remainder of this chapter is devoted to cutting the fog, or imprecision, out of speech. This is far more important to health than most of us realize. It's amazing how much energy we waste — and how much unnecessary tension and anxiety we accumulate — when we struggle to get our point across or get tangled up in misunderstandings with other people. Beginning right now, listen to yourself speaking. And listen to the messages you receive from those close to you — family members, friends, co-workers. Read the following examples and then begin applying the principles to your conversations in a gentle, positive manner. You'll feel the improvement right away.

Conversational Style

"Sometimes strains in a conversation reflect real differences between people; they *are* angry at each other; they really are at cross-purposes," says language and communications expert Deborah Tannen, associate professor of linguistics at Georgetown University. "But sometimes strains and kinks develop when there really are no basic differences of opinion, when everyone is sincerely trying to get along. This is the type of miscommunication that drives people crazy. And it is usually caused by differences in conversational style."[126]

Our conversational style seems self-evidently natural to each of us; yet ingrained habits — involving our choice of words, voice level and tone, the use of questions and certain phrases, and how much or how little we talk — differ from person to person, far more than we're aware. "Nothing is more deeply disquieting than a conversation gone awry," says Tannen. "To say something and see it taken to mean something else; to try to be helpful and be thought pushy; to try to be considerate and be called cold . . . such failure at talk undermines one's sense of competence and . . . can undermine one's feeling of psychological well-being."[127]

How do we become more aware of our own conversational style and that of others? First, we can learn to stop at that first moment we sense misunderstanding and remind ourselves that others may not mean what we thought we just heard them say.

Here's a key point: Each time we speak, the response we elicit reflects what we actually communicated, regardless of our intent. *You* are responsible for getting your message through, for finding a way — if at all possible — to make it clear to the listener. Use the active listening techniques, especially paraphrasing, to keep in better touch with what other people are saying and meaning. What are you doing when you communicate? How is your speaking style a response or reaction to the other person's way of speaking to you? Precise language skills can really pay off.

Receiving and Giving Feedback

To communicate better, you must ask for and encourage honest, constructive feedback. You can't take it for granted, since most people will tell you only *what they think you want to hear*. You might ask a close friend or relative to study with you, or use an audiocassette recorder to tape yourself speaking so that you can listen to yourself as an outsider and make improvements. If you aren't comfortable taping, or if the people you talk with aren't at ease being recorded, you can simply choose to be a keener conversational observer.

Precise Language

Precision in language — communicating with maximum clarity — deserves everyone's attention. Distorted thoughts twist our words and lead to conflict. One way to improve our communication is by improving our thinking. Chapter 44 identifies distorted thinking patterns and reviews ways to eliminate them.

Choose your words carefully. Certain words and phrases create instant resistance and damage rapport and friendship. A classic example is the conjunction "but." It is often used to negate everything said before it. While "but" and the similar conjunction "however" are usually spoken unconsciously and automatically, they still irritate and alienate almost everyone. Notice how these feel: "I agree with you, *but* . . ."; "That's true, *but* . . ."; "I respect your opinion, *but. . . .*"

According to communications experts, one way to solve this dilemma is something called an *agreement frame*. Certain phrases can be used to establish rapport, share honest feelings, and minimize resistance to the opinions of others, thereby avoiding many conversational conflicts. You first point out something positive and specific about what the other person said and add your comments or ideas with the connection "and."

Examples: "I agree with your basic idea (or a specific point you made), *and* here's another angle (thought, suggestion, resource) that might be helpful"; "I respect your intense feelings about (a problem), *and* here are several of my thoughts." The process works just as effectively in self-talk: "I want to solve this conflict, *and* (not *but*) that looks very challenging to do"; "I'm choosing not to get so upset over little things *and* (not *but*) it's taking me quite a while to learn how." Can you see — and feel — the difference?

In each case, you are establishing rapport by acknowledging the communication rather than blocking, ignoring, or denigrating it with trap words like "but" or "however." You are bringing attention to areas of mutual agreement, a process that tends to form a positive bond. And you are creating the opportunity to redirect the conversation by avoiding and overcoming resistance wherever possible.

The following are examples of imprecise word usage and suggestions for using precise language to avoid miscommunication.

Avoid Erroneous Limitations

Universal qualifiers. All; always; constantly; never; none; every; everybody; nobody. . . . These words imply categorical truth and wind up in many dialogues to hide ignorance or add emotional emphasis. Rarely are they true. Cut through the fluff and get down to specifics by repeating the absolute as a question. "All?" "Always?" "Everybody?" "Never?" This helps the speaker become more aware of the problem and helps you be clearer about the actual message.

Restrictives/rules. Must; can't; ought to; shouldn't; have to; forced to; no choice; must not; unable to. . . . These trap words imply impossibility or assume inevitability. It's easy for them to block change and to suggest that there is something wrong with the speaker or listener — you don't measure up. Step outside these words by posing simple consequence questions (in your mind or aloud), such as "What would happen if you did or didn't do that?" or "What causes or prevents you from doing that?" And begin substituting *choosing to* or *choose to* in place of *have to, can,* and *try to.*

Stop Errors in Information or Logic

Overloads. Too much; too many; too expensive; too complicated; too difficult. . . . To cut through the fog, ask, "Compared with what?" Be specific.

Deletions. "I disagree." Get at the real message by asking, "With what, exactly, do you disagree?"

Unspecified nouns and verbs. "*They* don't *understand* me"; "*It* always *gets me down.*" If left unclarified, references to unspecified nouns and the use of vague verbs foster helplessness. Get an exact frame of reference. Ask, "*Who* doesn't seem to understand you, and *how* do they make you feel misunderstood?" "Exactly *what* happens to get you down, and in what ways does it make you feel unhappy?"

Speak from the first person and collaborate with others. Expressing your thoughts and feelings with "I" statements ("I'd like to talk to you about something very important to me") bypasses the "you" comments ("You ignore me"; "You're never willing to hear what I say") that make listeners feel as if you are blaming them. And be sure to err on the side of inclusion — "we" statements make friends and co-workers feel part of the issues and activities at hand. It's a scientific fact: cooperative — not competitive — efforts are a key to success.

Judgments/comparatives/superlatives. Obviously; clearly; without a doubt; good; better; best; bad; worse; worst; more; less; least. . . . To clarify, ask, "Compared with *what* is it (good, bad, better, worse)?" "To *whom* is it clear or obvious?"

Change Problem-Focused Questions. When we habitually ask problem-focused questions — usually beginning with "why" — we often receive lengthy justifications and excuses rather than clear information. Whenever possible, choose outcome-focused questions — frequently beginning with "how" — since they tend to turn the attention toward solutions. Compare "*Why* did you make the mistake that caused this big problem?" with "*How* can we do that (specific task) better from now on?" And contrast "What's *wrong* with you/me/them?" with "What do you/I/ they *need?*"

The Bottom Line of Communication

Good communication comes down to listening attentively and speaking clearly, congruently, honestly, compassionately, and with good timing (knowing when and where to communicate). Clarify what you don't understand, and ask for what you want and need. Presuppositions, hinting, and expectations put listeners in a cloud of confusion or create conflict. Tell the appropriate truth (which means that the person you are talking to needs to know it, that you can give a fair representation of it, and that you can tell it kindly). This all takes regular practice and lots of attention to dialogue. Can you think of many better investments for your health and happiness?

RESOURCES

For more on listening and communication skills, see Chapter 44 as well as the following books.

- ▶ *"If You Could Hear What I Cannot Say": Learning to Communicate with the Ones You Love* by Dr. Nathaniel Branden (Bantam, 1983). A book of sentence completions designed to help overcome the communication impasses that block our ability to say what our heart really feels.
- ▶ *Language of the Heart: The Body's Response to Human Dialogue* by James J. Lynch, Ph.D. (Basic Books, 1985). An important self-care book.
- ▶ *Making Contact* by Virginia Satir (Celestial Arts, 1976). Summarizes communication techniques developed by this well-known psychotherapist and family counselor.
- ▶ *Messages: The Communication Book* by Matthew McKay, Ph.D., Martha Davis, Ph.D., and Patrick Fanning (New Harbinger Publications, 220

Adeline St., Suite 305, Oakland, CA 94607; 1983). A comprehensive handbook filled with on-the-mark advice.

▶ *People Skills: How to Assert Yourself, Listen to Others, and Resolve Conflicts* by Robert Bolton, Ph.D. (Prentice Hall, 1979). A good textbook on improving relationships by improving communication.

▶ *That's Not What I Meant! How Conversational Style Makes or Breaks Your Relationships with Others* by Deborah Tannen, Ph.D. (William Morrow, 1986). The best book yet on conversational style. The author is an international expert.

10 30-Second Rejuvenation-in-Motion Routines

DAILY WORK BREAKS. Most of us think of them as chances to escape from pressure — to stretch our legs, daydream, drink coffee, avoid the phone, or just plain stop rushing and sit still, numbly wrapped in a kind of recovery blanket.

Some of us seem to barely make it from this break to the next and the next. We survive one hour at a time, checking off days on the calendar. In contrast, a growing number of us are giving up on breaks entirely — we seem to never stop working at all.

Take a moment to look back at the work breaks you have taken over the past months. Chances are that at best they seem like a string of little pauses in your busy, often hectic, life.

Without realizing it, you have been letting a golden opportunity slip away. And this chapter can change that. Your work breaks can be turned into health-and-energy breaks, quick new steps on your inner staircase to success — the path of least resistance to your goals and dreams. How? With *rejuvenation-in-motion routines*.

Now, in as little as 30 seconds, you can release tight muscles and balance your posture; send a wave of relaxation through your body; replace nutrients and replenish fluids; revitalize your vision; lift your mood; and clear and refocus your mind.

Solving Persistent Problems

As the hours wear on during the day, it becomes more and more difficult for each of us to remain in complete control of our thoughts, feelings, speech, and actions. The more tension we pick up, the more anxious or fatigued we become, and the harder it is to feel enthusiastic about exercising and other self-care priorities. Everything turns into more of a struggle, and our resistance to disease goes down.

Let's get back to the source for a moment: where does the original tension come from? To a great extent from work — the effort of getting there, dealing with job challenges, coping with other people, fighting your way home through traffic, worrying about the next day's problems. And the stress load can be just as great if you work at home. Add relationship difficulties, and the stress burden nears maximum.

Let's face it, other than eating healthful snacks and planning a good lunch, most of us find it difficult to pay much attention to health and fitness on work breaks during the day and brief at-home breaks on evenings and weekends. And things may get so hectic that you're lucky to find more than a free minute or two here and there.

Even if you do have the time to spend 20 minutes in the middle of the morning or afternoon meditating or listening to a relaxation tape, scientists have discovered that while these techniques relieve muscle tension and provide other benefits, they can also have a detrimental effect on attention span, reaction time, and other aspects of performance and productivity.[128]

This is not to suggest that practicing meditation and deep relaxation (I do both) aren't valuable. But, by themselves, these self-improvement techniques aren't enough to make best use of your work breaks even if you do have the time for them. And neither is aerobic exercise, a power snack, weight training, yoga, a massage, or any other health factor, by itself.

The rejuvenation-in-motion routine includes the instant calming sequence (ICS) and goes beyond it, combining key health and fitness priorities in a commanding 30-second technique that can be used successfully on its own or added before or after your favorite relaxation, meditation, lunch, or exercise session. Either way, you have a winning formula. American, European, and Japanese research substantiates the need for short daily breaks to revitalize the body and mind, make it easier and faster to learn new skills, and increase productivity.[129]

Basic 30-second Rejuvenation-in-Motion Routine

The basic 30-second rejuvenation-in-motion routine includes 4 steps:

1 Instant calming sequence (ICS)
2 Mind moves
3 Body moves
4 Replenishment of nutrients

Step 1: Instant Calming Sequence (ICS)

Time required: 1 second or less.

The ICS is a powerful 5-step technique (see Chapter 7) to keep you calm and in control whenever stress strikes or you walk into a high-pressure situation. As the first step in the rejuvenation-in-motion routine, the ICS gives you a unique safety valve to release accumulated stress and shift your mind and senses into a state of calm, attentive present-moment awareness so you can take full advantage of every second in your break.

Once learned, the 5 steps of the ICS refocus you in an instant and make what follows more effective. Here is a summary of the 5 steps.

1 *Uninterrupted breathing.* Continue breathing in smooth, steady, diaphragmatic breaths. This prevents the sudden loss of oxygen — and rise in tension and anxiety — that occurs when you unconsciously halt your breathing in response to stress.

2 *Positive face.* Even the slightest smile (smiling inwardly with your mouth and eyes) increases blood flow to the brain and resets the nervous system so that it's less reactive to negative stress.

3 *Balanced posture.* With properly balanced posture you have an exhilarating sense of no effort in action, of moving buoyantly, comfortably in space.

4 *Wave of relaxation.* In one sweep of your mind, you find and release all unnecessary muscular tension in your body (from your scalp, face, jaw, tongue, neck, and shoulders to your fingertips and toes).

5 *Mental control: Acknowledge reality.* In a rejuvenation-in-motion routine this means becoming fully aware that you are choosing to revitalize your thoughts, feelings, and actions during this break.

Focus your mind. Choose an intent to learn instead of react — to pause for a moment, to listen with an open mind; to resolve rather than create or conflict; to apply your personal golden rule, ethical standards, and spiritual philosophy in place of anger, dishonesty, or anxiety; to be skilled enough to protect yourself without harming other people.

Step 2: Mind Moves

Time required: 3–4 seconds (more if you have it).

Through a lifetime of modeling others, much of what we think is automatic — and negative. Thoughts are brief electrical flashes in the brain. They happen so fast that we often don't even "hear" them. But we feel their effect because *our thoughts create or influence our perceptions, emotions, and behaviors.*[130] Why is our thinking so powerful? Because the brain is extremely precise in its interpretation of and response to incoming messages. That's why so much "positive thinking" is really negative. The more we focus on preventing and inadvertently magnifying what we *don't* want — anxiety, body fat, interpersonal conflicts, fear of speaking, fatigue, memory loss, or a disease — the more likely the dreaded results will occur.

As a unique individual, each of us sees reality differently — reality is what *appears* to be happening within us and around us at this moment. Our thoughts help formulate that reality. We each give acceptance and life to our thoughts. Accordingly, our perceptions, feelings, and behaviors are our own — they are not thrust on us by an outside force (other people, our job, or a particular situation). Only when we can learn to step outside our limited, habitual patterns of thinking can we view circumstances and other viewpoints with objectivity and without judgment. When we reach that point outside ourselves, conflicts diminish, productivity surges, and there's room for more happiness to fill our lives.

When our moods are positive, we feel optimistic, motivated, productive, and creative. Regardless of external events and stress pressures, when our consciousness or mood is high we have a general sense of wellbeing and hope for the future. We are more helpful and generous toward others and experience improved cognitive processes such as judgment, problem solving, decision making, and creativity.[131] We have a higher psychological vantage point from which to view the challenges and conflicts that enter our lives.

In contrast, negative feelings and emotions are a sharp signal that we're dropping into a lower psychological state of functioning — reverting into old patterns of negative thinking. We start attacking ourselves with our thoughts and lose our conscious ability to make commonsense decisions. We feel insecure and emotionally fragile and become poorer in various intellectual capacities.

Most of us have been led to believe that we can find solutions to our emotional distress if we think about it enough. But that is rarely true. Thinking about our difficulties and inadequacies — dwelling on them in our mind — is precisely what keeps most problems alive and growing.

When work stress starts to pile up, for example, it's easy to feel overloaded and anxious. Just as soon as our thoughts become negative, our mood drops. We begin to feel stuck, things start looking bleak, our work becomes more of a struggle. Our thoughts then become twisted, distorted, filled with presuppositions, jumping to conclusions, amplifying the negative, minimizing the positive, all-or-nothing statements, catastrophizing, blaming, "shoulds," labeling, and so on. (Chapter 44 takes a detailed look at ways to identify and eliminate these victimizing thoughts.)

We each have the natural ability to disengage ourselves from pointless, negative thinking. The fastest, surest way to do that is to raise our mood. Although we all experience mood fluctuations, some of us — many of us — get stuck in low moods. New research shows that that's usually unnecessary.

Psychologists have identified some fast, simple ways to elevate mood.[132] These techniques can be included in each rejuvenation-in-motion routine during the day. First, fully acknowledge your current circumstances in order to move forward. Shift your thoughts away from problems. Think about what you want, not what you don't want.

Second, choose not to take negative thoughts seriously if you happen to be in a lower mood. Third, take action — balance your posture, breathe deeply, think in a new direction, get up and move around, exercise, talk to someone new about something new. Taking action steps raises moods.[133]

Your choice of food for snacks and meals also influences your state of mind and emotion (discussed in step 4 on the next page).

One other mood-raising tool is mental imagery. Images occur when our thoughts are focused in a specific way. Rejuvenation-in-motion routines provide a great opportunity to use imagery to direct your mind in new directions, to stay in touch with your goals and dreams. Pictures in the mind often have two predominant emphases: the subject and the event. *Both* must be positive to avoid self-sabotage:

1 Is the subject of your attention (the specific person, group, place, feeling, action, or circumstance) positive and enhancing?

2 Does something good happen (the actual statement about the subject of your thought) once your concentration is focused there?

How do you tend to envision yourself and others throughout the day? Take several minutes right now to relax and examine some of your thoughts and statements in slow motion. When you say or think "I," do you automatically sense yourself at your best? Or do you tend to see a self-image that you don't like very much? What about patterns in your thoughts and images of other people, places, and circumstances? With some practice, you can teach your mind to choose the *most vivid, positive, competent view* of yourself (and most other subjects) every time you think or say the name or pronoun.

Now look at the predicate — which describes what is happening to the subject in each sentence. Choose accurate, empowering descriptions. To the best of your ability, surround yourself with people committed to doing the same. Start a mental campaign to cut out doom and gloom — the catastrophizing, generalizations, assumptions, pessimism, put-downs, and cynicism that lock us in stress closets. As discussed in Chapters 9 and 44, experts recommend choosing honest, specific statements that zero in on the positive — we need to think and speak in ways that prompt our best feelings, perceptions, and actions.

There's no doubt that it takes lots of practice to change automatic thoughts and deeply ingrained imagery habits. One of the most effective ways to do this is to choose a bright, productive mental image each time you go through a rejuvenation-in-motion routine. Picture the subject and predicate in a sensory-rich, constructive way. Remember: At the best, things are going well and you feel great; at the absolute worst, you are learning and growing by changing unproductive habits. When you think about life that way, it's impossible to lose.

Step 3: Body Moves

Time required: 10–15 seconds (more if you have it).

Get up, walk, and unstress by moving. This activity automatically helps to raise your mood. Make a quick assessment: what part of your body is in greatest need of attention right now? Choose a range-of-motion exercise to fit that need — such as gentle head nods or neck ovals; shoulder shrugs; pelvic-leveling exercise; "spheres of light" for your wrists, hands, and fingers; or any of the dozens of exercises described in Chapters 11–19.

Shift your visual focus. This activity relieves eyestrain and sharpens your vision. If you have been doing close work, take a few moments to blink your eyes and look at more distant objects. If you have been scanning faraway scenery at your job, switch to focusing on something nearby.

Step 4: Replenishment of Nutrients

Time required: 10–15 seconds (more if you have it).

Drink some cool pure water. As explained in Chapter 22, drinking water can reduce fatigue and improve health.

Eat several bites of a small, carefully selected snack every two to three hours. First, as described in Chapter 21, "small snack" means just that — *small;* and "carefully selected" means to take full advantage of the latest nutritional discoveries. Choose wholesome, fresh, contaminant-free foods that, overall, are high in complex carbohydrates and fiber, moderate in protein, and low in fat, cholesterol, and salt.

With these basic guidelines in hand, you're ready for a key decision: choosing foods that contribute either to increased mental alertness or to increased calmness. Researchers have found that food choices influence production of brain messenger chemicals called neurotransmitters, which affect mental alertness, concentration, attitude, mood, and performance. There is increasing evidence that you can help manage your mind and mood through food.[134] Here is a quick summary of two basic food choices for your small snacks.

Foods for increased mental alertness. Snacks that are low in fat and include a small amount of protein-rich food can often promote faster thinking, greater energy, increased attention to detail, and quicker reaction speed.

Several options: You can put a small amount of protein-rich food (such as skinless white meat chicken or turkey breast, low-fat fish salad, hummus/bean spread, tofu-cinnamon-raisin spread, vegetable-tofu spread, low-fat cottage cheese–fruit spread, grilled or steamed soy tofu) on top of low-fat, whole-grain, high-fiber bread, bagel, muffin, baked pita chips, or rice crackers. Other ideas include lentil soup; low-fat or nonfat yogurt or cottage cheese with fruit and a whole-grain cracker; vegetable pieces with tofu or bean dip; or a glass of skim milk with a piece of fruit and low-fat muffin, several nonfat, whole-grain crackers, or a bagel.

Foods for increased calmness. Snacks that are low in fat and protein but high in complex carbohydrates help many people produce a calm, focused state of mind and relaxed emotions (although in late afternoon these snacks make some people drowsy, so be certain to experiment to find which snacks are best for you). Options include very-low-fat pasta salad with fruit or vegetables, or low-fat, whole-grain, high-fiber bread, bagel, muffin, baked pita chips, or crackers topped with your favorite all-fruit preserve.

For more details on the mind-mood-food connection, see Chapter 27.

Note: Bring a glass or container of pure water (and the rest of your snack if possible) back to your desk or the vehicle seat next to you if you're traveling. Then you'll have a chance to sip some extra water and eat the remaining bites of food to further boost your performance until the next break.

Fitting the Rejuvenation-in-Motion Routine into Your Schedule

To accomplish these 4 steps in 30 seconds, it's obvious that you need to make advance arrangements to have the water and snack nearby (a lunch box and quick-pour Thermos work just fine). After some practice, you might try combining steps 2 and 3, going through the mind moves while your body is in motion. This gives you an extra 10–15 seconds of physical movement time.

I am the first to admit that you need to be well organized and to move at a calm but quick pace to complete this routine in 30 seconds. But the bottom line is that *it works*. And, in comparison, 60 seconds will seem pleasantly long — and several minutes can feel like a holiday gift. That's the fresh perspective this rejuvenation-in-motion routine can give. Let's face it: if you have 30 seconds, you probably have a minute or two. And most of us could convince our boss to allow us at least one 30- or 60-second break every half hour throughout our work shift. You can even do these routines while riding on a commuter train or in an airplane.

How often should you take time out for a rejuvenation-in-motion routine? Once every half hour or hour would be ideal, but begin with whatever increments you can manage. The small snack in step 4 is included only once every two to three hours (during your midmorning and midafternoon break). The other steps, including the drink of water, are included every time.

1-minute to 5-minute Rejuvenation-in-Motion Routines

You can expand the 30-second rejuvenation-in-motion routine into 1-minute, 2-minute, or 5-minute versions by adding other *Health & Fitness Excellence* recommendations that appeal to you.

Examples: Take more bites of your small snack; walk outside for fresh air and a moment of sunshine; add a breathing exercise (Chapter 12), several transpyramid abdominal exercises (Chapter 13), a flexibility and posture exercise (Chapters 14 and 15), a balance and agility exercise (Chapter 19), or some resistance exercises (such as dynamic isometrics or rubber tubing; Chapter 18); take a quick look at ways you might take better care of yourself over the next hour, improve performance, or support your co-workers; go through a sensory rejuvenation exercise for your sight, hearing, or touch (Chapters 36 and 37); read an inspiring quote or look at a beautiful photograph or painting; team up with a co-worker or friend for a quick seated massage (Chapter 36); walk over to someone who has been doing a good job and give him or her a pat on the back and a word of genuine appreciation; jot out a note of praise or a thoughtful reminder to catch small errors before they turn into big problems; call someone special for a brief "thinking of you" greeting; look over your to-do list to make sure you're on track with priorities; go through a mental exercise to boost creativity or problem-solving skills (Chapter 48); send a silent lighted thought or prayer to a person or group in need (Chapter 49); or do any other *Health & Fitness Excellence* option.

Why Small Steps Beat Big Leaps

How important are little successes — those daily handfuls of "minor" personal improvements? More and more of us have come to view life as an either/or situation: either we achieve big or we feel small. To a great extent our focus has shifted to winning the lottery instead of saving our dimes, to waiting for a once-in-a-lifetime trip around the world but missing the sunsets we can see from our own back porch.

Millions of us are living conditional lives — "Once I get through this hectic week, *then* I'll take better care of myself"; "Once I lose five pounds, *then* I'll calm down"; "Once I get this job promotion, *then* I'll spend more time with the children"; "Once the kids are out of high school, *then* we can rebuild our relationship." We put off right-now time, becoming numb to life's unvarnished golden moments.

We even wait to write or call loved ones "until we have the time" — as if we have to compose fifty-page letters or spend hours rehearsing for phone conversations. It's tragic, because for most of us that delay habit blocks communication with the very people we care about most. It's O.K. to be busy and it's even fine to feel rushed sometimes. But it isn't all right to stop staying in touch with ourselves and others in the midst of that busy-ness. Loved ones and friends will rarely be disappointed with quick, from-the-heart phone calls, simple cards, and short notes. Try it.

Rejuvenation-in-motion routines exemplify what the Japanese call *kaizen,* a revolutionary success formula. *Kaizen* means living your life with full awareness so that not a day goes by without one — and usually many — small improvements.

Kaizen is "the single most important concept in Japanese management" and an underlying reason for Japan's miraculous economic growth in recent decades, writes management consultant Masaaki Imai in *Kaizen: The Key to Japan's Competitive Success.*[135] Rather than focusing on big breakthroughs and breathtaking leaps — with the crash landings that characterize so many American efforts — *kaizen* aims at "constant revision and upgrading" in one's personal and work life.

Kaizen relies on open, clear communication and a deep sense of responsibility to notice opportunities and eliminate problems. A problem is defined as anything that inconveniences anyone downstream from you, in your work, family, anywhere. Individuals resolve to notice opportunities for improvement and to identify problems, which are solved immediately and corrected right where — and as — they are found.

This is possible only when you take control of your life from moment to moment and hour to hour. And lifestyle/workstyle habits like rejuvenation-in-motion routines make this not only possible but practical.

Rejuvenation-in-motion routines give us a new way to bring our lives into focus — to uplift our thoughts, perceptions, feelings, and actions in as little as half a minute. How many of these golden opportunities have slipped through your hands today?

Step 2

EXERCISE OPTIONS

11 Introduction

MYTH: As long as you stay "busy" and "active" during the day you don't need any special "exercise time."

FACT: The evidence is clear: If you want to be fit and reap dozens of health and performance benefits, you need to exercise an average of 25 to 35 minutes most days of the week. Here's the payoff: By learning the right exercises that are safe, fast, and enjoyable, you may increase your productivity by *20 percent or more*. Bottom line: If your career now demands 60 hours a week, you may, through enhanced mental and physical energy, stamina, and other benefits, accomplish as much in 50 hours as you now do in 60 — not only giving you the time to exercise but actually helping you gain six or seven free hours a week!

MYTH: If you exercise, you will want to eat more and that makes weight problems worse.

FACT: *Moderate* exercise — the kind recommended in this book — burns excess fat and helps stabilize blood-sugar levels. And scheduling your exercise sessions at the best times can help reduce or control your appetite.

MYTH: If you're tired most of the time, you might as well forget about exercise — you just don't have the energy to do it.

FACT: Exercise should help you *gain* energy, not lose it. Case in point: Lack of oxygen is a predominant cause of fatigue. The right exercises boost your body's ability to take in oxygen and use it in making new energy.

MYTH: Good breathing is automatic. You just breathe in as much air as your body tells you it needs.

FACT: Most of us take in an absolute minimum of air and breathe using only the upper chest rather than our full lung capacity. This shallow breathing contributes to fatigue, poor concentration, anxiety, and many other problems. You can learn how to change your breathing so that you bring plenty of oxygen-rich air to the lower part of your lungs. (*See Chapter 12.*)

MYTH: Traditional sit-ups and leg-lifts are the best exercises to flatten your abdomen.

FACT: To have a slim, strong waist you need to exercise five key muscles, including the little-known transversalis and pyramidalis. Sit-ups and leg-lifts don't work; in fact, they can create — or worsen — the lower-back pain that gives serious problems to three out of every four Americans. Answer? Easy, scientifically correct abdominal exercises. (*See Chapter 14.*)

MYTH: Exercise must hurt to do any good — "No pain, no gain" — and to get *great* results you need to spend plenty of extra time ("more is better").

FACT: That's ridiculous. More *isn't* better, and pain tells you only one thing: you're hurting — not helping — your body. *Health & Fitness Excellence* gives you scientific strategies for *exercising smarter,* for accomplishing the best results in the shortest amount of time.

MYTH: Aerobic exercise is simply a matter of picking an activity such as walking, jogging, swimming, dancing, cycling, or rowing and then doing it every day at a brisk pace.

FACT: Researchers have identified seven key guidelines for aerobic exercise. If you don't know them, there's a good chance you're wasting time and risking needless injuries. Worse, you may be missing many — even most — health and productivity benefits. (*See Chapters 16 and 17.*)

MYTH: To be flexible you need to take regular yoga classes or go through runners' stretches such as those you learned in school.

FACT: European researchers have discovered quick, safe ways to develop flexibility for the entire body in less than 10 minutes a day. (*See Chapters 14 and 15.*)

MYTH: Strength exercises are for bodybuilders and serious athletes, not for people who just want to get into good shape.

FACT: Strong, toned muscles are healthy muscles. No matter what your age and whether you are an athlete or nonathlete, no exercise program is complete unless it includes basic strengthening exercises. Depending on your needs and goals, you can design your own "bare minimum" muscle-toning program that becomes part of your other exercises and takes *no* extra time; or go through a full-body workout in which all you need are some ankle weights, light dumbbells, a flat bench, and two chairs; or select the best values in strength-building "home gyms"; or choose a health club with equipment that produces fast, safe results. (*See Chapter 18.*)

MYTH: Balance and agility are automatically developed in all types of exercise. The only people who need more than that are dancers, martial artists, gymnasts, and tightrope walkers.

FACT: Brain scientists have discovered what martial arts experts have known for centuries: balance and agility exercises help develop the body and mind in ways no other fitness activity can. Best of all, these exercises are fun and take as little as six minutes a week! (*See Chapter 19.*)

"I've never liked exercise." "I don't know where to begin." "I'm not an athlete." "I get tired too quickly." "I'm not young enough anymore." "It's too easy to get hurt."

These are just a few of the reasons people give for not exercising. Don't believe them. It's time to stop thinking about exercise as difficult, painful, or for young athletes only. The right program can be safe and fun, and it can give you a surge of new vitality. You can exercise with a group, a friend, or solo; in the comfort of your own home or a local fitness club, a neighborhood park, or your own back yard. Even in moderate amounts — beginning *anywhere* in this program — exercise will improve your health and performance if you know the right way — the *scientific* way — to do it.

This, the second step to *Health & Fitness Excellence,* takes the mystery, fear, and drudgery out of exercise. I want you to discover how easy it is to exercise and how varied your choices are. If you've been injured or have hated some kind of exercise and sworn off *all* fitness programs, it's time to give exercise another chance. I believe that with enough choices and a plan to make it fun and safe, you'll love it and stick with it.

If you flip through the following chapters, you'll find exercises that not only are easy to learn but don't require any special athletic ability. Best of all, because they're fun, you're not going to count the seconds until they're over.

The "Golden Circle"

Exercise is a central thread of the golden circle of *Health & Fitness Excellence.* And there's another golden circle *within* exercise itself — integration, which goes well beyond the fitness fads, gimmicks, and traditions that emphasize a single area or go off on a tangent. Such fragmented approaches are as inadequate — and sometimes as dangerous — as ever. A new scientific focus has emerged in recent years: *total fitness,*[1] which is based on a comprehensive approach. And this is why *Health & Fitness Excellence* integrates six types of exercise:

1 Breathing enhancement
2 Abdominal fitness
3 Flexibility and posture
4 Aerobics
5 Muscular strength and endurance
6 Balance and agility

Here's the bottom line: *Every one of these six kinds of exercise is vital.* The benefits you receive from each one of them improves, and is improved by, all the others. Within each of the six areas you have a wide variety of options. Best of all, you can combine all six in a daily plan that *will take less time than most people spend doing any one of these types of exercise alone.*

Scientific Guidelines for Exercise Programs

As an All-American athlete, I have known firsthand the training intensities demanded by serious sports. As a martial arts instructor for more than two decades, I have come to appreciate the tremendous capabilities of the human body and mind. As a performance researcher and fitness consultant since 1970, I have observed remarkable transformations by people of all ages when they added a balanced exercise program to their lifestyles. And after certification as a Health and Fitness Instructor by the American College of Sports Medicine and as a Fitness Specialist by the Institute for Aerobics Research, I am more convinced than ever about the need for up-to-date scientific guidelines when designing exercise programs — and *Health & Fitness Excellence* provides just such guidelines.

Benefits of Exercise

Chances are that you're not reading this chapter while panting to dash out and exercise. You're reading it because you think it's important that you read it. First, you want to be convinced that it's true: exercise will make you feel, look, and perform better. Then you want to know that it can be enjoyable and worth the small amount of time it takes.

In the past decade, I have reviewed hundreds of scientific and medical studies on various aspects of exercise. In the following brief summary of benefits, I've noted several of these references for each area. For in-depth presentations, see *Exercise Physiology: Energy, Nutrition, and Human Performance* by Drs. William McArdle, Frank Katch, and Victor Katch (Lea & Febiger, 1986), a preeminent exercise text; *Resource Manual for Guidelines for Exercise Testing and Prescription* by the American College of

Sports Medicine (Lea & Febiger, 1988), the most definitive guidebook to date for health/fitness professionals; and *The Sports Medicine Fitness Course* by David C. Nieman, D.H.Sc., M.P.H. (Bull Publishing, P.O. Box 208, Palo Alto, CA 94302; 1986), written for the American College of Sports Medicine Fitness Instructor Workshop.

Physical Benefits of Exercise

Cardiovascular and respiratory benefits. Recent studies suggest that physical inactivity is a serious health hazard — similar in magnitude to such primary coronary heart disease risk factors as uncontrolled hypertension, high blood cholesterol, and cigarette smoking.[2]

Regular, moderate exercise increases circulation, reduces resting heart rate and blood pressure, strengthens the heart, increases lung capacity and transport/utilization of oxygen, improves blood cholesterol ratios (cholesterol is discussed in Chapter 22), increases protection against heart attacks and strokes, and may decrease the risk of certain cancers.

Neuroendocrine and musculoskeletal benefits. Your brain, nerves, muscles, bones, and glands depend on regular balanced exercise for peak function. Research at New York University Medical School and other centers suggests that more than 80 percent of all lower back pain may be due to muscular deficiency rather than pathology.[3] Exercise — especially aerobics and strength training — increases bone density and helps prevent osteoporosis.[4]

Exercise also provides a powerful antidote to fatigue, says Dr. Per-Olof Åstrand, one of the world's leading exercise physiologists.[5] Other documented benefits include increases in mental alertness, cognitive (thinking) abilities, sensory awareness, reaction speed, and physical coordination.

Metabolic benefits. Regular exercise, especially aerobics, is one of the keys to losing excess body fat and maintaining balanced metabolism (see Chapters 16, 17, and 30).

Immunological benefits. Studies suggest that regular exercise can boost the body's resistance to a wide range of illnesses and diseases.[6]

Sexual benefits. Recent national surveys report that enhanced fitness improves sexual well-being and intimate relationships.[7]

Psychological Benefits of Exercise

"Vigorous . . . exercise is the best antidote for nervous and emotional stress that we possess," says Dr. Paul Dudley White, the dean of American cardiologists, "far better than tranquilizers or sedatives to which, unhappily, so many are addicted today."[8]

Current studies report that regular exercise is associated with a significant increase in self-esteem, boosts overall psychological well-being, decreases depression, and helps relieve negative stress.[9]

Learning, Performance, and Career Benefits of Exercise

A number of reports associate regular exercise with improvements in learning abilities, job performance, and career advancement.[10]

Longevity (Anti-Aging) Benefits of Exercise

It should come as little surprise that scientists are linking exercise to a slowing down of the aging process and to an extended life span.[11] A 20-year study of nearly seventeen thousand Harvard University graduates was recently completed by Dr. Ralph S. Paffenbarger, Jr., and reported in the *Journal of the American Medical Association* and the *New England Journal of Medicine*. Major finding: There is significant evidence that regular exercise helps prevent heart disease, lowers the risk of respiratory illness, and extends life.[12]

Preliminary Issues Involved in Exercise

It bears repeating: The golden circle of *Health & Fitness Excellence* makes it essential for you to keep your sights on all seven major areas of this program, not simply exercise. Stress management, good nutrition, balanced posture, a well-designed living environment, and the ability to fully relax your body and focus your mind each contribute to exercise success. There's a tendency in America to charge off on tangents and overdo things. That overdoing exacts a price, especially when it comes to exercise. Here's an example.

Researchers at the University of California at Berkeley[13] and other institutions[14] have discovered that exercise produces a large number of *free radicals,* highly reactive and potentially dangerous molecule fragments (discussed in Chapter 22), inside the cells of the body. Even though exercise stimulates your body to produce more of certain anti-free-radical protective enzymes, this often doesn't appear to be enough to handle all the free radicals produced by exercise.[15] Bottom line: some of these free radicals may damage body tissues unless your diet (and perhaps a balanced, low-dosage vitamin-mineral supplement) provides an adequate supply of anti-free-radical nutrients such as vitamins C and E and the trace mineral selenium. As detailed in Chapters 20–28, this type of diet can be simple and inexpensive to plan, but it does require an accurate, basic knowledge of nutritional facts and dietary priorities.

The exercise-is-everything fanatics are, it turns out, at even greater risk than previously thought. Be certain you capture *all* the advantages of the golden circle of *Health & Fitness Excellence*.

Safety

Is exercise safe? The answer is a conditional yes. "Some people don't believe in moderation and feel they have to do as much as possible to get the best results," says Dr. Richard Birrer, a professor specializing in exercise and activity at the State University of New York at Brooklyn. "More people are showing up with overuse injuries, and ironically, many . . . should know better."[16]

"We're a compulsive society that believes you can't do anything fast enough or take it far enough; you have to keep pushing for more," adds Bryant Stamford, director of the exercise physiology laboratory at the University of Louisville School of Medicine. "There's an attitude that if a little is good for you then a lot has got to be great. But that mentality is hurting people."[17]

Some exercise critics have claimed that too much of certain types of exercise, or the wrong kind of exercise, may increase the risk of heart attacks. In very rare cases, this may be true. But the benefits of intelligent, balanced exercise programs *far* outweigh the risks, says Dr. Kenneth H. Cooper.[18]

Common causes of exercise injury include inadequate warm-up and cool-down and faulty technique or form. Another risk factor is overtraining, spending *too much time* in fitness activities.

The *Health & Fitness Excellence* program enables you to *exercise smarter,* keeping your options open, enjoyment high, and risks low and finding every way to get the greatest benefits from the smallest investment of your time.

When to Seek Medical Advice About Exercise

Do you need a medical examination and exercise tolerance test (ETT) or maximal graded exercise test (MaxGXT) before beginning an exercise program? The answer, say the experts, is maybe. It depends on which medical authority you listen to and on the common sense and balance of the program you choose.

The National Heart, Lung, and Blood Institute advises that if a person is at low risk for heart disease and has no symptoms, he or she does not need to see a physician before starting a moderate exercise routine.[19] The American Heart Association in 1981 simply stated that "older sedentary individuals may . . . wish to seek medical advice."[20]

According to the American College of Sports Medicine, apparently healthy individuals under age forty-five with no major coronary risk factors — family history of high blood pressure, heart attack, or cardiovascular disease prior to age fifty; history of high blood pressure above 145/95; elevated total cholesterol/HDL cholesterol ratio (above 5 for males or 4.5 for females); abnormal electrocardiogram; cigarette smoking; or diabetes mellitus — can usually begin exercise programs without undergoing an ETT or MaxGXT "as long as the exercise program begins and proceeds gradually and as long as the individual is alert to the development of unusual signs or symptoms."[21] Individuals at higher risk (above age thirty-five with one or more coronary risk factors) or individuals at any age with symptoms suggestive of metabolic, pulmonary, or coronary heart disease should undergo a physician-supervised exercise tolerance test.

"People often ask, 'Should I have a medical check-up before I start training?'" says Dr. Per-Olof Åstrand, a leader in sports medicine. "The answer must be that people who are in doubt about the condition of their health should consult their physician. But as a general rule, moderate activity is less harmful to the health than inactivity. You could also put it this way: a medical examination is more urgent for those who plan to remain inactive than for those who intend to get into good physical shape!"[22]

Certainly you should consult your physician if you have any medical symptoms, are undergoing treatment for any ailment, or have one or more major coronary risk factors.[23] Dr. Kenneth H. Cooper says that it's advisable for those over forty "to undergo a thorough medical examination and a maximal performance treadmill stress test before [beginning] any vigorous exercise program."[24]

The American College of Sports Medicine and the Institute for Aerobics Research advise that if your physician calls for an exercise stress evaluation, strict and specific testing methods must be used to maximize reliability and accuracy. There are a number of accepted protocols. Here is a summary of Dr. Kenneth Cooper's Cooper Clinic Protocol, which reports a remarkable 80 percent accuracy rate in identifying coronary artery disease with stress testing:[25]

1 *Get a thorough pretest screening.* This includes a medical history (noting any family history of heart disease); physical exam; a check for any medications you're taking that may affect the results of an electrocardiogram (ECG); and a thorough evaluation of a resting ECG. The resting ECG includes four twelve-lead ECGs: two ECGs taken with the patient in the supine position (one with leads in the normal places and one with leads located where they'll be placed for the treadmill test), then one ECG standing up, and one after hyperventilation.

2 *Monitor a minimum of nine ECG leads, with seven chest electrodes.* (Technicians at the Cooper Clinic monitor fifteen leads, using fourteen electrodes.)

3 *Use the proper treadmill procedure.* The Cooper Clinic prefers a modified version of the Balke Protocol. The speed is held constant at 3.3 miles per hour (90 meters per minute) until the 25th minute. Thereafter, the speed is increased 0.2 mph per minute. The treadmill is flat the first minute, and then its angle increases by 2 percent. Each minute thereafter it is increased by 1 percent until the 25th minute. After that, with the incline at 25 percent, only the speed increases. This uses more of a warm-up than other tests and is therefore safer. The patient at no time holds on to the treadmill bar and keeps exercising to his or her maximum heart rate. The test continues up to the point of exhaustion. As soon as the test is completed, the patient spends a 3-to-5-minute period doing low-intensity walking. Finally, the patient lies down and rests — the physician should monitor blood pressure and ECG at 2-to-3-minute intervals until they have returned to normal.

4 *Ask your doctor for a detailed blood evaluation.* The evaluation should especially note the various cholesterol (lipoprotein) levels and ratios (discussed in Chapter 22). For top accuracy, your doctor may want to average three separate cholesterol test measurements taken a month apart. In addition, be certain that your physician or laboratory is using the reference standard established by the Centers for Disease Control. To learn more about the cholesterol issue, see *Controlling Cholesterol* by Dr. Kenneth H. Cooper (Bantam, 1988).

Listen to Your Body

Perhaps more than any other exercise guideline, "Listen to your body" is a cardinal rule. The best guide to safety in fitness activities is your self-awareness. Listening to your body takes practice — you have to sharpen your senses and think about how you feel. Appropriate exercise shouldn't make you feel unusually fatigued or sick in any way. If it does, pay attention to the feelings and stop exercising until you can determine that nothing is wrong with your health.

Is a Health Club Right for You?

The next few chapters will help you design a comprehensive exercise program that you can do right at home, alone or with a friend or group. Or you can use this book to help you undertake a program at a health club or fitness center. The best of these establishments provide three primary advantages: companionship and motivation; supervision and instruction; and equipment and facilities.

These days, fitness clubs range from traditional YMCAs and YWCAs to large sports complexes to specialty centers (strength training or aerobic dance only, for example), and from spartan warehouse-like decor to sleek chrome-and-velvet, computer-monitored exercise emporiums. The best clubs are usually multipurpose facilities that offer a variety of organized group classes, a diversified equipment collection, and supportive accompaniments (massage therapists, showers, saunas, whirlpools, health and fitness libraries, restaurants). If you enjoy sports, added features such as running tracks, racquetball and squash courts, a swimming pool, and tennis facilities are a bonus.

Personal instruction is particularly valuable for those at either end of the fitnesss continuum — individuals who are out of shape and haven't exercised before and dedicated athletes training for competition. If you opt for one-on-one guidance, choose it wisely.

Ask about the credentials and experience of anyone you consider as a private coach. Insist that your fitness instructor have a health-related educational background and will tailor recommendations to your personal goals, condition, and abilities. *Never* assume that a "staff member" polo shirt or a good physique signify professional competence.

The most competent fitness specialists and exercise leaders are usually certified (through comprehensive practical and written examinations) by one or more of the following organizations (listed alphabetically): Aerobics and Fitness Association of America (15250 Ventura Blvd., Suite 802, Sherman Oaks, CA 91403); American College of Sports Medicine (P.O. Box 1440, Indianapolis, IN 46206); Institute for Aerobics Research (12330 Preston Rd., Dallas, TX 75230); International Dance-Exercise Association (6190 Cornerstone Ct. East, Suite 202, San Diego, CA 92109); National Strength and Conditioning Association (P.O. Box 81410, Lincoln, NE 68501); or the YMCA (101 N. Wacker Dr., Chicago, IL 60606).

Long-Term Exercise Success: Going Beyond Good Intentions

There's no question about it: a regular exercise program takes organization and commitment. Here are three considerations to planning your program.

Selecting the Right Program

Aim for variety in the types of exercise you choose. This will keep your motivation and enjoyment high and, on a medical note, this "cross training" (as it is called) gives solid health benefits since you are using muscles in different ways with each varied activity. The result is what we discussed early in this chapter — *balanced* or *total* fitness — and you avoid problems such as the strong legs–weak upper body syndrome found in single-sport specialists like many runners, skaters, and cyclists.

"We cannot stress too strongly that lack of variety is one of the major stumbling blocks along the bumpy road to fitness," write Dr. Irving Dardik and Denis Waitley in *Quantum Fitness*. "Somewhere along the way you lost *mental* flexibility and got locked into jogging or weightlifting or some other less-than-complete form of exercise. You lost sight of the fact that our wonderfully complex bodies can move in wonderfully complex ways; that fitness means coordinating muscles and limbs, which are capable of an infinite variety of effective movements; that the body must be continually challenged with a wide variety of physical tasks or it will cease to grow. Just as variety in food choices can ensure satisfaction of the body's nutrient needs, variety in exercise can satisfy the body's requirements for movement."[26]

Warming Up and Cooling Down	To maximize progress and enjoyment, precede every exercise session with a gradual, appropriate warm-up (usually lasting 2–5 minutes) and follow each activity with a progressive cool-down (3–5 minutes).
Setting a Clear Direction	One of the reasons that most people don't reach their fitness goals is that they didn't bother to set them in the first place. Put your goals in writing and schedule specific step-by-step progress markers. Give yourself positive reinforcement — some kind of small personal reward — *every step of the way*. And begin today. A "do it now" attitude paves the way for long-term success.
Sticking with It	Over half (and perhaps three-quarters or more) of all adults who start an exercise program quit within a short period of time.[27] Beyond obvious adherence problems caused by poor attitude, poor exercise choice, pre-existing injuries, and frequent complaints of lack of time, the underlying problem is simply not sticking with it. One predominant reason is that major benefits — in terms of self-esteem and visible fitness "results" — often don't become evident for ten to twelve weeks.[28] So once you begin your program, keep it going.

Finding the Time and Establishing Your Schedule

Those who think they have not time for bodily exercise will sooner or later have to find time for illness.

— EDWARD STANLEY, EARL OF DERBY, 1873

Another key component of your exercise program is a commitment to set aside a certain period of personal fitness time each day. Don't view it as a task. Instead, think of it as a break from your heavy workload and as a chance to do something positive for your body; it will help you feel better, more energetic and productive. Focus on the sheer joy of movement, the welcome break in your busy routine. Remember, all that's required is a commitment of between 1 and 2 percent of your time, and the other 98–99 percent will be more enriching because of it.

Sample Weekly Schedules	Here are four sample weekly exercise schedules — two at the beginning level and two at the intermediate level — that incorporate the variety of fitness activities recommended throughout *Health & Fitness Excellence*. The average time investment is between 20 and 38 minutes a day for the entire program. Start by pinpointing your own interests and begin anywhere. Then, over the upcoming weeks, create your best personal schedule.

Note: Choices 1, 2, and 3 for aerobic exercise mean that you should choose several *different* aerobic exercises to include in your weekly schedule.

EXERCISE OPTIONS: Sample Weekly Schedules

Beginning Level I: Example A

Every Day:	Breathing exercises — free moments throughout the day	
Monday:	Flexibility and posture exercises, phase I	5 minutes
	Aerobics: Choice 1 (with warm-up/cool-down)	35 minutes
	Balance and agility exercises	2 minutes
	Abdominal exercises	3 minutes
Wednesday:	Flexibility and posture exercises, phase I	5 minutes
	Balance and agility exercises	2 minutes
	Aerobics: Choice 2 (with warm-up/cool-down)	35 minutes
	Abdominal exercises	3 minutes
Friday:	Flexibility and posture exercises, phase I	5 minutes
	Aerobics: Choice 3 (with warm-up/cool-down)	35 minutes
	Balance and agility exercises	2 minutes
	Abdominal exercises	3 minutes

Tuesday, Thursday, Saturday, and Sunday: Off

Average daily time investment: 20 minutes

Beginning Level I: Example B

Every Day:	Breathing exercises — free moments throughout the day	
Monday:	Flexibility and posture exercises, phase I	5 minutes
	Aerobics: Choice 1 (with warm-up/cool-down)	25 minutes
	Balance and agility exercises	2 minutes
	Abdominal exercises	3 minutes
Tuesday:	Flexibility and posture exercises, phase I	5 minutes
	Aerobics: Choice 2 (with warm-up/cool-down)	25 minutes
	Flexibility and posture exercises, phase II	5 minutes
	Balance and agility exercises	2 minutes
Thursday:	Flexibility and posture exercises, phase I	5 minutes
	Aerobics: Choice 1 (with warm-up/cool-down)	25 minutes
	Abdominal exercises	3 minutes
	Balance and agility exercises	2 minutes
Friday:	Flexibility and posture exercises, phase I	5 minutes
	Flexibility and posture exercises, phase II	5 minutes
	Balance and agility exercises	2 minutes

Saturday:	Flexibility and posture exercises, phase I	5 minutes
	Aerobics: Choice 2 (with warm-up/cool-down)	25 minutes
	Balance and agility exercises	2 minutes
	Abdominal exercises	3 minutes

Wednesday and Sunday: Off

Average daily time investment: 22 minutes

Intermediate Level II: Example A

| *Every Day:* | Breathing exercises — free moments throughout the day | |

Monday:	Flexibility and posture exercises, phase I	5 minutes
	Aerobics: Choice 1 (with warm-up/cool-down)	35 minutes
	Balance and agility exercises	2 minutes
	Abdominal exercises	3 minutes

Tuesday:	Flexibility and posture exercises, phase I	5 minutes
	Strength and endurance exercises (upper body)	30 minutes
	Flexibility and posture exercises, phase II	5 minutes
	Balance and agility exercises	2 minutes

Wednesday:	Flexibility and posture exercises, phase I	5 minutes
	Aerobics: Choice 2 (with warm-up/cool-down)	35 minutes
	Abdominal exercises	3 minutes
	Balance and agility exercises	2 minutes

Thursday:	Flexibility and posture exercises, phase I	5 minutes
	Strength and endurance exercises (legs)	20 minutes
	Flexibility and posture exercises, phase II	5 minutes
	Balance and agility exercises	2 minutes

Friday:	Flexibility and posture exercises, phase I	5 minutes
	Aerobics: Choice 3 (with warm-up/cool-down)	35 minutes
	Abdominal exercises	3 minutes

Saturday and Sunday: Off

Average daily time investment: 30 minutes

Intermediate Level II: Example B

| *Every Day:* | Breathing exercises — free moments throughout the day | |

Monday and Thursday:	Flexibility and posture exercises, phase I	5 minutes
	Aerobics: Choice 1 (with warm-up/cool-down)	25 minutes
	Flexibility and posture exercises, phase II	5 minutes
	Abdominal exercises	3 minutes
	Balance and agility exercises	2 minutes

Tuesday and Friday:	Flexibility and posture exercises, phase I	5 minutes
	Strength and endurance exercises (upper body)	30 minutes
	Balance and agility exercises	2 minutes
Wednesday and Saturday:	Flexibility and posture exercises, phase I	5 minutes
	Aerobics: Choice 2 (with warm-up/cool-down)	25 minutes
	Strength and endurance exercises (legs)	15 minutes
	Flexibility and posture exercises, phase II	5 minutes
	Abdominal exercises	3 minutes
	Balance and agility exercises	2 minutes
Sunday:	Off	

Average daily time investment: 38 minutes

Over the past 25 years, I have come to appreciate the power and value of a written exercise schedule. I also think it's a great idea to keep a notebook and calendar so you can enter each accomplishment and any observations or questions that come to mind. This recordkeeping aids in modifying the program to fit your personal needs. Post your schedule in a conspicuous place at home and at work. Take full advantage of this tool to stay on track, have fun, reach your goals, and avoid overtraining. One other tip: Take a week or two off from formal exercise several times a year.

Shattering the All-or-Nothing Myth

Fitness comes from more than formal exercise. The fact is that just being more active brings rewards too. Experts report that, in addition to exercise sessions, a wide range of informal activities also provide fitness benefits:[29] taking the stairs instead of an elevator; walking or cycling to and from work or on errands; actively gardening with hand tools; cutting, splitting, carrying, or stacking firewood; doing household chores; getting out of your chair and moving around on work breaks; taking early morning or evening strolls; doing light, impromptu calisthenics while talking on the phone; playing half-court basketball games; taking weekend hikes; and so on. An active lifestyle is a cornerstone of lifelong good health.

Family Fitness: Make It Fun

For adults, exercise programs are a personal choice, an option. But when it comes to our children, fitness is a family issue. Research shows that we can't leave it to the schools. "The physical fitness of American public school children has shown virtually no improvement in the last 10 years, and in some cases, has greatly deteriorated," the President's Council on Physical Fitness and Sports reported in 1986.[30] Study after study shows that today's students, aged five to seventeen, tend to have more body fat and symptoms of heart disease than students a decade ago. And performance levels on various tests of endurance, agility, coordination, and fitness have been steadily declining too.[31]

New school programs are part — and only part — of the solution. By contacting your local education officials, school board members, and government representatives, you can help ensure that *high-quality* health and fitness take on added emphasis in our schools. Three top-rated programs merit everyone's attention: *Feelin' Good* (Fitness Finders, 113 Teft Rd., Spring Arbor, MI 49283), *FitnessGram* (Youth Fitness, Institute for Aerobics Research, 12330 Preston Rd., Dallas, TX 75230), and *Know Your Body* (American Health Foundation, 320 East 43rd St., New York, NY 10017). Write for details.

Just as important, how can we, as parents and friends, best help youngsters improve their fitness? First, we can respect our younger children's natural play initiatives. Play areas planned around what children need from play — and how children actually play together — can keep them playing happily and safely for hours.

In *Make Your Backyard More Interesting Than TV* (McGraw-Hill, 1980) and *How to Design and Build Children's Play Equipment* (Ortho, 1986), home playground consultant Jay Beckwith shows how to build a variety of play structures that will engage children's interest and provide countless opportunities for them to develop physical fitness. He includes plans for everything from sandboxes to complex modular play areas that incorporate climbers, rope devices, elaborate slides, and treehouses. Using simple hand tools and low-cost materials, you (and your children) can construct one piece at a time or everything at once. Modification ideas are included for easy adaptations and expansions as your children grow up.

Second, we can set good fitness examples for our children. Numerous studies confirm that the "Do as I say, not as I do" adage doesn't work with kids.

Third, we can learn about and implement a regular and enjoyable family exercise program that includes a variety of *Health & Fitness Excellence* options. There's no doubt that getting kids to work out for sustained periods of time isn't easy. They love pursuing lots of different activities rather than sticking to just one. Too much regimentation leaves many kids resentful, especially those under age ten.

To get children to exercise for a full 20-to-30-minute period you'll have to make it entertaining. Here are some ideas:

Nothing beats a parent's enthusiasm and participation for getting young children interested in physical activities. Fun but vigorous daily aerobic "play times" can really pay off. Games like aerobic softball, volley-ball, badminton, soccer, and basketball, where you simply keep the ball in play and everyone keeps moving — usually with lots of laughter — make the exercise time pass more quickly. Cycling, aerobic dancing, rope skipping, swimming, skating, and mini-trampolining are other fun options for kids, especially if the parents like the activity too. Music can make any activity even more entertaining. You might also permit television viewing while exercising, so long as your child, for example, pedals comfortably and steadily on a stationary cycle for an entire 20-to-30-minute show.

How do you tempt reluctant kids? There are many ways to share fitness time with your children in ways that can be fun for you too. Dust off your sense of adventure — if kids see that this is a chore for you, they'll quickly lose interest. Make sure each child has good-quality foot-wear and appropriate, comfortable clothing.

Create a home and back yard environment that encourages fitness play. Set aside several hours each Saturday or Sunday as "family fitness time" and let each family member take turns choosing the activity for that day. This is a great time for hiking, canoeing, cycle touring, throwing and chasing a Frisbee, orienteering, swimming, basketball, skating, cross-country skiing, folk dancing, and walking (nature walks, beach walks, neighborhood walks, farmer's field walks, and museum walks).

If you take bike rides or long walks through the country, plan a des-tination reward such as a low-fat frozen yogurt treat, a special movie, or a snack at Grandma's house. Take along your camera (or video camera) and take lots of pictures. Post them — or have a special showing — where everyone can see.

Participate in local fun walks and group bike tours or organize your own, going at the kids' pace and making the focus fun, not just fitness. Set off to go bird watching, star gazing, window shopping, collecting pine cones or leaves, or looking for animal tracks in the snow — taking a book along to identify what you find. Take a trip to a local lake and rent canoes (and life jackets) with paddles for everyone.

Consider fun-oriented exercise videos for kids. Plan your children's birthday parties at a local roller rink, ice skating arena, swimming pool, or beautiful park where nature hikes are safe and fun.

If your children are interested in organized sports, contact your local YMCA or YWCA. Groups like Jazzercise (2808 Roosevelt, Carlsbad, CA 92008) offer special programs for kids based on body awareness, dance routines, and low-impact aerobics.

If you are handicapped, contact the National Handicapped Sports and Recreation Association (P.O. Box 33141, Washington, DC 20005; 202-783-1441). This group sponsors fitness clinics across the nation and recently produced a videotape series entitled "Fitness Is for Everyone!"

designed to help disabled persons participate in a full range of exercise activities.

There are three keys to creating total fitness. First, make it a personal and family priority, something positive and special in your daily life. Second, learn all you can about it and design your own balanced program incorporating all six exercise elements. That's what the next chapters of *Health & Fitness Excellence* are all about. Third, while you're learning, get started — anywhere, right now.

12 Breathing Enhancement

He lives most life whoever breathes most air.
— ELIZABETH BARRETT BROWNING

Are You "Just Barely Alive" or "Fully Alive"?

We each breathe about twenty thousand times every day — and we assume that we take in plenty of oxygen. But the fact is that most of us breathe just deeply enough to keep from falling over unconscious. Neuroscientists have reported that although we remain technically "alive," we don't supply our brains with optimal levels of oxygen.[32] This chapter presents easy breathing exercises — quick ways to energize the body, calm the emotions, and sharpen the mind.

Optimal Breathing Must Be Learned

Optimal breathing is a *skill*, not something automatic or programmed into the body. "In day-to-day life few basic physiological functions have escaped the attention of modern man to the degree that breathing has," says Dr. Alan Hymes, professor of cardiovascular and thoracic surgery at the University of Minnesota School of Medicine.[33] It's unfortunate that so few fitness programs in America teach breathing exercises. With just a small amount of practice over the next few weeks, you can *permanently improve the way you breathe* — and you'll never have to think about it again. At least one-fourth of the oxygen in every breath you take is needed to fuel the central nervous system.[34] With poor breathing habits, you silently strangle yourself.

According to experts, vital lung capacity decreases about 5 percent with every decade of life, mostly as a result of lost elasticity of lung tissue.[35] Most — perhaps nearly all — of this loss can be prevented with proper breathing habits, good posture, and regular aerobic exercise. Research at the Baltimore Gerontology Research Center of the National Institute on Aging (NIA) shows that it's common to find a huge drop in the amount of oxygen taken in by the lungs as we age.

NIA studies indicate that the circulating blood of a twenty-year-old man takes up an average of nearly 4 liters of oxygen per minute.[36] In contrast, because of shallow breathing and loss of lung elasticity, a seventy-five-year-old man takes up only 1.5 liters a minute. This is typical — but *it isn't inevitable*. Worldwide research suggests that a fit seventy-five-year-old can take in as much oxygen as a fit twenty-year-old.

So why is the problem so widespread? Because of a common habit — shallow, upper-chest breathing (explained in a moment). Here's a startling estimate: Blood is flowing at the rate of about one tablespoon (0.07 liter) a minute at the top area of your lungs, about one pint a minute in the middle area of your lungs, and about one quart a minute at the bottom of your lungs.[37] Upper-chest breathing automatically leaves you under-oxygenated. Poor posture, tense muscles, and a general lack of fitness further restrict blood flow to the brain. The result is fatigue, diminished brain power, and weakened health.

Here's another surprise: Poor breathing contributes to high blood pressure. "If we don't take in enough oxygen by breathing, our blood has to circulate more rapidly to compensate and carry the same amount of oxygen," reports Dr. James J. Lynch of the Center for the Study of Human Psychophysiology at the University of Maryland School of Medicine, after studying more than one thousand people over a five-year period. "This can result in an increase in blood pressure, because our blood has to move faster to maintain the oxygen supply."[38]

Breathing Is Tied to Emotions

Since breathing is under both voluntary and automatic (autonomic) nervous system control, it acts as an important "mind-body bridge" and a key to relaxation. Throughout history, martial artists, yoga practitioners, and meditators have viewed breath control as a key to mastering life's challenges and elevating mind and mood.[39]

"As the link between body and mind, breath can intervene in the activities of either level," says Dr. John Clarke in *Science of Breath*. "With an increased awareness and control of the subtle aspects of breathing, these interventions can affect deep physical and psychological changes. . . . [Optimal breathing], then, opens up new avenues of being to the conscious mind, providing a powerful tool in the pursuit of [wellness] and personal growth."[40]

There is also growing evidence that breathing patterns are tied to personality traits. Sheila Sperber Haas, psychologist at New York University, conducted a recent study of 160 healthy adults. Haas discovered differences in breathing patterns that were unexplainable through variances in oxygen demands or body build. Her conclusions: Slow, deep breathers tended to be "strong, stable and adventurous, intellectually and physically in control of their lives," and rapid, shallow breathers tended to be "shy, passive, fearful and dependent on others for a sense of self and security."[41]

As we free our breath through diaphragmatic breathing, we calm our emotions and can more easily let go of body tensions. "Learning to monitor and control your breathing gives you the ability to maintain appropriate rhythms, thus ensuring optimal oxygenation for proper brain- and muscle-cell efficiency," says performance researcher Charles Garfield. "In addition to increasing the amount of oxygen in the blood, there is considerable evidence that full diaphragmatic breathing strengthens weak abdominal and intestinal muscles. Furthermore, once you establish a habit of abdominal breathing, your heart rate will tend to decelerate. Mental concentration is increased and the ability to create mental imagery . . . is greatly enhanced."[42]

Four Breathing Patterns: Which Is Yours?

Chest Breathing

By far the most common breathing method is called *chest breathing* or *upper-chest breathing*. Chest wall muscles, rather than the diaphragm, act to take in air, filling the upper and middle portions of the lungs but ineffectively reaching the lower, more gravity-dependent lung areas where most blood exchange takes place.

Consequently, chest breathing "wastes" more energy and demands more work from the heart to achieve the same blood/gas mixing provided by diaphragmatic breathing.

Paradoxical Breathing

This is even more inefficient than chest breathing since it combines chest breathing with tensing of the abdominal muscles, which drives the diaphragm up against the lungs, reducing air intake. Paradoxical breathing is often triggered by mismanaging stressful situations. You feel stress, tense your abdomen, and interrupt your breathing. It soon becomes an unconscious habit.

"After being accustomed to this abnormal pattern the very real danger exists . . . [that] . . . relatively minor stresses may then also begin to initiate the same response," says Dr. Hymes, "and can, in turn, reinforce or recreate the original emotional atmosphere — a vicious cycle ensues."[43]

Clavicular Breathing

This respiration pattern involves the uppermost portions of the lungs and comes into use only when the body's oxygen demands are especially great, such as during intensive exercise activities.

Diaphragmatic Breathing

Here's the key: Diaphragmatic breathing is vastly superior to the other choices. It requires only about 1 percent of the body's ongoing energy consumption to bring air in and out. In comparison, chest breathing takes at least twice as much energy to accomplish the same work,[44] and paradoxical breathing even more.

Training yourself to use diaphragmatic breathing is, then, of tremendous importance. The diaphragm, as it contracts, provides an added benefit: it gently pushes the internal organs down, massaging them and, some researchers suggest, improving circulation and digestive-eliminative function.

In diaphragmatic breathing, the diaphragm muscle moves downward, creating a natural pressure vacuum that draws air into the lower lungs. This is quickly followed by a slight expansion of the abdomen and lower ribs. Finally, as the inhalation cycle is completed, the chest expands and the upper lung areas are filled with air.

One of the most effective ways to develop diaphragmatic breathing is through simple awareness exercises. Here is an example.

Breathing Exercise 1: Diaphragmatic Breathing Patterns

Technique: Sit or stand with head up, neck long and relaxed, chin slightly in, shoulders broad and loose, back straight. Place your hands lightly around the sides of your lower ribs with the fingertips pointing in toward the front centerline of the body (navel) with your thumbs to the rear. Slowly inhale through the nose.

As the abdomen expands slightly downward and forward (with the lower back staying flat), feel your lower ribs move out to the sides. Then, as you complete the breath in, feel your chest expand comfortably. Exhale slowly through the mouth, feeling a wave of relaxation flood the abdomen, chest, throat, and face.

Touching the outside of the lower ribs gives the brain a tactile (touch) "biofeedback loop," which improves your results. Repeat the exercise. Become more and more aware of the exact sensation of breathing correctly. With practice, it will become your automatic breathing pattern.

Frequency: Perform this simple exercise often throughout the day. (You will need to hold your ribs only the first day or two; after that your other senses should tell you that you're doing it correctly.)

Find a convenient way to remind yourself to regularly practice proper breathing. You might use the same idea recommended for the instant calming sequence in Chapter 7: stick some small brightly colored circular stickers in key places at home and at work — on the bathroom mirror, corner of the TV screen, remote control, refrigerator door, car dashboard, watchband, telephone receivers, bookmarkers, bedroom nightstand, a noticeable spot on your lunch box, purse, or briefcase, and so on. Each time you see this bright dash of color, remind yourself to check your breathing. Breathing techniques can also be used in other ways to calm the body and energize the mind, as illustrated in the next two exercises.

Breathing Exercise 2: Revitalization Breaths

Technique: Standing with feet about shoulder width apart and knees slightly bent, extend both arms up over your head as you slowly inhale a full, natural breath (don't hyperventilate). As you begin an easy, steady exhalation, bend your knees and smoothly roll forward from the hips and bring your arms and entire upper body into a relaxed position with head and arms pointing down, keeping the knees bent. Release *all* tension from your neck, forehead, face, scalp, jaw, tongue, shoulders, arms, and hands. Stay down for several moments and then inhale as you slowly return to the upright position.

Revitalization breaths gently direct the force of gravity to help improve circulation in the upper body, including the neck, face, eyes, and brain.[45]

Frequency: Revitalization breaths may be performed several times each day, more often as desired. Don't do this exercise without your physician's approval if you have a history of respiratory, cardiovascular, visual, or equilibrium disorders.

Breathing Exercise 3: De-tensing Breath

Whenever you're under pressure, feeling tense, or in a rush, let your breathing help you survey the situation and keep things under control. You can stop anxiety before it starts and be more patient and pleasant. Here's the basic technique: Loosen your shoulders and neck, relax your tongue, jaw, and face muscles, and feel your breath come in and out *smoothly, evenly, fully*. Imagine it reaching and calming every muscle in your body, evaporating tension. Use your mind to guide each breath to any tight spots you notice in your body, releasing them. For another version of this de-tensing technique, see Chapter 4. And for an exciting, instantaneous technique for calming the body and focusing the mind, see Chapter 7.

Don't get so involved with any of these exercises that you hyperventilate — that is, take in more oxygen than your body can comfortably handle. If you become dizzy or lightheaded during the exercises, hyperventilation is probably why and it will soon pass. Over the next days and weeks, your lung capacity will grow and your body will be able to process more and more oxygen.

Aerobic exercise (Chapters 16 and 17) also helps improve respiratory capacity and cardiovascular health. In addition, certain flexibility and strengthening exercises (Chapters 14, 15, 33, and 34) can be used to enhance breathing by increasing your chest elasticity and improving your posture.

13 Abdominal Exercises

A STRONG, SLIM WAISTLINE: it's the most sought-after symbol of fitness success for millions of Americans. Yet it almost always remains only a dream. The reason: Most people base their abdominal fitness efforts on myths, not facts.

The two most popular abdominal exercises, traditional sit-ups and leg-lifts, don't slim the waistline — no matter *how many* you do. And worse, they contribute to poor posture and back pain.[46]

"More than 30 million Americans are afflicted with lower back pain, and an estimated 80 percent [24 million] of these problems are due to improper posture, weak muscles, or inadequate flexibility," says Brian J. Sharkey, author of *Physiology of Fitness*. "Weak abdominal muscles cannot prevent the forward tilt of the pelvis, which displaces the vertebrae and causes pain. . . . Most cases of lower back pain can be prevented by assuming good posture and adhering to a regular program of flexibility and abdominal exercises."[47]

When strong and balanced, the abdominal muscles help stabilize your lower back at its most vulnerable point — the lumbosacral angle of the pelvis. Weak muscles promote abdominal distention (a "pot belly"), lordosis (an exaggerated inward curvature in the lower back), kyphosis (a pronounced bend or "hump" in the upper back), and other problems.[48]

"Muscles flatten the abdomen and hold the abdominal organs in place," writes Dr. Elizabeth M. Mensendieck, founder of the Mensendieck system of posture and movement developed in the Netherlands. "Many [people] . . . are disturbed by the bulge of their abdomen. Yet

few realize that this is basically a problem of muscle development. . . .
[The abdominal muscles] serve as a wall, holding the abdominal organs
such as the digestive tract and the reproductive organs in place. The
weight against this wall is heaviest at the lower end. If the muscles become weak from inadequate use, they can no longer hold the contents of
the abdomen in place. The result, a bulging abdomen. This also affects
the functioning of the abdominal organs."[49]

This chapter teaches three of the best exercises for lifelong abdominal fitness, exercises that quickly help develop all key abdominal muscles,
including the rectus abdominus (from the breastbone to the pubic bone),
the transversalis (which surrounds the deep abdominal area and attaches
at the lower front of the abdomen), the pyramidalis (at the lower front
of the abdomen), the internal obliques (the lower four ribs and the sides
of the waist to the top of the pelvis), and the external obliques (the lower
eight ribs and the sides of the waist to the top of the pelvis).

At the same time, it's important to stretch and strengthen the lower-
back muscles — and that's taken care of by the flexibility and posture exercises in Chapters 14 and 15.

Abdominal exercises may be performed as often as four times a week
(see sample schedules in Chapter 11). A number of authorities recommend these exercises as part of a warm-up for aerobics or muscular strengthening activities. Do each abdominal exercise slowly and
smoothly. You should not experience any pain; stop immediately if you
do. Begin with 5–10 repetitions of each exercise and gradually work up
to 25 or more.

Transpyramid Exercise   The transversalis and pyramidalis muscles play an important role in maintaining a flat lower abdominal wall. However, they are rarely exercised
effectively. Unlike the other abdominal muscles, the transversalis and pyramidalis are not involved with spinal flexion and therefore receive little
or no benefit from traditional waist exercises. To strengthen these muscles, you must practice deep and forceful exhalations.[50]

Starting position: Sit or stand with balanced posture — head up,
neck long, chin slightly in, shoulders broad and relaxed, back flat.

Movement performance: Slowly exhale and, as you reach the place
where you normally finish exhaling, smoothly and forcefully breathe out
more, lifting up with the abdominal muscles. Use your hands to help
push up on the lower front abdomen during this forced exhalation; you
should be able to notice the transversalis and pyramidalis muscles helping
push the air out.

Relax and take several normal breaths. Then repeat the transpyramid
exercise. Be careful not to hyperventilate and become dizzy. Perform a
maximum of 5 transpyramid exercises at any given time. It's best to do
2–5 repetitions at several different times during the day.

Abdominal Roll-ups

Abdominal roll-ups are excellent for developing the upper abdominal area.[51]

Starting position: Lie on your back with knees bent and legs and feet free. (Do *not* secure the feet or legs under a heavy object or have them held by a partner since this lets the powerful hip-flexor muscles take over the movement and stress your lower back.) You can bend your legs at the knees and place them over a bench or chair as shown in Figure 13.1. Cross your arms on your chest or clasp your hands lightly behind your head. Don't let your arms whip upward since this may cause injury to the neck.

Movement performance: Leaving your middle and lower back flat on the floor, slowly raise your head and shoulders off the ground about 20 to 30 degrees, as shown in Figure 13.2. Pause for 1 second at the top of the motion and then slowly lower yourself to the original position. Do repetitions at slow speed.

Note: To increase the intensity of this exercise, you can perform 5–10 roll-ups at extra slow speed and come up a bit higher — to perhaps 40 degrees (the shoulder blades may come up off the floor but the lower

Figure 13.1

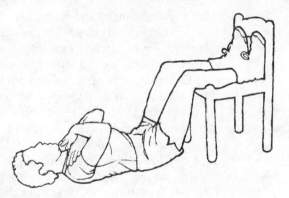

Figure 13.2

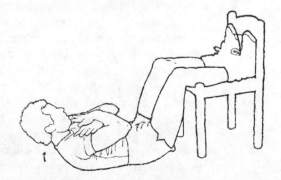

back should always remain on the floor for safety). A second way to increase intensity is to add "holds" at one or more angles of the movement. For example, curl up to 10 degrees, hold that position for 2–5 seconds, curl up farther to 20 degrees, hold for 2–5 seconds, and then very slowly return back down to the starting position. A third variation is to add rotation, curling up to the 10-to-20-degree height and rotating your torso to the side, keeping your pelvis stationary and drawing your opposite shoulder up and around to emphasize abdominal rather than back muscles. Hold this position for several seconds, rotate to the other side, hold again, then return to center and smoothly lower your torso back down to the starting position.

Reverse Trunk Rotations

The reverse trunk rotation is one of the most useful and beneficial exercises for abdominal fitness and good posture, experts say.[52] It involves the external and internal obliques, a set of midsection rotation muscles that help keep your abdomen slim and toned. This exercise also strengthens the deep spinal muscles (multifidus and rotatores), posterior spinal surface muscles (erector spinae), and an important lower-back muscle, the quadratus lumborum.

The full range of motion of this exercise builds both flexibility and strength in the waist and lower back, an ideal combination for helping to prevent injuries and back pain.

Starting position: Lie on your back in a supine, face-up position on the floor. Extend your arms out to the sides, perpendicular to your torso so that, viewed from the ceiling, your body forms the letter *T*. Raise your knees up in a sharp angle (pulling your heels toward the buttocks) and hold the legs together as shown in Figure 13.3. If you're certain you're already in great shape, raise your legs to a 90-degree angle, vertical to the floor (see Figure 13.4).

Movement performance: Maintain your leg-trunk angle as you slowly lower your legs to the right and touch the floor with the outside of the knee and foot of the lower leg (see Figure 13.5 or 13.6, depending on your starting position). Smoothly raise the legs back up to the starting position and repeat the movement to the other side.

Your arms and shoulders should remain in contact with the floor throughout the exercise to stretch and strengthen the internal and external obliques.[53] If your shoulders come off the ground as you lower your legs to the side, you may wish to have a friend *gently* hold your shoulders down as you do the exercise. If you still find the exercise difficult, use more knee bend and, as rehabilitative medicine authority Dr. Rene Cailliet suggests, you may also wish to bring the knees up toward your shoulder as you gently lower them to the side.[54] If you have any doubt about being able to do this exercise effectively, begin by having a partner support your knees as you gently lower them down to one side and then the other to test your current strength and flexibility levels.

Figure 13.3

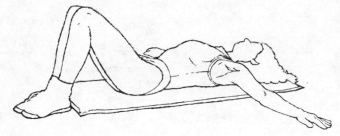

Figure 13.4

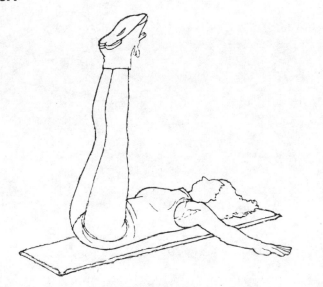

Over time, gradually straighten your legs (to the positions shown in Figures 13.4 and 13.6) as you do the exercise. Once the straight-leg reverse trunk rotation has become easy, you may want to incrementally add very light ankle weights to increase resistance.

Contrary to the myths and fads ("Revolutionary No-Effort Device Melts Tummy Fat") that steal perhaps a billion dollars a year (and injure and frustrate countless people), all the gadgets and wishes in the world won't give you a slim, toned waistline — or keep it that way. A scientific formula for bona fide, *lasting* results includes a good diet with frequent small meals and light snacks that, overall, are high in complex carbohydrates and fiber, moderate in protein, and low in fat, cholesterol, alcohol, and salt (see Chapters 20–26), regular aerobic exercise, balanced posture, and scientifically correct abdominal exercises (each performed 5–25 times three or four times a week). You don't need special equipment, so there's no expense and no reason to wait any longer to receive the benefits.

Figure 13.5

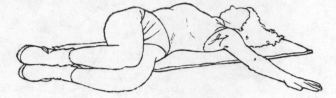

Figure 13.6

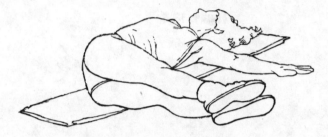

14 Flexibility and Posture Exercises, Phase I

IT'S EASY TO BE an incomplete exerciser, to miss the golden circle and be left with only a fragment or two in your hands, to charge off toward utmost strength but overlook flexibility, or to train for cardiovascular endurance and have deteriorating posture. And so on. This chapter presents flexibility and posture exercises for lifelong fitness.

Over the years, exercise authorities have recommended many different ways to increase flexibility. Ballistic stretching (bounce-stretching), ballistic and hold, passive lift and hold, prolonged stretch, active PNF (proprioceptive neuromuscular facilitation), passive PNF, and relaxation methods of stretching have all been popular to varying degrees. Some work well in specific therapeutic circumstances. Others don't work at all. Some, rather than relaxing the body, make it more tense.

Beyond that, the most commonly taught stretching exercises in America are dangerous. These gymnastic-type "bounce-stretches," also called ballistic stretches, include bouncing toe touches, side bends, and traditional hurdler's stretches.

"The rapid bounce-stretch releases a nerve reflex that signals the muscle to contract," explains Dr. Sven-A. Sölveborn, sports medicine expert from Sweden and author of *The Book About Stretching*. "This stretch-reflex is a protective mechanism that prevents the joint from getting hurt when a stretch is going too far. Every bounce-type stretch activates the stretch reflex. Since the created muscle contraction works against the stretching movement, the muscle fibers are torn. When they heal, scar tissue is created which makes the muscle elasticity worse. The muscle becomes sore and stiff."[55]

A number of exercise specialists now recommend two basic types of stretching exercises for developing and maintaining flexibility: dynamic flexibility exercises and static tighten-relax-stretch exercises.[56] We will make use of both types in this chapter and the next.

Dynamic flexibility exercises are smooth, easy movements that increase ranges of motion for the joints of the body. Tighten-relax-stretch exercises tense a muscle or group of muscles for 10–30 seconds, followed by 2–3 seconds of relaxation, and then a gentle stretching action for 10–30 seconds. This stretching method gives a surprisingly fast and effective increase in flexibility and works well for people of all ages.

Dynamic Flexibility Exercises

Dynamic flexibility exercises — performed slowly and smoothly, without any bouncing movements — are often included as part of a general exercise warm-up. Do each exercise at least twice. With practice, all ten exercises can be completed in 3 to 5 minutes a day. If you have a history of back injury or pain, have your physician approve these exercises.

1. Neck   Three simple exercises are especially helpful for stretching and strengthening many small but important neck muscles.

Neck Ovals

Starting position: Assume a comfortable sitting or standing position with neck and shoulders relaxed. Use your hands to lightly support your neck, jaw, and base of the skull.

Movement performance: *Smoothly* and *slowly* move your head in clockwise and then counterclockwise ovals (with the far points out to the sides) of varying radii, starting with tiny ovals where your neck remains almost vertical and then making the ovals wider. Don't attempt to stretch to the maximum in any direction, but if you feel any minor points of tension, pause a moment or two as you let the muscles relax. Do *not* extend your neck straight back, since this can place excessive stress on the cervical spine area.

Head Nods

The little-known rectus capitus anterior muscle is attached to the top spinal vertebra and base of the skull. It flexes and rotates the head. Perhaps most important, it helps you maintain good neck posture. Without having this muscle in shape — and some postural therapists believe that very few Americans do — it's difficult to have the relaxed, erect neck position necessary for best blood flow to the brain and senses.

Starting position: In a comfortable sitting or standing position, place your hands (thumbs facing to the rear) on the rear base of the skull just behind and above your earlobes.

Movement performance: Let your neck lengthen, gently extending upward as if lifted by an imaginary sky hook attached to the top of your skull. With your neck in this slightly lifted position, nod your head as if in agreement, bringing the forehead a little forward and chin slightly in. Repeat the nodding motion several times. Take a moment to become more aware of your neck alignment. (Chapters 33 and 34 cover posture and neck alignment in detail.)

Neck Isometrics

These exercises, which need to be performed only every other day or every third day, use isometric tension to improve neck strength and resiliency.[57] In each exercise it's important to be sitting or standing straight, with your head and neck in a vertical "best posture" position. During these exercises, your head and neck *don't actually move* — the brief resistance is isometric, provided by your attempt to move your head in the direction indicated in the instructions while resisting equally with tension in the muscles of the arm(s) and hand(s).

Starting position: As shown in Figure 14.1, place both hands against your forehead.

Movement performance: Slowly, smoothly push forward with your head as you simultaneously push back using equal pressure with your hands. Do not exceed about two-thirds of your maximum tensing strength. Hold the tension position for 2–5 seconds. Then release and

Figure 14.1

Figure 14.2

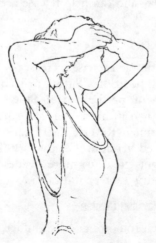
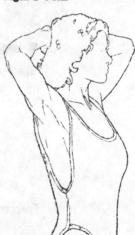

relax. Next, place your hands behind the center of your head with fingers interlaced (Figure 14.2). Slowly, smoothly push backward with your head as you simultaneously pull against your head with equal pressure from your hands. Hold the tension for 2–5 seconds. Release and relax.

Advanced version: Vary the resistance angles like points on a compass — instead of straight ahead and straight back, you may add left-right angles and half-right/half-left variations. You may also choose to provide hand resistance to *turning motions* with the head — again, not actually moving but using carefully controlled isometric tension. At no point should this exercise be the least bit painful.

2. Shoulders

"Hanging in There"

A "brachiated stretch" is a simple exercise in which you hang by your hands from a pull-up bar. This action relaxes the midsection muscles, gently stretches and aligns the spine, and brings welcome relief to over-taxed back muscles.[58] This can be a good home exercise, using a door-frame pull-up bar (available in sporting goods stores). Select one with strong brackets that can be installed in any door frame.

Starting position: Stand beneath a secure pull-up bar and reach up to hold on firmly with your hands. If you're not certain whether your grip is strong enough to hold your body weight, keep your feet on the floor (or on a sturdy chair if the bar is high) and bend your knees, shifting as much weight to your hands as you can comfortably handle.

Movement performance: As shown in Figure 14.3, hang by your hands (in the down position of a pull-up exercise) for up to 10 seconds, then rest. Repeat several times. This exercise feels wonderful toward the end of the day and can help release accumulated tension in the shoulder area.

Shrugs and Rolls

This quick, simple exercise increases shoulder flexibility.[59]

Starting position: Sitting or standing with your arms relaxed.

Movement performance: Slowly roll your shoulders up toward your ears, down in back, then forward and up toward the ears again in a circular manner. Reverse the direction and repeat.

Advanced version: Gently vary the circular angles from front-back and back-front circles to more inside-outside (toward the midline/away from the body's center) and outside-inside circles.

Freestyle Swimming Circles

This exercise promotes good shoulder flexibility.[60]

Figure 14.3

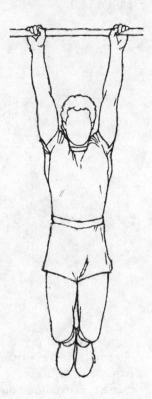

Starting position: Begin in a standing position with balanced posture and knees slightly bent.

Movement performance: Bend the torso slightly forward at the hips, *with knees bent*. Smoothly perform a swimming motion using the shoulders, similar to the freestyle or "crawl" stroke (see Figures 14.4 and 14.5). As your arms circle with the center of axis at the shoulder joint, let your knees bend and hips shift to help make each circle as smooth and flowing as possible. Then "swim backwards," reversing the direction of the arm motions for variation.

3. Chest and Upper Back: Ribcage Lifts and Expansions

This exercise helps increase the elasticity of your ribcage,[61] complementing the breathing exercises presented in Chapter 12.

Starting position: Sit up or lie supine, face up, on the floor. Relax your body as you flatten your lower back and keep your head properly aligned, with neck long and chin slightly in. Place your hands on either side of the ribcage, with palms and fingers pressing lightly against the ribs.

Figure 14.4   Figure 14.5

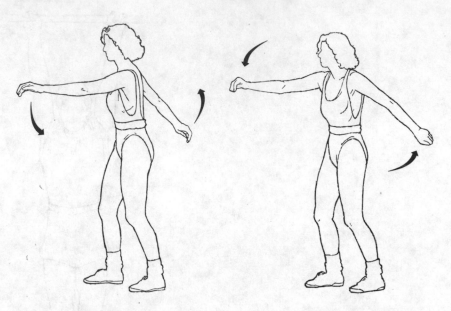

Movement performance: Inhale slowly and deeply, using your diaphragm. Lift and expand the chest fully as you maximize the inhalation. Exhale slowly. Rest for several moments, breathing normally. Repeat the exercise, expanding your chest out against some light hand pressure, lifting the ribs a little higher. Some people find this exercise more effective if they inhale using a series of short in-breaths until the thorax is completely expanded.

4. Arms: Elbow Circles

Starting position: In a sitting or standing position with neck and shoulders relaxed, hold the upper right arm out to the front of the body; support it under the elbow with the left hand.

Movement performance: Begin a series of slow clockwise and counterclockwise circular rotations at the elbow joint, gently turning and twisting your right forearm, wrist, and hand. The motion looks a bit like the circular action of washing a small window at face height. When finished with your desired number of repetitions (two or more) with the right arm, switch to the left.

5. Wrists: Wrist Circles

Starting position: This exercise is best performed by using your left hand to hold your right forearm just back from the wrist.

Movement performance: Move the free right hand smoothly in clockwise and counterclockwise circles of varying diameters, with the movement originating at the wrist joint. Repeat with the other hand and wrist.

6. Hands and Fingers: "Spheres of Light"

Starting position: In a comfortable standing or sitting position, hold your right hand out in front of you and gently grasp the right wrist with your left hand.

Movement performance: Be creative, performing a series of circular finger movements to increase the flexibility of your hands and fingers. Imagine gently touching every point in a small sphere or globe surrounding each finger. Repeat with the left hand.

7. Waist and Lower Back: Tibetan Circles

This unique exercise has been used for centuries by martial artists to develop flexibility and strength in the waist and lower-back area — the upper-body/lower-body "bridge" — which assists in many fitness movements and is essential to good posture. Variations are recommended by a number of exercise scientists.[62] Seek your physician's advice before doing this exercise if you have a history of back injury or pain.

Starting position: Assume a comfortable standing position with back erect and straight, neck relaxed, and head aligned with the spinal column, feet spread at shoulder width or a little wider, *with knees moderately bent*. Lightly clasp your hands together and extend your arms over your head as shown in Figure 14.6.

Movement performance: Inhale a normal breath, and then *slowly and smoothly* begin to exhale as you rotate the torso down and to the right as if you were lightly swinging an ax in slow motion (Figure 14.7).

Allow your torso to bend as your arms swing in a slow, gentle arc toward the floor and then on up to the left and back to the hands-overhead starting position. As you move, your knees should bend to eliminate stress on the lower back. Pause for a moment with a natural inhalation at the top of the arm motion, and then repeat the circle in the opposite direction — down to the left and back up to the right.

Don't swing too hard or too fast. This exercise should be comfortable and you must remain in full control at all times.

As you become proficient, try varying the arc of the circle. For example, begin the exercise in the same position (Figure 14.6) and then swing down to the right but more to the front of your body than to the side (that is, at a more oblique angle) and then continue the circle from the bottom of the motion in front of the right knee back past the left knee and then more to the rear of the body as the circle completes itself with the arms passing near the left hip and up to the top of the motion once again. After pausing briefly, repeat this motion in a complementary manner, going down and to the left.

8. Hips and Knees

Alternate Leg-ups

Starting position: Standing on a padded surface (suspended hardwood floor, grassy lawn, or carpet).

Figure 14.6   **Figure 14.7**

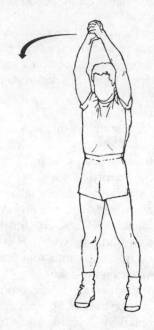
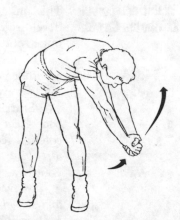

Movement performance: Slowly jog in place, using high, smooth pull-ups of the knees and with the heels gently touching the buttocks at the top of the motion.[63]

Imaginary Pedaling

Starting position: Stand, holding on to a countertop or other secure object for stability.

Movement performance: Go through a slow series of smooth circular movements centered at the hips. Lift one leg and move it as if pedaling an imaginary bicycle from the hip. Then vary the leg motion as if the pedaling circles were shifted a little toward the right or the left (keeping your torso in the original position). Rest for a moment and then repeat with the other leg. Be gentle and creative, progressively expanding the flexibility of your hips and knees.

9. Ankles, Feet, and Toes: "Spheres of Light"

Some of the simplest exercises for developing flexibility in your ankles, feet, and toes approximate those for the wrists, hands, and fingers.

Starting position: Sitting in a chair, lift your right leg several inches off the ground and extend it to the front about 6 inches. You may wish to support your right knee by cradling it in your right and left hands, fingers intertwined.

Movement performance: Perform slow circular movements, clockwise and counterclockwise, for both ankles, flexing and extending the foot. Move your toes in as many directions as comfortably possible. Repeat for the other ankle, foot, and toes.

10. PC Exercise

This little-known exercise takes just 2 or 3 seconds and can be done almost anywhere, anytime. Medical evidence indicates that it enhances sexual wellness and helps prevent some common pelvic and reproductive system disorders.[64]

It's called the PC (pubococcygeal) exercise, or Kegel (*kay*-gill) exercise, named after the physician who discovered and developed it in the late 1940s and early 1950s, Dr. Arnold H. Kegel.

The important muscles of the base of the pelvis are not contracted by normal exercise or sports routines. These pelvic floor muscles consist of several layers. The outermost layer is composed primarily of sphincters, circular closing or clamping muscles that act to close the openings of the urinary passage, rectum, and vagina. These muscles are very weak in most people and can progressively atrophy from disuse throughout our lives.

One key pelvic muscle, present in both men and women, is the pubococcygeus (*pew*-boh-cox-ee-*gee*-us), abbreviated PC. It runs from the pubis (the bony prominence in front of the pelvis) to the coccyx at the base of the spine. The PC is more than two finger widths thick and is designed to be very strong, yet medical studies have found that in most people it isn't.

Studies report that, compared with women who have strong, toned PCs, women with weak PCs experience more difficulty in childbirth, are more frequently troubled with incontinence (involuntary urination),[65] and are more often sexually dissatisfied.[66]

Weak PCs in men can contribute to incontinence, poor ejaculatory control, and problems related to the seminal vesicles and prostate gland.[67] PC exercises have been proven helpful to women who have difficulty achieving orgasm and can assist men with easier erections and more control of orgasm.[68]

To become toned, the PC must be exercised regularly, and this is very simple to do. However, before beginning PC exercises it is important to learn how to consciously control this muscle. Among other functions, the PC can control the voiding of urine.

Technique: Dr. Kegel found that to learn the sensation of the PC contracting, you can start by interrupting urination. He recommended that to help the PC do most of the work itself, you should at first leave the knees spread wide when urinating and, once flow has begun, make an effort to stop it, let it start again, stop it, and so on.

After a few trials, most people can consciously tense the PC by simple mental command, anytime and anywhere, and then should use the occasional interruption of urination only as a simple check.

Practice doing the PC exercise a number of times during the day. However, there is some evidence to suggest that performing it on first awakening and before urinating while the bladder is very full may not be beneficial. Any other time is fine. Tense the PC strongly, holding for 1–2 seconds. Relax for several seconds. Repeat this cycle so that you complete 5–10 contractions in a set. You may also include quick flexing and relaxing sequences. As you gain strength and control, progressively increase the intensity of PC exercise contractions, holding some for more than the usual 1–2 seconds.

At first, the muscles may fatigue quickly. Don't overdo it. For many people, 60–100 contractions in a day is a reasonable goal in sets of 10 contraction-relaxation sequences performed six to ten times during the day. You may want to use small colored dots, posted in conspicuous places, as a reminder for both breathing improvement, postural awareness, and PC exercises. Favorite times and places to do these exercises include while sitting at a desk, driving (one good plan is to do the exercises at each stoplight or mileage marker on short trips), watching television, working at a counter, waiting in line, brushing your teeth, first getting into bed, and so on. Make PC exercises a regular habit in your daily routine.

15 Flexibility and Posture Exercises, Phase II

THIS SECOND PHASE of flexibility and posture exercises is designed to promote extra ease of movement in commonly tight areas of the body and to strengthen muscles that improve posture. A number of experts suggest scheduling these exercises immediately following an aerobics or muscular strength and endurance session.

As with the exercises in Chapter 14, the exercises in this chapter should be performed slowly and smoothly, without abrupt or bouncing movements. Once you're familiar with them, you should be able to complete the entire series in about 5 minutes, one to four times per week. On a beginning level, perform one set of two to five repetitions of each exercise.

Too Much Stretching Is as Bad as Too Little

Here is an important note for fitness enthusiasts who think that the more flexible you are, the better. These individuals would have us stretch before we get out of bed; stretch before we walk, run, or lift weights; stretch after we walk, run, or lift weights; and again before bed at night. Live to stretch, stretch to live.

Is all that stretching really necessary? Maybe not, says Dr. Michael Yessis, training consultant to United States Olympic teams and author of *Secrets of Soviet Sports Fitness and Training*. "Yes, increased flexibility will help prevent injuries, but only to a certain extent. . . . Too much flexibility by itself can backfire. . . . Research has shown that flexibility exercises initially stretch the muscle and connective tissues. Once they've been stretched to their [natural] limits, however, the only way to achieve more flexibility is by stretching the ligaments . . . which don't have the elasticity of the muscles and tendons. Thus, when the ligaments are stretched, they remain stretched. As this happens, the joints they hold together will weaken, making you even *more* susceptible to injury."[69]

The bottom line: Don't overdo it. Balance stretching with strengthening exercises and other fitness steps in the golden circle of *Health & Fitness Excellence*.

Posture: Key to Health

Good posture is prerequisite to good health. The stretching and strengthening exercises in this chapter have a lot to do with preventing the weary shoulders, caved-in chests, stiff necks, and tense stomachs that we see in people around us every day. (Chapters 33 and 34 deal with other aspects of posture.)

Dynamic Flexibility and Posture Exercises

1. Modified Knee Bends   Modified knee bends, sometimes called squats or half-squats, can be a simple and valuable exercise. Though maligned through years of misunderstanding, when correctly performed they are an effective way to develop pelvic balance and tone and strengthen the muscles of the legs, buttocks, lower back, hip joints, and knee joints.[70]

Starting position: As illustrated in Figure 15.1, start in a comfortable standing position, feet about shoulder-width apart, toes pointed forward and slightly outward. Maintain balanced posture with neck long, back straight, shoulders broad and relaxed. Your weight should be evenly distributed on both feet.

Cross your arms in front of your chest, hands on opposite shoulders, elbows high and pointed out to the sides. During the exercise, do *not* drop your head or look down at your feet as this may cause you to lose your balance.

Movement performance: *Slowly* bend your knees and lower your body into a squat position. At first, limit the depth of the squat to about the height of a chair seat (see Figure 15.2). At no time during the movement should your knees extend in front of your toes. As your capabilities

Figure 15.1   **Figure 15.2**

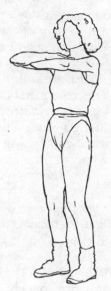   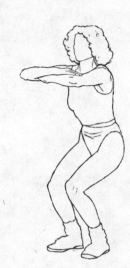

expand, you'll be able to slowly lower your body until your thighs are below the horizontal position. Your feet (including the soles and heels) should remain flat on the floor throughout the entire exercise, although at first this may be difficult. (To make it easier, try some of the tighten-relax-stretch leg stretches presented later in this chapter.)

As you move downward into the squat, your knees will come forward several inches, your buttocks will move to the rear and your trunk-torso line will incline slightly forward (your back is straight — the slight bend comes from the *hips,* not the waist). This position enables you to maintain solid balance over both feet.

When you reach your lowest squatting position, gently reverse the movement and, keeping your chest and head up, slowly raise your body back up to the original standing position.

"By keeping your whole foot in contact with the floor, you develop flexibility in the ankle joint and, more importantly, keep your body in good alignment," explains Dr. Yessis. "When the squat is done correctly, your knees are directly above your toes or slightly in front of your feet when in the lowest position. In this position you don't place additional stress on the knees and the exercise is not dangerous. . . . Another potential danger to avoid is the 'bounce' in the bottom position. This happens when you lower your body too quickly, which forces your joints to go to their maximum range of flexion (bending) and then 'rebound' upward. . . . This puts great strain on the ligaments and tendons and usually results in injury. . . . Move at a slow to moderate rate of speed and prepare yourself to rise up as you approach the bottom position."[71]

Individuals with osteoarthritis or a previous injury should begin by using a chair to restrict the extent of this exercise; sit down and rise up from the chair until leg strength improvements make this support unnecessary.[72]

As an athlete and martial arts instructor, I have been concerned with developing *multi-angular* strength and flexibility. Once you reach an advanced level with this exercise, consider performing modified knee bends using a narrow stance; using a wide stance; with the toes pointed inward, straight ahead, or outward; and varying the depth of the squat.[73] When first performing these advanced variations, hold on to a secure object for balance. Always move slowly and smoothly.

2. Side Bends

Lateral flexion, or side bending, exercises help develop a strong, flexible back by stretching and strengthening the oblique muscles of the waist and lateral muscles of the spine.[74] Side bends also help tone the sides of the waist.

Starting position: Stand with the knees slightly bent.

Movement performance: Slowly, smoothly raise your right arm over your head and relax your left arm down at your side or cross it in front of your abdomen, stretching as far to the left as is comfortable (see Figure 15.3), holding the position for a count of two. Then reverse the motion to the other side. *Don't bounce.*

3. Torso Turns

This simple martial arts exercise has been performed for centuries. Variations are endorsed by a number of fitness experts.[75]

Starting position: As shown in Figure 15.4, stand in an upright position with good posture, legs spread shoulder width, knees bent for good balance, arms out to the sides, and elbows at about mid-chest height.

Movement performance: *Smoothly* and *slowly* rotate your torso to the right, leading the motion by circling your left elbow and shoulder to the front — parallel to the ground — while your right elbow and shoulder circle back to the right (Figure 15.5). Move as far as you comfortably can. Then repeat the motion to the left side. As long as there are no abrupt or fast movements, you may either hold your head in a face-forward position or allow it to turn smoothly to the left and right to follow the torso rotation motions.

4. Pelvic Leveler

For many years, postural therapists and rehabilitative medicine specialists have advocated exercises to reduce the common sway (lordosis) in the lower back and help align and balance the pelvis. One of the most effective of these is called the pelvic leveler or pelvic tilt.[76]

Figure 15.3

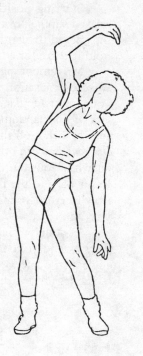

Figure 15.4

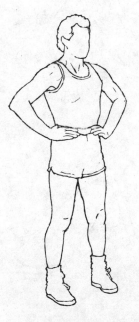

Figure 15.5

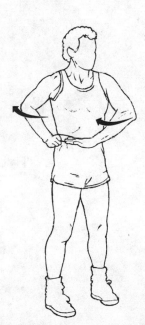

Starting position: As shown in Figure 15.6, lie on your back in a relaxed supine position, with the feet flat on the floor and both knees and hips flexed (bent). Relax and press the lower back gently to the floor and hold it there for a few seconds.

Movement performance: *Breathe* into the lower back to send a wave of relaxation there. Repeat. Next, as shown in Figure 15.7, leave your lower lumbar spine area firmly on the floor while you use the muscles of your abdomen, legs, and buttocks to very slowly curl your pelvis several inches off the floor, lifting your coccyx and buttocks *without arching your back* (in other words, avoid pushing your belt-buckle up into the air while your buttocks sag down). This movement will help flatten your lower back to the floor. Hold this upper position for 1 second and then slowly return your coccyx and buttocks back down to the starting position and relax.

As your pelvic muscles are strengthened, you will be able to gradually extend your feet farther away from your buttocks (decreasing the angle at the knees), but never fully straighten the legs (so that the backs of the legs touch the floor).

Figure 15.6

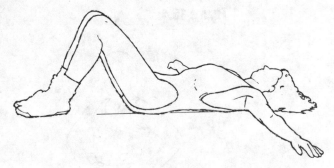

Figure 15.7

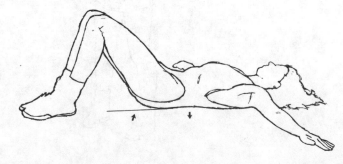

5. Pelvic Lifts   This exercise develops firmer buttocks and a stronger spine.[77] When performed correctly, it also aids postural balance and helps prevent back pain.

Starting position: Begin in the position shown in Figure 15.6.

Movement performance: Keeping your upper back on the floor, slowly raise your buttocks until there is an imaginary straight line from your shoulders to your knees, as shown in Figure 15.8. Then slowly lower your pelvis back to the floor as shown in Figure 15.6. *Don't arch your back.*

6. Back Ups and Downs   There are several safe exercises that build strength and flexibility to the columns of spinal muscles. Do these exercises slowly and smoothly, with no bouncing motions or undue pressure.

Forward Roll-ups

This simple exercise stretches and relaxes the lower back.[78]

Starting position: Sit in a chair, knees apart, back straight, feet spread about shoulder width and flat on the floor.

Movement performance: Slowly bend forward as far as you comfortably can (Figure 15.9). Hold the down position for several seconds, then return to the upright position.

Figure 15.8

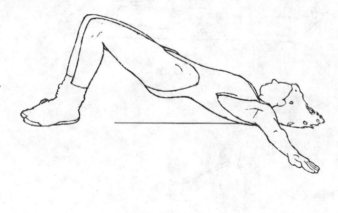

Figure 15.9

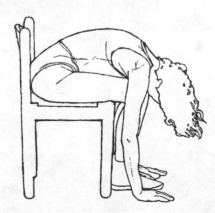

Cat Stretch

"Cat back." "Mad cat." Whatever the name, this simple exercise is recommended by many back-care specialists.[79]

Starting position: Kneel on your hands and knees.

Movement performance: Relax and lower your head and neck as you exhale, and *gently, slowly* arch your back upward like a cat stretching. As you complete this comfortable stretching motion, shown in Figure 15.10, hold for several seconds, then inhale and come back to the starting position. Then, as you exhale again, gently relax the center of your back down toward the floor as you smoothly bring your head up — without straining (see Figure 15.11). Hold this position for several seconds. Then return to starting position.

Figure 15.10

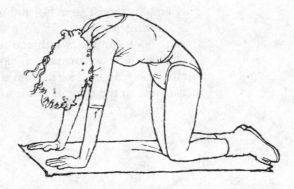

Figure 15.11

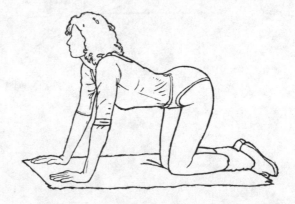

Back Raises

Correctly performed, back raises, often called back extensions or hyperextensions, are a wonderful exercise for strengthening and balancing the muscles of the spine.[80]

Starting position: As illustrated in Figure 15.12, begin by lying face down on a padded surface with your legs extended and chin resting on your folded arms. Some authorities recommend extending the arms out in the direction the eyes are facing; others suggest placing a pillow under the hips for comfort.

Movement performance: Keeping your legs on the floor, slowly and smoothly raise your head and shoulders in a rolling-up motion from the floor, as indicated in Figure 15.13. *Lift gently — only as high as is fully comfortable* (not more than 10–20 degrees). Hold this extended position for a second or two and then slowly return to the starting position. Relax. Repeat.

Advanced option: An advanced version of this exercise (not recommended for beginners or without a physician's approval for those with a history of back injury or pain) uses an adjustable piece of equipment called a Glute-Ham-Gastroc Developer, designed by sports fitness expert Dr. Michael Yessis (available from BiggerFasterStronger, Inc., P.O. Box 20612, Salt Lake City, UT 84120).

Figure 15.12

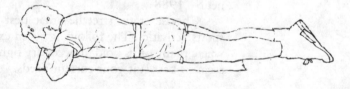

Figure 15.13

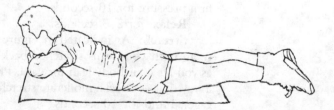

A Word About Yoga

Hatha yoga (one of the most popular of more than twenty yoga systems) teaches physical postures and breathing exercises. The *asanas* (postures) are designed to stretch and relax the body, and the overall theme is a spiritual discipline, not simply calisthenics. For people willing to devote the time — in addition to, rather than in place of, a balanced fitness program — yoga practice can be very rewarding. The leading periodical for yoga practitioners is *Yoga Journal* (P.O. Box 6076, Syracuse, NY 13217), and one often-recommended introductory book is *Bikram's Beginning Yoga Class* by Bikram Choudhury (J. P. Tarcher, 1978).

Tighten-Relax-Stretch Exercises

Another valuable way to increase flexibility and improve posture is by doing tighten-relax-stretch exercises. One very useful reference guide is *The Book About Stretching* by Sven-A. Sölveborn, M.D. (Japan Publications, 1985). Dr. Sölveborn describes more than fifty specific stretches covering major muscles of the body and provides stretching sequences for eighteen popular sports, from bodybuilding and soccer through tennis, cycling, and swimming. Another useful book is *Stretching* by Bob Anderson (Shelter Publications, 1980). For a more technical view of flexibility exercises, see *The Science of Stretching* by Michael J. Alter, M.S. (Human Kinetics, 1988).

Choose static stretches that best match your exercise sessions or sports activities. The following seven exercises increase flexibility in areas where many of us hold unnecessary tightness. Begin with one or two that seem to best suit your current needs.

1. Chest

Tense: As shown in Figure 15.14, extend your arms straight out in front of your torso, clasp your hands (you may squeeze a ball between them if desired), and press them against each other from left to right with firm pressure for 10 seconds.

Relax for 2–3 seconds.

Stretch: As indicated in Figure 15.15, stand facing the corner of a room with your arms stretched back and palms holding on to the walls as you let your body lean forward. Press inward against the walls in such a way that you feel a moderate stretching in the front of your thorax (ribcage). Hold for 10 seconds.

Figure 15.14

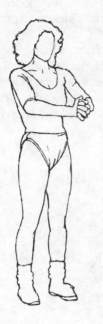

Figure 15.15

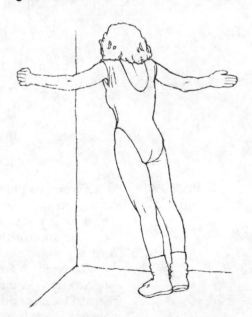

2. Shoulders   **Tense:** As shown in Figure 15.16, stand, keeping your elbows bent and within six inches of your sides. Clasp your hands (you may squeeze a ball between them if desired) and press them together with firm pressure for 10 seconds.

Relax for 2–3 seconds.

Stretch: As illustrated in Figure 15.17, with a partner (or, if you are exercising alone, in a corner of the room or a door frame), move your arms back as far as comfortably possible, keeping the upper arms fairly close to your sides. Hold the stretch for 10 seconds.

Figure 15.16

Figure 15.17

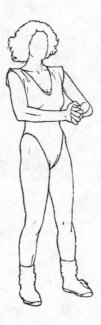

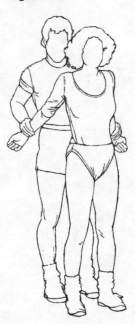

3. Hamstrings   **Tense:** As illustrated in Figure 15.18, stand with one foot resting on its heel on a stool or other sturdy object (the exact height may be varied to fit your comfort level and needs), keeping your knee straight. Bend the knee of the supportive leg slightly. Press your heel down as hard as possible into the stool, pushing toward the floor for 10 seconds.

Relax for 2–3 seconds.

Stretch: As shown in Figure 15.19, maintaining good upper-body postural balance with your head up, bend forward at the hip while keeping your hands behind you. Hold the stretch for 10 seconds.

Figure 15.18

Figure 15.19

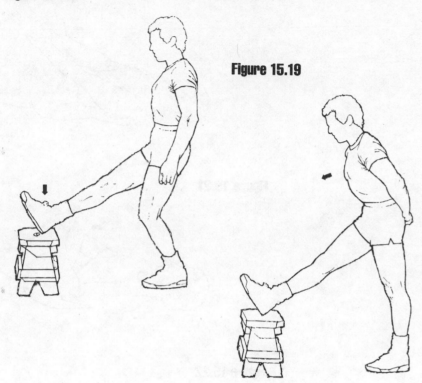

4. Hip, Lower Back, and Buttocks

Tense: As indicated in Figure 15.20, lie on your back with the lower back straight and flat (see Pelvic Leveler exercise), bend one leg, raise it toward your head and grasp it with clasped hands. Press the leg away against your hand pressure for 10 seconds.

Relax for 2–3 seconds.

Stretch: As shown in Figure 15.21, with your lower back remaining straight and touching the floor, pull the bent leg up toward your head as much as comfortably possible with assistance from your clasped hands. Hold the stretch for 10 seconds.

5. Outside Hips and Thighs

Tense: As shown in Figure 15.22, lie on your back, raise one leg, and bend the knee to a 90-degree angle, leaving your foot flat against the floor. Press your thigh out to the side (away from the centerline of your body) while you resist this motion as much as possible with your hands. Hold for 10 seconds.

Relax for 2–3 seconds.

Stretch: As illustrated in Figure 15.23, pull the leg you just tensed

Figure 15.20

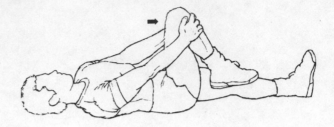

Figure 15.21

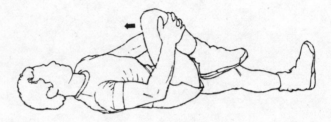

Figure 15.22

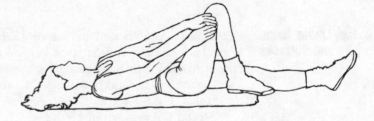

Figure 15.23

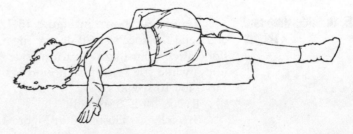

over the other leg and press it down toward the floor with the opposite hand. Turn your head in the direction opposite the leg and extend the corresponding hand and arm out to the side. Hold the stretch for 10 seconds.

6. Groin and Inner Thighs

Tense: Sit on the floor with your knees bent and feet pulled toward your buttocks. Hold your knees apart with a ball (kickball size) or your forearm (see Figure 15.24) and then set up a resistance by pressing your knees in toward each other against the ball or arm. Hold the tension for 10 seconds.

Relax for 2–3 seconds.

Stretch: As shown in Figure 15.25, draw your heels in toward your buttocks, bend your upper body forward slightly as you push down moderately on your legs with your elbows to stretch your knees out to the sides as far as possible. Hold the stretch for 10 seconds.

7. Lower Legs

Tense: As shown in Figure 15.26, with a wall or counter for hand support, stand as high as comfortably possible on your toes. Hold for 10 seconds.

Relax for 2–3 seconds by letting your heels come back down on the floor.

Stretch: Stand facing a solid object (such as a wall) with one foot forward and one foot back, with knees slightly bent. Slowly lean forward against the wall, leaning far enough that you can feel a stretching in the calf at the back of the leg (Figure 15.27). Hold the stretch for 10 seconds. Alternate leg positions and repeat.

Figure 15.24

Figure 15.25

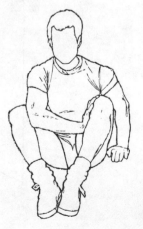
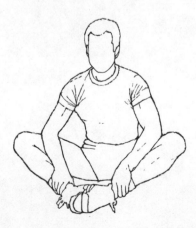

Figure 15.26

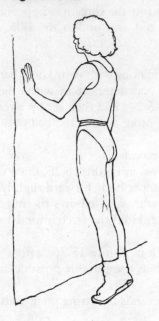

Figure 15.27

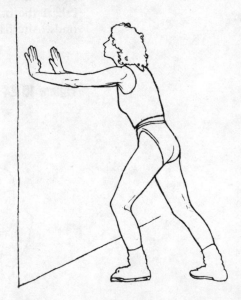

16 Aerobic Exercise: Introduction and Outdoor Options

AEROBIC EXERCISE can give you a gold mine of health and performance benefits. In this chapter, we focus on three key issues: how to do aerobic exercise right, how to make it fun, and how to capture the full rewards in the least amount of time.

It may surprise you to learn that many — even most — of the people now following "aerobic fitness programs" are unknowingly wasting time and missing benefits. Why? Because they're unaware of some simple scientific guidelines. In this chapter, you'll learn them.

What Is Aerobics?

In the mid-1960s when I first began studying exercise science, this kind of workout was called "cardiovascular fitness." Then it became "cardiorespiratory exercise," and today we call it "cardiovascular endurance" or "aerobics." The term *cardiovascular endurance* signifies the sustained ability of the heart, lungs, and blood to perform optimally. *Aerobics* means that oxygen uptake, transport, and utilization are improved with regular training.

Preventive medicine specialist Dr. Kenneth H. Cooper, founder and president of the Aerobics Center, Cooper Clinic, and Institute for Aerobics Research, is responsible for much of the attention and popularity that now surround aerobics. Under the supervision of his research team, more than 1.25 million exercise hours have been recorded and assessed over a fifteen-year period with nearly fifty-two thousand participants.[81]

Aerobic exercises are those that safely, comfortably increase your breathing and heart rates for an extended period of time (usually at least 20 minutes) without disturbing the balance between your intake and use of oxygen. In contrast, activities that require sudden, excessive bursts of energy — such as sprinting — are anaerobic.

Benefits of Aerobic Exercise

Dr. Cooper has written extensively about aerobic exercise. Here are several of his summary comments:

> Aerobic exercise increases the amount of blood in your system and increases the amount of oxygen-carrying hemoglobin in your blood. Your blood becomes, in a word, richer: it can bring in more oxygen to each cell and can take away more CO_2 and other wastes than it could before you started exercising. Your muscle cells, also, improve their ability to process the oxygen and eliminate wastes more efficiently. . . .
>
> With each breath, you take in more air and get rid of more CO_2 than you did before. . . . Aerobic exercise makes your blood vessels more flexible, so that they don't tend to accumulate atherosclerotic deposits as readily. The result? Less resistance in the blood vessels and again less work for your heart. . . . Aerobic exercise increases the number of those tiny blood vessels that form a network throughout the cells of your body. New vessels may appear from nowhere perhaps because of the physical stimulus of the vigorous circulation or perhaps by some chemical trigger.[82]
>
> The capacity of the lungs increases, and some studies have associated this increase in "vital capacity" with a greater longevity; the heart muscle grows stronger, is better supplied with blood, and with each stroke, the heart can pump more blood (increased stroke volume); high-density lipoprotein (HDL) [discussed in Chapter 22] increases, the total cholesterol:HDL ratio decreases, and thus there is a reduction in the person's risk of developing atherosclerosis, or hardening of the arteries.[83]

One of the first noticeable signs of improved aerobic fitness is a lowered *resting heart rate*. Elite athletes in endurance sports can become so well conditioned that they have resting heart rates between 30 and 45 beats per minute. People who have developed good cardiovascular fitness from regular aerobic exercise will generally have a heart that beats 45 to 50 times a minute when at rest, pumping at least the same amount of blood as does an unconditioned person's heart beating 75 to 80 times a minute. Result: Over the course of a day, the unconditioned person's heart must beat 50,000 times more than a conditioned person's heart.[84] In a year, that's a workload of 17 *million* extra beats that an unfit person's heart must provide!

Seven Aerobic Exercise Guidelines

The basic principle in exercise is *Do it*. Get up and move more. Be active in every reasonable way every single day. The easiest way to start is to go for walks of all kinds, choose stairways over elevators, distant parking spots over close ones. There's little value spending your money and time doing a formal regimen you detest. But that's no excuse to stop looking for, and trying, new kinds of exercise. If you do that, you'll soon find a fitness activity you can truly enjoy. This chapter and the next are filled with options for outdoor and indoor aerobic activities.

Since the focus of this book is *excellence,* it's my responsibility to share scientific priorities you need to know to receive greatest benefits from aerobic exercise — in the least amount of time and with the most fun doing it. The following are seven key guidelines for aerobic exercise programs.

1. Good Technique and Rhythmic Performance

The best aerobic exercise is performed with correct technique and at a steady, moderate pace, using large muscle groups.

2. Correct Intensity

Once you have a rhythm going, the next consideration is intensity. Studies indicate that it's advisable to exercise within an "aerobic training zone," working just hard enough to have your heart rate cross over an "aerobic threshold" into a *target heart rate zone* (*THRZ*).

If you work too hard, you'll cross over an upper "anaerobic (without oxygen) threshold," sometimes called the "ventilatory threshold," where the ability of the heart and lungs to supply oxygen to the muscles becomes limited. The higher you push yourself above this threshold — as in sprinting — the more quickly you become exhausted and must stop exercising.

Exercising at or above the anaerobic threshold will be perceived as strenuous. To a certain extent, the anaerobic threshold is also an endurance threshold, since it's difficult to exercise above it for very long.

Your body's maximum aerobic capacity or power is called VO_2 max by physiologists. It's the laboratory measurement of your ability to deliver maximal amounts of oxygenated blood to exercising muscles and the effectiveness of the muscles in extracting oxygen from the blood to provide energy for your body during exercise. If you have a high VO_2 max you are considered to be in excellent aerobic condition.

With regular aerobic exercise, your VO_2 max will increase. It is measured in sports medicine laboratories while an individual undergoes a graded maximal exercise test — while running on a treadmill or pedaling a bicycle ergometer. Although a laboratory test of your VO_2 max is the most accurate way to determine your present cardiovascular fitness level, the target heart rate zone formula is generally considered a safe and reliable substitute that you can perform at home or in the gym.

Monitoring your heart rate is especially important in the beginning months of an aerobic exercise routine. There are three respected formulas for calculating your target heart rate zone:

▶ The Institute for Aerobics Research recommends a THRZ of 65 to 80 percent of your maximal heart rate.[85]
▶ The American Heart Association recommends a THRZ of 60 to 75 percent of your maximal heart rate.
▶ The American College of Sports Medicine suggests a THRZ of 65 to 90 percent of your maximal heart rate.[86]

To determine your THRZ, first calculate your predicted maximal heart rate (PMHR). There are several widely accepted formulas. Here is the formula recommended by the Institute for Aerobics Research:

▶ For physically inactive men and for women regardless of activity level:

220 minus your age = PMHR

▶ For well-conditioned or physically active men:

205 minus one-half your age = PMHR

For example, if you are forty years old and (a) a woman or (b) a man who is presently out of shape, you would have a PMHR of $220 - 40 = 180$ beats per minute (bpm). A very fit man of the same age — for example, someone who has exercised aerobically on a regular basis for a year or more — would have a PMHR of $205 - 20 = 185$.

Once you've determined your PMHR, you can calculate your target heart rate zone (THRZ). If you want to choose a THRZ that falls within the general guidelines of leading fitness organizations, choose 65 to 75 percent of your PMHR.

Here is an example: Forty-year-old females or inactive males would multiply 0.65 times their PMHR of 180 for a lower threshold heart rate of 117 beats per minute (bpm). Then, choosing the conservative anaerobic threshold of 75 percent PMHR, they would multiply 0.75 times the PMHR of 180 for an initial upper threshold heart rate of 135 bpm. Thus the THRZ for aerobic exercise in this case would be approximately 117 to 135 beats per minute, and those individuals should strive to exercise at a pace that maintains a steady heart rate within this zone.

In general, aerobic exercise should not exceed an upper limit of 75–80 percent of PMHR for most people. However, as you reach a high level of fitness or pursue serious athletics, you can probably train effectively above the 75–80 percent level of PMHR. The precise upper limit of your THRZ may be best determined by a qualified fitness professional.

Monitoring procedure. Most experts recommend monitoring your heart rate during exercise, especially when beginning a new program. You can do this by taking your pulse with your finger, not your thumb, at the radial artery in your wrist. The radial artery is easily located at the thumb side of the wrist about one-half inch up from the heel of your palm toward your elbow. Pressing on the carotid artery of the neck can cause dizziness or even worse effects, so it's usually discouraged. With a little practice, taking your pulse at the wrist will be easy.

Using a watch, count your pulse for a full 15 seconds (the first beat is 0, not 1) and then multiply by 4 to arrive at your heart rate per minute. Counting heartbeats for 6 seconds and multiplying by 10, or for 10 seconds and multiplying by 6, may leave too much room for mathematical error.

With practice, you won't need to check your heart rate because you'll know how it feels to be in the THRZ. The "conversation pace" or "talk test" can be a good way to double-check whether you're within your THRZ: as you exercise you should be able to carry on a normal conversation without sounding out of breath.

Start by taking your pulse just after the warm-up period, then about one-third of the way into your aerobic workout, once more about two-thirds through, and then take a final pulse check right after the cooldown period to assess heart rate recovery. Do not keep interrupting your workout to check your pulse every minute or two; this stop-and-start pattern interferes with aerobic training.

Electronic monitors. You may want to invest in an electronic heart rate monitor. While not necessary for most people, these high-tech devices can be very helpful. The best pulse monitors have sensing mechanisms that attach with a comfortable elasticized strap directly to your chest and feature a remote, wristwatch-type monitor. At the time of this writing, top-quality units included the CIC Uniq HeartWatch and Pro Trainer (Computer Instruments Corporation, 100 Madison Ave., Hempstead, NY 11550; 800-227-1314) and the Vantage Performance Monitor (Polar Electro Inc., USA, P.O. Box 920, Hartland, WI 53029).

These heart rate monitors are accurate and are easily programmed to monitor your upper and lower THRZ limits, sounding a warning beep when you drop below the lower threshold or exceed the upper.

What about low-intensity aerobic exercise? Do you always need to reach the aerobic (lower) threshold of your THRZ to receive aerobic benefits? No.

Dr. Steven Blair, director of epidemiology for the Institute for Aerobics Research, conducted a study of low-intensity exercise programs showing a significant improvement in aerobic fitness for young, healthy male subjects who exercised at only about 50 percent of their PMHR for 30 to 40 minutes five days a week.[87]

In other words, you may set your heart rate at less than your aerobic threshold and, by exercising less vigorously for longer periods than those listed in the following section, still achieve some aerobic benefits.

3. Duration and Frequency

How much should I exercise? When people ask that question, they usually mean, How little exercise can I get away with? Here's the generally accepted minimum:

The Institute for Aerobics Research recommends exercising *four times per week for 20 minutes each session* or *three times per week for 30 minutes each session.*

The American Heart Association suggests "properly regulated sessions [in the THRZ] *at least three days a week."*[88]

The American College of Sports Medicine (ACSM) recommends aerobic exercise sessions with *15–60 minutes* of "continuous aerobic activity" in the THRZ *three to five times per week.*[89] (The ACSM states that cardiovascular endurance conditioning is most readily and safely attained in low-intensity, longer-duration programs. Therefore a practical minimum guideline in most cases is 20–30 minutes per session three to five times per week.)

For guidelines on how to take greatest advantage of aerobic exercise for burning excess body fat, see Chapters 29–30.

4. Warm-up and Cool-down

It is very important to precede aerobic exercise sessions with a 2-to-5-minute warm-up and then follow the workout with a 3-to-5-minute cool-down safety period.

Don't stretch. A good warm-up increases circulation to your muscles and makes them more pliable and relaxed. Many people begin workouts with stretching exercises as the warm-up. This is a mistake. Stretching cold muscles is difficult and can result in injuries.[90] Even if stretches were successful, some authorities believe that you end up loosening and relaxing your muscles and joints just when you need them to be strong and stable.[91]

The best warm-up is one that mimics your sport, moving around at an easy pace doing whatever you're going to do for aerobic exercise that day — walking, jogging, swimming, rowing, and so on.[92]

A 3-to-5-minute cool-down period is generally recommended after you stop exercising. Then check your pulse. Dr. Kenneth Cooper's research team suggests that if your heart rate isn't below 120 beats per minute (or less than 100 if you're over fifty years old) after 5 minutes, then your workout was too strenuous.

The cool-down period, brief though it is, is critical from a health safety standpoint because it allows the body to return gradually to its pre-exercise state. The basic guiding principle is to *never stop exercising suddenly*. The drop in blood pressure that occurs during the cool-down period should take place gradually, so keep moving, swiftly at first and then at a slower pace.

Don't stand still, sit down, start talking to a friend, or get distracted in any other way from a sensible cool-down period of up to five minutes — longer if you end your aerobic workout with a final burst of speed. Keep moving. When you take your pulse, learn to check it while moving rather than standing motionless.

5. Avoid Competitive Thoughts

Here's a surprising finding: Competitive thoughts during exercise can increase harmful stress. According to a study at Shippensburg College in Pennsylvania, levels of stress hormones such as norepinephrine, which normally increase a moderate amount during strenuous activities, rise dramatically when you mentally drive yourself with words like "harder" and "faster."

Psychologist Kenneth France studied the effects of thoughts on norepinephrine levels. During identical workouts, athletes (in dancing, running, walking, cycling, and swimming) were given alternate sets of mental cues, first using the words "calm," "relaxed," and "steady" and then using the more competitive words "faster," "harder," "better." Both types of mental signals produced equal pulse rate changes, but the aggressive words caused norepinephrine levels in the urine to more than double. After completing the study, France recommended that people "abandon competitive thinking during workouts. Performance may even improve when you take pressure off yourself."[93]

Make your exercise fun. "Fun" is a word seldom heard in exercise circles. But from a scientific perspective, it's essential. Begin thinking of exercise as time for something special for yourself, and include friends in your fitness sessions if that's enjoyable to you. And beyond trying a wide variety of activities and sports to choose your favorites, consider adding background music to some of your workouts.

Researchers at Ohio State University have found that music helps many people relieve the mental stress of exercising.[94] In separate studies, researchers at Stanford University Medical Center and the Massachusetts Department of Public Health concluded that, in many cases, music can stimulate movement and improve coordination.[95] The Medical and

Sports Music Institute, Inc. (1200 Executive Pkwy., Eugene, OR 97401; 503-344-5323) offers more than fifty audiotapes for various athletic activities. Music in Motion (Box 2688, Alameda, CA 94501; 415-521-1224) conducts ongoing research on applications of music in exercise programs and provides tapes to many fitness centers.

6. Keep Replacing Fluids

Replenishing body fluids is essential to good health. From an exercise standpoint, it can make a big difference in your performance. Losses of only 1 percent of body fluid from sweating can cut strength, speed, endurance, and the heart's output capabilities.[96]

Drink extra fluid — preferably pure water — *before* you begin to exercise. The Sports and Cardiovascular Nutritionists (a specialty group of the American Dietetic Association) recommend drinking up to 20 ounces of water in the hour or two preceding exercise.[97] Add another 3 to 6 ounces every 10 to 20 minutes during the exercise session (be sure to plan ahead so that pure water is accessible). Studies recommend cool water, since it enters the digestive tract faster than tepid or warm liquids.

You should also plan to drink extra fluid *after* exercising. You can lose up to 2 quarts of water before becoming thirsty, so don't rely on thirst alone as your signal to replace fluids.

7. Progress Gradually and Cross Train

People often increase exercise intensity or duration too rapidly. A sensible general rule is to progress in increments not greater than 2 to 3 percent per week. Aerobic "cross training" means varying your weekly exercise choices. Example: walking or dancing on Monday and Thursday and bicycling or swimming on Tuesday and Friday. Cross training develops a more balanced state of fitness by exercising different muscles. It also helps reduce injury risks and prevent boredom.

Summary of the Seven Guidelines

1 Warm up for 2–5 minutes preceding and cool down for 3–5 minutes following aerobic exercise.

2 Use good technique and exercise rhythmically at a moderate pace.

3 Monitor your heart rate to stay within your target heart rate zone (THRZ), which is generally 65 to 75 percent of your predicted maximum heart rate (PMHR).

4 Exercise for at least 20 minutes four times per week or 30 minutes three times per week.

5 Think noncompetitive thoughts: "calm," "relaxed," "steady."

6 Drink plenty of pure water before and after exercise.

7 Progress gradually and cross train by performing at least two different aerobic activities during each week of exercise.

And most of all — enjoy!

Primary Aerobic Exercise Options: Outdoor

Outdoors, you're exercising for more than exercise. A special sense of joy is added to the health benefits. You feel the sunlight and breeze and get in closer touch with the cycles of nature all around you. This section of *Health & Fitness Excellence* highlights seven of the most popular and easy to learn outdoor aerobic sports. I love them all.

"When we're swimming, we pity the sweaty walkers making their way down summery city streets," say sports medicine authorities Dr. Ronald M. Lawrence and Sandra Rosenzweig in *Going the Distance: The Right Way to Exercise for People Over Forty* (J. P. Tarcher, 1987). "When we're walking, we're sorry for the poor swimmers who can't smell the roses or feel the wind in their hair. When we're kayaking, we don't understand why anyone would want to struggle with two oars instead of one light paddle, and when we're rowing, we can't fathom why anyone would paddle an inefficient glorified canoe. When we're cycling, we really feel for the poor souls bound by their two feet when they could be exploring miles and miles of countryside in the same amount of time. And when we're [cross-country] skiing, we can't imagine anything more glorious."[98]

It's a matter of cross training, but it's something more. It's different tastes, the magic of variety. Don't get stuck in an exercise rut. Read through the outdoor and indoor aerobic options on the following pages. Whenever something captures your interest, make plans to try it. Or best of all, try everything. Put together your own collection of favorites.

One more message: Even though exercise may at first seem to invade your established routine, find time to fit it in. If necessary, walk before breakfast or after dinner. Bike, swim, or jog during your lunch break. Cycle to and from work or on errands. Exercise indoors while you read (by using a bookstand), watch a favorite television show, or listen to educational audiotapes or music. Pick the best times of day for you, match the activities to the weather and your mood, and savor the changes that start to happen.

Go it solo if that gives you some extra time with yourself in the middle of a hectic daily schedule. Or invite your spouse, children, best friend, work associates, or your entire neighborhood to join you. Exercise in the same place or following the same route if that comforts you, or unfold the map and explore all points of the compass. Identify what you love, and do it.

Cross-Country Skiing

Cross-country skiing is an elegant, gliding sport for snowy meadows and quiet country lanes. It's safe and easy to learn and can involve the whole family. Every part of your body gets an exhilarating workout, and your psyche gets rejuvenated. Sound hard to beat? It is.

Your movements flow easily, rhythmically calling upon the muscles of the arms, shoulders, back, chest, waist, hips, and legs. There's none of the jarring you experience in many other aerobic sports. Exercise scientists call it the best all-around workout. In fact, of all the athletes in the world, those that are most highly conditioned and in the best cardiorespiratory shape are cross-country skiers.[99]

Equipment choices make a difference. To cross-country ski, you need skis, bindings, boots, socks, gloves, and poles with wrist straps. Whether you rent, borrow, or buy, this equipment must fit your body measurements, technique, and ability level (see "Resources" at the end of this section). Cross-country skis perform two opposing functions: gripping the snow and gliding across it. Skis are therefore manufactured with a bowlike arch or camber with gripping surfaces in the center and gliding areas at the ends.

There are two basic types of cross-country skis: waxable and waxless. Waxable skis require application of various types of wax to match weather and snow conditions. Waxing is a fairly easy process. Waxless skis have patterns along the bottom surfaces that grip and glide on the snow without wax. Waxless skis require less care and generally perform well for noncompetitive skiers. Beyond deciding between waxed and waxless, it's important to select skis for in-track skiing (following preformed tracked trails), off-track skiing (creating your own path), or a bit of both.

Cross-country ski boots are made of leather or synthetic materials, and newer models combine advanced designs with running shoe comfort; get the best-fitting ones you can. The boots are clamped at the toe to the ski in a binding. The rear half of the boot sole anchors into a groove or gripping surface when your weight shifts back to the heel.

For traditional cross-country skiing, poles are usually at least as long as the distance from the ground to your armpit. For the newer, advanced "skating" techniques, poles are chin height or higher.

Clothing choices are important, too. The clothes you wear for Nordic skiing are of prime concern, since you'll be perspiring in cold temperatures — and may feel like wearing a T-shirt — and then when the workout is over your cool-down can get really *cold*. Check the local weather conditions and determine the length of your planned outing. If skiing far from a warm shelter, carry a light backpack or fanny pack with warm clothes for emergencies. Layering — including head-to-toe underwear that wicks perspiration away from your skin — is a must; also valuable is a warm cap, toasty socks, comfortable gloves, sunglasses, skin sunscreen lotion, and a belt pack with water and a snack. High-tech breathable outer shells are worth considering, as are waterproof gaiters to keep your feet dry.

Basic Techniques   While it's ideal to learn cross-country skiing from a qualified instructor, you certainly don't need to. Here are some guidelines that can have you up and gliding your first day out. Beginners usually learn the traditional diagonal-stride technique used worldwide by recreational skiers. It's a smooth, steady Nordic skiing style that looks like fast walking and is easy to learn.

To get the feel of your skis, the first thing to do is walk in them. Keep your knees slightly bent, just enough to keep you stable over the center of the ski, with your weight a little more on the balls of your feet than the heels. Notice how the heel comes off the ski on your trailing foot. Use your poles for balance. Push off a little, gliding forward first with one ski and then the other.

Next comes the kick-and-glide motion of traditional Nordic skiing. In place of just pushing off, lift your leg and foot slightly from the hip, unweighting the ski as you push it forward in the glide. This kicking action uses your buttocks, hamstring muscles, and lower back. If your right foot is trailing, then your left arm is back and your right arm forward, elbow bent, planting the pole on the outside of the right ski. Then push off lightly with the right trailing foot as you put some oomph into the right pole with your arm and shoulder.

Once you've pushed off, relax your grip on the pole so your arm is free to move forward to plant the pole again. Some ski instructors paint the picture of using the right pole to pull the distance toward you as your right ski glides into it. The same then happens on the left side.

Lean forward at about a 30-to-45-degree angle with good posture. Keep your head up and eyes focused 10 to 20 feet ahead of you.

The left and right poles and skis are activated alternately; that is, as the right ski trails and the right pole plants to the front on the right side, the left ski is gliding forward and the left pole pushes; as the left ski trails and the left pole moves ahead to plant to the front on the left side, the right ski glides forward while the right pole pushes. And so on.

Your weight shifts smoothly from side to side. Right-left. Right-left. The motion feels almost like roller skating or ice skating, but the heel comes up off the ski as your foot moves behind you. As your heel comes off the ski, put your weight on the ball of your foot and push the ski forward, at the same time pushing with the pole on that side. Once you've given yourself a little forward momentum, slide the trailing foot to catch up. Alternate sides, pushing the rear ski and forward pole in the opposite hand to set up a rhythm.

As a beginner, try to avoid hills; if you can't avoid them, at least don't ski down them. Instead, take your skis off and walk down. Banzai charges down even the smallest of hills invite injuries.

The next skills to learn include single- and double-poling techniques, snowplow stops, sidestepping, various turning methods, and herringbone uphill strides (see "Resources").

Advanced techniques, such as the marathon skate, double-pole V skate, and single-pole V skate methods used by world-class experts can be fast and exhilarating once mastered. More and more intermediate-level skiers are learning them. During recent trips to Europe, I've observed Nordic skiers of all ability levels using skating techniques. Skating can be used alone or combined with diagonal striding in different terrains.

Touring the World on Skis

One great way to cross-country ski is to take your vacation at a beautiful spot with a ski tour. It's a great fitness holiday for couples and families. The Ski Touring Council, Sierra Club, vacation tour groups, local ski clubs, and many ski resorts offer organized half-day, full-day, and weekend ski tours in many parts of Europe and North America, even in Hawaii (on the mountain elevations of the big island).

RESOURCES

Organizations and Publications

▶ *Cross-Country Skier Magazine* (P.O. Box 1203, West Brattleboro, VT 05301).

▶ *Cross-Country Skiing* by Ned Gillette and John Dostal (Bantam, 1984). A good basic book on cross-country skiing.

▶ *Cross-Country Skiing* with Jeff Nowak (Sybervision, Fountain Square, 6066 Civic Terrace Ave., Newark, CA 94560; 800-255-9666). A cross-country skiing video that teaches diagonal-stride skiing plus turns, stops, and ways to climb hills. Uses muscle-memory programming techniques that make learning fast and fun.

▶ *Skating for Cross-Country Skiers* by Audun Endestad and John Teaford (Leisure Press, 1987). A book for serious skiers by an Olympic cross-country team member and international speed skater.

▶ *Skating with Gunde Svan* (available from Eagle River Nordic and New Moon Ski-Shop; see next page). An instructional video by one of the world's top cross-country ski champions from Sweden.

▶ *Ski Faster, Ski Better* by Lee Borowski (Leisure Press, 1986). An up-to-date book in the U.S. Ski Team Sports Medicine series. Includes skating techniques.

▶ Ski Touring Council (West Hill Rd., Troy, VT 05868). Promotes noncompetitive cross-country skiing and touring.

▶ Sierra Club (530 Bush St., San Francisco, CA 94108).

Suppliers

▶ Eagle River Nordic (P.O. Box 936, Eagle River, WI 54521; 800-423-9730). A mail order cross-country skiing supply company that uses a computerized system to help customers make the best equipment choices.

▶ New Moon Ski-Shop (P.O. Box 132, Hayward, WI 54843; 715-634-8685). Another reliable mail order cross-country skiing supply company.

Swimming

When you swim, you glide serenely through the water, with the feeling of being cushioned on a cloud. You're alone in a quiet world of personal thoughts and refreshing, calming water. Swimming is the second most popular sport in America (walking tops the list), for a number of good reasons. Anyone can swim. It's a tremendous aerobic sport for the whole body, exercising the shoulders, arms, chest, back, trunk, hips, and legs. The water's buoyancy avoids weight-bearing stresses and helps prevent injuries to bones, muscles, and joints. This makes it easy to be invigorated without becoming exhausted.

Recent research shows that — like weight-bearing exercises such as walking and running — swimming helps retard mineral (especially calcium) loss.[100] For years doctors have recommended swimming to ease the stiffness and pain of lower-back problems and arthritis. The smooth, rhythmic motion stretches and strengthens the body.

Swimming was among my favorite sports while growing up, and I spent lots of time swimming just for the fun of it — in pools, lakes, ponds, and rivers. As an All-American competitive swimmer, I have also seen this sport from the inside edge of five-hour-a-day training sessions for months on end.

To maintain a steady, rhythmic pace for 30 minutes in your target heart rate zone (THRZ), you need good technique, not erratic or struggling strokes. To be an efficient swimmer, you must float high and flat in the water parallel to its surface, evenly distributing your weight and offering a streamlined form for minimal resistance. There's no need to waste energy trying to remain buoyant.

The THRZ Is Lower in Swimming

"If swimming . . . [is] used for training, an adjustment should be made in estimating maximum heart rate," reports exercise physiologist William D. McArdle, coauthor of *Exercise Physiology: Energy, Nutrition, and Human Performance.* "Maximum heart rate . . . averages about 10 to 13 beats per minute lower than running in both trained and untrained subjects."[101]

When calculating your predicted maximal heart rate (PMHR) for swimming, subtract 10 to 13 from the higher number. For example, use 207 minus your age = PMHR (instead of 220 minus your age). If you're very fit, use 195 minus one-half your age = PMHR (instead of 205 minus one-half your age).

Why the difference? "Swimming," explains McArdle, "uses a smaller muscle mass, since you use mostly the arms. You can still get a good aerobic workout, but unless you're an Olympic swimmer, you can't generate the same heart rate." Since swimmers are horizontal in the water, the heart has an easier time pumping more blood with each beat. The volume of blood pumped by the heart in swimming is more important than heart rate in determining aquatic aerobic fitness.

Some electronic heart rate monitors (mentioned previously in this chapter under "Electronic Monitors") are available in waterproof versions for swimmers.

Swimming Alone or with a Coach

If you already know how to swim, you probably don't need lessons. Just get in the water and begin swimming laps. At some point, however, it's advantageous to have a swimming instructor help perfect your form and technique. You'll enjoy swimming more than ever and your aerobic benefits will be greater, too. Swimming is difficult to learn from a book, although some good books are listed under "Resources." Here are several highlights and guidelines.

Swimming provides a variety of opportunities for varying speed and resistance. It involves different muscles in different movements than those used in jogging, skiing, and cycling. Resistance can be varied by alternating body position, changing movement directions, or using supplemental equipment such as air tubes, hand paddles, and fins.

Proper Freestyle Stroke for Maximum Benefit

The freestyle, or crawl, is considered the premier aerobic swimming stroke. Little energy is wasted, and its rhythmic movements maximize aerobic benefits. In aerobics ratings, freestyle is followed by the backstroke, breaststroke, and sidestroke. These latter three strokes can be used to break the monotony of long training periods.

Some coaches recommend that in the freestyle stroke the waterline be at mid-forehead. If you have difficulty staying flat in the water, you are probably arching your neck and head for air on each breath, forcing your legs to sink. Proper breathing in the freestyle stroke depends on a smooth rolling motion along the long axis of the body, reducing resistance to the front by pulling first one shoulder and then the other out of the water with each stroke. This helps keep your posture relaxed and aligned as you bring your face up to the surface for each breath in.

If you've accomplished flatness in the water, are rolling far enough (usually 45 degrees) to each side and are turning (not lifting) your head to clear your mouth, but are *still* experiencing breathing problems, your timing may be off. With each breath cycle you're probably not emptying your lungs early enough but are attempting to force in new air before the exhalation is complete. You may need to practice forceful underwater exhalations to help time the breathing pattern more efficiently.

Use of Snorkels, Face Masks, and Float Belts

If you have a history of back trouble or lack confidence in your swimming ability, consider using a snorkel and face mask. While this may look amateurish to pool speedsters, the Institute for Aerobics Research has found that it's advisable to *first* get flat in the water — keeping your head down and breathing through the snorkle while avoiding overarching your back. Later, you can learn proper breathing techniques. Some dedicated aerobic swimmers never abandon the snorkel and mask, enjoying the unlimited air supply.

Float belts — adult versions of around-the-waist inner tubes — help some people keep their trunk high in the water when swimming.

Other Tips About Swimming

Biomechanical tips. Many freestyle swimmers experience problems by not finishing each arm stroke or by kicking inefficiently. Freestyle arm strokes must complete a full cycle. Roll the shoulder into the water as you reach fully forward with the elbow remaining slightly bent, then smoothly pull downward and to the back (*not* up). The arm pull should extend back to pass your hip joint near the bottom edge of your swimming suit.

Your kick in the freestyle swimming stroke provides about 20 percent of the power and helps stabilize the body against unwanted rotations while maintaining forward motion. Top swimmers kick with their entire leg, with knees and feet relaxed, toes pointed, kicking about half as high with the leg motion as in a brisk walking stride and using smooth hip and thigh actions to provide most of the power.

Training options. If you enjoy swimming continuous laps for aerobic exercise, then laps are a good choice. If you begin to lose interest in swimming or simply want more variety, create a training routine with "broken swims," a technique suitable for swimmers of all ability levels. It's recommended by Jane Katz, professor of health and physical education at the City University of New York and author of *Swimming for Total Fitness*. The format is simple: Briefly pause to rest after each lap or set of laps for 1 minute or less so that you can recover oxygen without your heart rate dipping below the target zone. By varying the length and frequency of the breaks in the swimming routine — and continually staying within your THRZ — you can add extra enjoyment to your fitness sessions.

Masters programs. Many local swimming pools have "masters" programs, a national competition network for people age twenty-five and older. Masters swimmers like recruiting new team members but also enjoy helping aerobic fitness swimmers get started in a productive program. To locate the group nearest you, write to U.S. Masters Swimming, Inc. (5 Piggott Lane, Avon, CT 06001).

Miscellaneous tips. For daily exercise, it's best to swim in a heated pool, which helps ensure smooth water, premeasured distances for pacing, and water temperature between 75 and 80°F.

A good-fitting, streamlined swimming suit — which doesn't have to be expensive — can increase your comfort in the water and boost aquatic efficiency.

Goggles have become a virtual necessity for protecting the eyes from chlorine in pools and irritants in lakes, ponds, and rivers. Try several designs and models to find a pair that fits your face securely and comfortably. Opticians can now put eyeglass prescriptions into plastic watertight swimming goggles.

Bathing caps can be helpful for keeping your hair out of your eyes, minimizing water resistance, insulating your head in cool water, and protecting your hair and scalp from the irritating effects of chlorinated water. Tight-fitting nylon cloth caps don't pull hair the way rubber caps do.

Ear plugs are available in a variety of designs but their use is controversial from a health standpoint. For certain people, they *contribute* to ear problems rather than prevent them. If in doubt, consult your physician. Nose clips are often recommended for practicing diving skills and flip turns, but they interfere with breathing efficiency.

A recent study by the Centers for Disease Control in Atlanta found that acidic chlorine in swimming pool water can erode tooth enamel and cause gum irritation for some people.[102] To help avoid those problems, learn to breathe correctly and try not to hold water in your mouth as you swim.

When swimming in outdoor pools or lakes, plan to avoid high-intensity midday sun and protect your skin from sunburn by applying a water-resistant sunscreen with a protection factor (SPF) of 15 or more (discussed in Chapter 37).

Other Water Sports

Aquaerobics, also called water aerobics and aquatic exercise, is a form of aerobic dancing in water that is taught by most YMCAs and YWCAs and many health clubs. Classes can combine swimming strokes, aerobic dance movements, synchronized swimming, and calisthenics, sometimes with music. The National Institute for Creative Aquatics (12 Washington Ln., West Milford, NJ 07480) is one group involved in promoting this type of exercise. Some routines are outlined in *The W.E.T. Workout* by Jane Katz (Facts on File, 1985).

Two recent studies have shown that *hydro-walking* — walking on a treadmill submerged in water about waist deep — can give an effective aerobic workout.[103] It is especially valuable for injured athletes.

"Water supports your body weight so there is virtually no stress on the joints while you run," says Dr. Jack Taunton, professor at the University of British Columbia School of Medicine and president of the Canadian Academy of Sports Medicine. "The fact is, many runners are nonswimmers or have poor swimming technique, making it impossible for them to swim laps long enough to get an aerobic benefit. Even runners with good swimming technique find lap swimming difficult. They haven't trained their muscles for continuous swimming so they become fatigued after just a few laps."[104]

In an effective aquatic running program, you are capitalizing on the water's buoyancy and using a running motion similar to treading water. Always run in water deeper than your full height and maintain good posture as if running on dry land, with your head out of the water.

You may want to try a water-ski belt, swimmer's armpit pull-buoys, or rubber flotation ring. A product called Wet Vest is specifically designed for running in water (see "Resources").

RESOURCES

Publications

▶ *I Can Swim, You Can Swim* by Tom Cuthbertson and Lee Cole (Ten Speed Press, 1979). Good basic book on learning to swim.
▶ *Staying with It* by John Jerome (Viking Press, 1984). Award-winning book for late-blooming athletes, written by a masters swimmer.
▶ *Swim* magazine (P.O. Box 45497, Los Angeles, CA 90045). For adult fitness-oriented swimmers.
▶ *Swimming Faster* by Ernest W. Maglischo (Mayfield, 1982). Textbook for improving swimming strokes and planning a training schedule.
▶ *Swimming for Total Fitness* by Jane Katz, Ed.D. (Doubleday Dolphin, 1981). Offers an enthusiastic fitness program centered around swimming.
▶ *Swimming Technique* magazine (P.O. Box 45497, Los Angeles, CA 90045). A quarterly publication for coaches and swimmers, it discusses the latest trends in stroke mechanics and sports medicine.
▶ *Swimming World* magazine (P.O. Box 45497, Los Angeles, CA 90045). The most complete coverage of aquatic sports.

Suppliers

▶ The Finals (21 Minisink Ave., Port Jervis, NY 12771; 800-431-9111). A mail order fitness clothing source, with a good selection of swimwear, warm-ups, and other supplies.

▶ Wet Vest (Bioenergetics, Inc., 5074 Shelby Drive, Birmingham, AL 35243). An exercise vest designed for running in water.
▶ Worldwide Aquatics (509 Wyoming Ave., Cincinnati, OH 45215; 800-543-4459). "The Swimmers Mail-Order Supermarket."

Walking

Walking is for everyone. It's the most popular aerobic exercise of all — an estimated 40 million Americans now walk for fitness. Walking can find a way into most schedules and can be done anywhere, anytime, and in just about any attire. You can walk around the block, walk to work or on errands, hike through the woods, explore new neighborhoods or a local museum, or walk in indoor shopping malls. Walking is a low-impact exercise and injuries are therefore rare. Cardiologists recommend it for its safety, convenience, and cost-effectiveness.

Walking's Great, but It Takes More Time

All types of walking promote better fitness. But it takes a commitment to turn walking from a stop-and-go activity or casual stroll into an aerobic fitness option. You need to walk far enough and fast enough to get results.

The Institute for Aerobics Research suggests working up to walking about 3 miles in 45 minutes (20 to 30 minutes isn't enough for full aerobic benefits) and following this routine four to five times a week (three isn't enough) if you plan to use walking as your sole aerobic exercise.[105]

The Right Shoes

The wrong pair of shoes can turn fitness walking into sheer torture. The right pair make it a joy. Athletic shoe companies are now producing hundreds of different walking shoes based on modifications of the running shoe design.

When buying a pair of shoes for walking, look for padded insoles, midsoles, and heel counters. A good arch is essential, and there should be room for you to wiggle your toes. You need a firm, thick sole to protect your feet from rocks and pebbles and a flexible forefoot area where the ball of the foot meets the toes. The bottom sole surface should provide good traction. The uppers should be made from sturdy supportive material such as leather, canvas, or nylon, be reinforced at stress points, and be properly ventilated to let perspiration escape. Lace-up shoes make it possible to adjust snugness for maximum comfort. The back of the shoe, called the heel counter, should firmly support the heel.

Posture and Technique

As you walk, hold your head high, with your neck and shoulders relaxed and lower back flat. Poor posture will shorten your stride, throw you off balance, cause back pain, or exhaust you long before the workout is over. Walk with your heel coming down lightly on the ground first, rolling your weight forward across the sole of your foot, and then gently pushing off with your toes. Keep your feet pointed straight ahead and don't hyperextend the leg (let it lock straight). Use a "heterolateral" walking pattern, moving your left arm forward as your right leg advances, and the right arm forward as the left leg steps, and so on.

Choosing Fitness Walking, Speed Walking, or Power Walking

Conventional fitness walking, as described above and when performed in your target heart rate zone, is an excellent lifetime aerobic exercise. If you reach the point where walking gets too easy, there are several options for intensifying the workout.

First, go faster. This pays off until you reach the 12-minute-mile level, at which you use more energy to walk than to jog or run.

Second, intensify your workout. This can be accomplished by lengthening your stride, lifting your feet a little higher with each step, and swinging your arms more vigorously (a full, strong arm swing keeps you balanced and helps you breathe more regularly).

Third, include some hill training to increase the workload of your walking exercise, although it's difficult to find hills with a gradual incline long enough to sustain a full aerobic workout.

Fourth, carry hand weights. One technique, called power walking, incorporates hand weights or weighted vests to increase resistance and intensity, using more muscle groups to contribute to the exercise movements. Start with small hand-held, strap-on, or slide-on weights (usually one-half to two pounds in each hand or a balanced weight vest of several pounds). If the weights are hand-held, don't grip them too tightly (this restricts blood flow in the arms). Whichever weights you choose, use smooth, rhythmic motions to pump, push, and pull them as you walk; don't just carry them. A word of caution: Do *not* walk using ankle weights — they stress the knee and ankle joints and contribute to injury.

Fifth, if you're really excited about advanced-level walking, look into speed walking (also called race walking or striding) at walking clubs or fitness centers such as the YMCA.

Hiking and Trekking

Once you can comfortably walk 4 miles without stopping, consider taking scenic treks or hiking trips in local, state, and national parks. These activities are great for families and groups of friends and can last from a few hours to several months. Travel agencies now book exotic treks across all continents — group trips where all you need to do is walk at a moderate pace and carry a light knapsack. The tour guides carry all other luggage and handle meals and lodging. For ideas, check with the Sierra Club, local community groups, or a travel agent.

RESOURCES

▶ *Fitness Walking* by Robert Sweetgall (Perigee Books, 1985). Basic book on aerobic walking.

▶ *Race Walking: A Safe and Healthy Alternative to Jogging* by William Finley and Marion Webster (Stephen Greene Press, 1985).

▶ Sierra Club (530 Bush St., San Francisco, CA 94108).

▶ The Walkers Center (733 15th St. N.W., Suite 427, Washington, D.C. 20005). A clearinghouse for information and news about walking. Publishes the *WalkWays* newsletter and *The WalkWays Almanac*.

▶ The Walkers Club of America (445 E. 86th St., New York, NY 10028). Organizes health walking and race walking events. Contact the club for affiliate chapters in your area.

▶ *The Walking Magazine* (711 Boylston St., Boston, MA 02116).

Outdoor Cycling

Outdoor cycling puts the power of the wheel beneath you, providing a great opportunity to breeze along enjoying beautiful scenery and covering distances far greater than by walking or running. And cycling can be good aerobic exercise, less traumatic to the bones and joints than jogging. You can cycle to and from work, on errands, or to break away from the work site or home confines. It can also be a great family outing.

But you need to pay attention to cycle rhythmically and stay in your target heart rate zone. The Institute for Aerobics Research has found that cycling at speeds less than 10 miles per hour is of limited aerobic benefit. In contrast, cycling over 20 miles per hour is racing speed. For the average person, a cycling speed just above 15 miles an hour seems to give best aerobic benefits.[106]

There's also more to cycling these days than two wheels; that's why it's now often called *cycling*, not *bicycling*. New human-powered wheeled vehicles — adult tricycles and quadricycles — feature high-tech designs and handle like a dream. They'll be widely available in the next decade and may transform short-distance transportation. There are even some ingenious new canoe-cycles with a recumbent seat and foot pedal design for breezing across the water. What fun!

Selecting the Right Bicycle

An outdoor cycle is a relatively expensive investment. At first, it's best to borrow a bike or buy a cheap used one until you're certain you love the sport. When choosing a bicycle, there are several prime considerations.

There is no such thing as a one-size-fits-all bike, and there shouldn't be. It's important to match the model and size to your cycling routes, fitness abilities, and terrain. Investigate touring, recreational-sport, and mountain bike (all-terrain) models. Take test runs over your local cycling paths.

First, the bicycle frame size should be proportioned to your height and leg length. When you are seated, both feet should just barely touch the ground, and your leg should be slightly bent when your foot reaches the bottom of the pedaling movement.

Second, decide what position you want to ride in. There are three basic choices. Upright models let you sit erect, arms relaxed, head held high. They're great fun to ride. Bent-over (racer's crouch) models with dropped handles project the body in a forward tuck position — a stress to everyone's posture. Recumbent models — a new design — let you ride leaning back as if in a reclining chair with your feet propped up on an ottoman. With surprisingly little practice, the recumbent models are easy to ride, and new models are soon to be marketed in three- and four-wheel versions. They make sense but cost a lot. At the time of this writing, the best overall choice is an upright bike.

Third, there's the tire width decision. Racer's models come with skinny tires, whereas uprights can have skinny, medium-width, or wide tires. The wide ones give the softest ride and best grip on the road.

Fourth, you need to choose how many gears the bike has. Shifting from one gear to another lets you keep pedaling at a steady speed when faced with ups and downs of the road. You need at least three gears (to let you handle small hills with some degree of elegance); ten is ideal for most uses, and more than ten is fine but you probably won't use them all.

The mountain bike is an upright, wide-tired bicycle. It can take you charging up and down big hills or cruising with sure-handling ease on city streets. It weighs about the same as a racer's model ten-speed yet is ten times sturdier. Mountain bikes promote good breathing and posture (they're a good choice for people with a history of back pain) and provide more of a full-body workout, say sports medicine experts.

Other considerations: Few things hurt more than hard, poor-fitting bicycle seats (also called saddles). Select a comfortable seat that fits the shape of your pelvic bones and behind. Then pad it. Sheepskin or chamois seat covers are a good comfort investment. Best of all may be a variation of the Hydroseat (see "Resources"), a leather-covered seat that uses a water-filled polyurethane sack that shifts as you move to form a well-contoured cushion for racing, touring, and stationary cycle seats.

For long-distance riding, toe clips help you provide power to the up stroke when pedaling. But be careful. If you fall, they tend to keep you attached to the bike — a dangerous situation. If you use your cycle for commuting, shopping, or touring, choose a saddlebag or basket arrangement to conveniently carry essentials as you ride.

Cycling Posture and Technique

Cycling posture is determined by proper technique and must match the design of your cycle. If the frame size is too large or too small, you'll experience tension and probably pain. Adjust the seat and handlebars to a comfortable position, being certain that your leg is almost fully extended as the pedal reaches the bottom point of its circle. Bend forward at the hips (not the waist) when you ride, with your back straight, neck and shoulders relaxed. Don't stretch your neck forward, cave in your chest, or slouch your shoulders. When gripping the handlebars, keep your elbows slightly bent — for better leverage, shock absorption when going over potholes or bumps, and less fatigue. On long rides, change your hand positions often.

If you haven't ever ridden a bicycle, the first thing to do is practice getting on and off. Then practice sitting in the seat and looking backward through the rearview mirror(s). Start by riding on the flattest possible terrain. To beginning cyclists, downhill rides feel like a hurtling roller coaster and uphill routes are just too hard to be fun. Use smooth, gliding pedal strokes and ride in a straight line. Before you start picking up much speed, learn how to stop smoothly and with confidence. As you go into turns, lean a little bit into the direction in which you're turning. Work into practicing tight turns around broken glass, potholes, and obstacles in the road.

Cadence and Gearing

Experienced cyclists usually pedal at a high rate but in a low gear, giving them power while reducing fatigue. Choose the gear that best permits you to stay within your target heart rate zone. Shift gears to match changing terrain and wind directions.

When you cycle uphill, lean farther forward to give yourself better momentum. For extra stroking power on touring and racing bicycles with toe clips, imagine pedaling as a continuous pull-up, push-down motion. With constant pressure on the pedals and toe clips, your legs can work like pistons, driving the pedals up and down.

Spin is a term indicating wheel revolutions per minute (rpm). Generally, a spin between 80 and 90 rpm is recommended; it creates less fatigue by increasing speed without pushing into higher gears. The only ways to increase speed are to increase gear ratio with the same pedaling cadence or keep the same gearing while increasing the speed of your leg movements.

The Institute for Aerobics Research recommends giving yourself at least ten weeks to work up to a 15-mph cruising speed — about 1 mile every 4 minutes. Cycling 5 miles in 20 minutes four or five times a week is an effective and challenging training program.[107]

Safety Concerns

Safety is a paramount concern for cyclists. As a rider, you have to maneuver your bike through traffic, and you're always at risk of an accident. In addition, stop-and-go city traffic makes it very difficult to stay in your target heart rate zone. The likelihood of falling off a bike or getting into an accident is magnified by bad weather conditions, potholes in the road, and sudden distractions such as a barking dog charging at your wheel.

Buy and wear a good-fitting protective hard-shell helmet. Be certain it meets or surpasses the standards set by the American National Standards Institute's specifications. Most serious cycling injuries are to the head. Reflective rearview mirrors should be mounted on the handlebars, not on your helmet.

Keep your bike in good repair. Inspect it every time before you ride. Check the tires, brakes, gears, and lights. Attach a loud horn to the handlebars and use it whenever necessary. Don't ride at night unless you have no alternative; and then use safety reflectors, headlights, and reflective clothing.

Touring the Planet on Wheels

It's now possible to tour most of the world by bicycle. Clubs all across America and Europe schedule outings lasting from an afternoon riding the paths of a local park or nature reserve to an entire holiday vacation just about anywhere on the globe. You can pedal across America, Mexico, Europe, most of India, and huge tracts of China and Australia, covering about 50 miles a day. Cycling, travel, and outdoor magazines list all kinds of cycle tour options.

RESOURCES

Organizations and Publications

▶ *Anybody's Bike Book: An Original Manual of Bike Repairs* by Tom Cuthbertson (Ten Speed Press, 1980). A beginning-level instruction book.
▶ *Bicycle Guide* magazine (128 N. 11th St., Allentown, PA 18102).
▶ Bicycle USA (The League of American Wheelmen, Suite 209, 6707 Whitestone Rd., Baltimore, MD 21207). A nonprofit national organization for tourists, club riders, commuters, families, local clubs.
▶ *Bicycle Rider* magazine (29901 Agoura Rd., Agoura, CA 91301). Emphasizes touring and trekking.
▶ *Bicycling* by John Marino, Lawrence May, M.D., and Hal Z. Bennett (J. P. Tarcher, 1983). Provides good information on purchasing, riding, and repairing your bicycle.
▶ *Bicycling Magazine* (Emmaus, PA 18049).
▶ Bikecentennial (P.O. Box 8308, Missoula, MT 59807). A nonprofit, member-supported organization for touring cyclists.
▶ *Bike Touring: The Sierra Club Guide to Outings on Wheels* by Raymond Bridge (Sierra Club Books, 1979).
▶ The Consumer Product Safety Commission (Washington, DC 20207) offers a free "Fact Sheet No. 10" on bicycle safety, selection, and maintenance, along with a *Sprocket Man* comic book on bicycle safety for teenagers.

▶ *Cycling: Endurance and Speed* by Michael Shermer (Contemporary Books, 1987). A book for racers.
▶ *Cyclist Magazine* (P.O. Box 907, Farmingdale, NY 11737).
▶ *Greg LeMond's Complete Book of Bicycling* by Greg LeMond (Putnam's, 1987). For serious recreational road riding and racing.
▶ *Mountain Bike* magazine (Emmaus, PA 18098).

Suppliers

▶ Hydroseat (Hammacher Schlemmer, 147 E. 57th St., New York, NY 10022; 800-543-3366).
▶ Palo Alto Bicycles (P.O. Box 1276, Palo Alto, CA 94302; 800-227-8900). A mail order cycling supermarket.
▶ Performance Bicycle Shop (P.O. Box 2741, Chapel Hill, NC 27514; 800-334-5741). Another good mail order source.

Jogging and Running

If walking is such a good aerobic activity, why jog or run? Good question. Although the higher intensity of jogging and running give you aerobic benefits in less time than walking, the injury risk is greater. In fact, nearly three-quarters of all sports injuries seen by physicians are reportedly caused by running.[108]

Still, running — with proper shoes and technique — is one of the fastest ways to get into good aerobic condition and lose excess fat. And some people absolutely love to run, finding it a joy and a release from tension. What is the difference between running and jogging? Jogging is often classified as movement slower than 9 minutes per mile; running is faster. For the purposes of this book, I'll refer to them both as running.

Running Surface

A fairly flat running course helps you maintain a smooth rhythm and prevent injuries. Concrete is the worst running surface, with asphalt or blacktop close behind. A properly maintained cinder track is better, an even dirt road better yet, and a level grassy field superior to that. The best surface is a synthetic cushioned indoor track.

Most runners, however, spend most of their exercise time on outdoor paved surfaces because they're most accessible. No matter what road surface you choose for running, alternate the side of the road you train on. Many roads and tracks are banked, and if you continually run on only one side, your body posture must adapt. This creates stress and fatigue and leads to injuries.

Choosing the Proper Shoes

Selecting the proper shoes for running is critical to injury prevention and enjoyment. Jogging or running on a hard surface transfers tremendous shock waves from your feet up through your body to your head at speeds of more than 200 miles per hour. You need good shock absorption systems — found in your healthy muscles, joints, and bones and secondarily in your running posture, technique, and shoes. Without these factors on your side, there's a pretty good chance that sooner or later you'll get injured — suffering from stress fractures, tissue tears, strains, sprains, or perhaps degenerative joint diseases.

Long-term problems can be minimized by wearing top-quality shoes, using smooth and balanced running technique, and cross training with other aerobic activities so you don't run every day.

Meteoric advances have occurred in athletic footwear technology over the past two decades. New viscoelastic polymers hold their shape and absorb shock with remarkable efficiency, cutting the magnitude of skeletal shock waves by more than 40 percent.[109] If you plan to run regularly, don't economize on footwear.

Women require special shoes. Until recently, shoe lasts (specially designed forms that create shoe fit) used by major manufacturers were identical for both sexes and were based on traditional designs for male foot shape. But women require significantly different athletic shoes than men. Fortunately, research findings and consumer pressures are leading to an industry-wide change. Studies also show that children strike the ground with an average force three and a half times their body weight (adults average only two and a half times their body weight).[110] Kids need good-fitting, good-quality athletic shoes, even if they outgrow them before they outwear them.

Lacing techniques. Different lacing techniques can improve weight distribution when running, reducing foot slippage inside one or both shoes and varying the angles of support on different parts of each foot.[111]

Socks make a difference, too. Many fitness walkers, joggers, and runners choose great shoes but overlook their socks. That's a mistake. The fit and quality of your socks have a lot to do with foot comfort. The best socks are made with cushioning at strategic locations (which vary with different activities and sports). The fiber you choose should reduce friction between sock and skin and be able to wick perspiration away from the surface of your feet, conducting it through the sock material where it can evaporate.

Cotton, wool, and silk are good fibers for use in dress socks but poor choices for running socks since they trap moisture next to the skin and reduce cushioning power. This contributes to blisters and foot infections. Synthetics like Orlon, rayon, and polypropylene are considered superior because they draw sweat away from the foot through their fibers and stay drier.

To ensure perfect fit, choose the right size: about one-half inch longer and one-quarter inch wider than your foot. Don't wear socks more than once between washings; rotate them each workout. Salt from perspiration dries in the socks after a single use and, if not removed by washing, can contribute to blisters in subsequent workouts.[112]

Athletic Bras

It's important for women runners to wear a good-quality athletic bra. A recent medical study indicates that during running, female breasts are pulled on the spatial planes that provide the only support the breasts have besides the skin. If unrestricted, the bobbing motion not only throws a woman off-balance but can cause bruising and soreness. Over time, this can create problems ranging from endocrine hormone imbalances to sagging breasts.[113]

Sports bras should limit the motion of the breast relative to the body (so that the breasts and body move together), support from below, have adjustable straps that are nonelastic, have no metal hooks, fasteners or irritating seams, completely cover the breast, and be at least half cotton.

Running Form and Efficiency

Your form and efficiency in running and jogging are very important. The precise biomechanical analysis of running form is beyond the scope of this book. Nonetheless, here are several basic guidelines to help you increase your running efficiency.

Peak running form depends on two primary factors: postural balance and smooth ballistic (movement-related) technique.

For postural balance, keep the spine erect, back flat, pelvis vertical, chest suspended and slightly elevated, neck long, head poised and high, shoulders relaxed, and arms free.

Correct foot placement enables the midtarsal arch of the foot to evenly distribute weight forces rather than centralizing them. The best biomechanical foot plant is usually composed of an outward heel strike, smoothly rolling (pronating) into a flat midstance where the foot accepts all of the body's weight.[114] Then the midtarsal joint tightens, and propulsion (also called toe push-off) transfers to the front of the foot. All of these actions must occur in a smooth, fast sequence.

Each complete running stride has a drive or power phase, a float phase, and a contact or compression phase, with the legs alternating in support and nonsupport functions. Most running energy is used for the forward motion, which includes the foot strike, pronation-compression, and push-off. Many athletes and their coaches overemphasize the push-off phase (with corresponding drive and leg extension). For maximized efficiency, however, all three phases require smooth, equal speed without "braking" (an abrupt deceleration-acceleration technique that causes fatigue).[115]

The arm movements in running should match leg movements in rate of speed, with complementary actions and counteractions. Become aware of your arm position when you run. If one arm swings farther out to one side than the other or crosses over the midline of your body, your form is probably unbalanced. Heterolateral (right arm forward, left leg forward; left arm forward, right leg forward) motions are the most efficient. Smooth, coordinated arm swings develop power and help keep the body level and balanced, absorbing rotational stresses.

Hand Weights

For increased aerobic efficiency when jogging or running, a number of authorities recommend light hand weights, generally of 1 to 5 pounds each. They are held in the hands or worn as wrist weights and then are smoothly pumped, pushed, and pulled — not just carried — as you go through your aerobic workout (see the walking section earlier for details).

RESOURCES

▶ *Runner's World Magazine* (Emmaus, PA 18099).
▶ *Running Times Magazine* (P.O. Box 6509, Syracuse, NY 13217).
▶ *Galloway's Book on Running* by Jeff Galloway (Shelter Publications, 1984).

Outdoor Rowing

Outdoor rowing, once the exclusive sport of the Ivy League, is finally available to fitness-oriented people all across America. Yet most of us haven't realized how exhilarating and easy rowing can be as an aerobic activity.

You don't need any special talents and can pick up the basic skills in a matter of minutes from an instructor or experienced friend. Nearly every town has some rowable body of water — a river, inlet, bay, lagoon, pond, or lake. Local rowing clubs can put you in touch with places to rent equipment and receive instruction.

Rowing uses muscles in the arms, legs, back, abdomen, torso, and buttocks. Well-conditioned rowers are superbly fit from a cardiovascular endurance standpoint. An added dividend from this form of aerobic exercise is the sense of relaxation and euphoria that comes from gliding across open sparkling water with a light breeze in your face.

Rowing strengthens and tones the body without overtaxing muscles, bones, or joints because there's no jarring action. Your movements are smooth and parallel to the water. Many people with a history of pain or injury that bars them from running, walking, or skiing can sit down and row.

Goodbye to the Rowboat

The modern rowing shell is a lightweight, streamlined vessel that skims across the water surface at speeds of 8 miles per hour and sometimes more. Unlike the rowboat of yesteryear, the rowing shell has a sliding seat that enables you to use your whole body in the rowing motion. Your legs push the boat through the water as you pull the oars with your arms, adding your abdomen, thighs, calves, and buttocks to the standard rowing force.

Rowing has become more and more accessible with the advent of lightweight fiber glass shells that are easy to handle yet are stable enough for coastal waters as well as inland lakes, rivers, and streams. In addition, many colleges, universities, and local rowing clubs offer public access to their facilities and equipment, along with instruction for beginners.

One drawback: In most parts of the country, rowing is at best a seasonal exercise, dependent on weather and water conditions for enjoyment and safety. Therefore, be certain you have other aerobic activities to substitute whenever needed. Since most rowers take an occasional spill into the water, it's also essential to wear a U.S. Coast Guard–rated type II or III life vest if you're a good swimmer or a type I or II life vest (those with the highest flotation quality) if you're not a good swimmer.

Fitness rowers usually select a "single scull," a shell for one rower. Most recreational models available in America are built for moderate speed and long-distance travel and are constructed to handle relatively choppy water.

Balance and Stroke

Aerobic exercise in a rowing shell depends first and foremost on your ability to remain balanced. Be sure your body is centered in the craft and that the oars are level with each other throughout the stroke. Practice on a calm, predictable body of water. Even moderate turbulence can be too much to handle at first.

Each rowing cycle consists of two phases: drive and recovery. The drive phase depends on the oars catching water — called "hitting the catch" — as you push off with your legs and finish with your back and arms to propel the shell in a smooth, quick glide. The oars are then "released" — pulled out of the water — and you recover for the next drive phase.

During recovery, your body weight slides toward the stern of the shell, adding to the acceleration. Generally, the recovery should be longer than the oar time in the water.

Throughout each stroke, your body should remain free from unnecessary tension. The legs do the early drive work as the arms, shoulders, and back transfer the pressure to the oar, followed by the smooth motion of the torso toward the bow.

During the drive phase, the oar blades are squared, perpendicular, to the water surface. The oars are feathered, just out of the water with the blades turned parallel to the water surface, to move back toward the stern in the recovery phase.

Familiarity with and Adjustment of Equipment

It is very important that beginning rowers become familiar with their rowing shell and make adjustments to the equipment so that the aerobic activity is safe and enjoyable.

Before going out in any shell, check all nuts and bolts on the oar riggers to see that they are tight. Make sure that the foot stretcher allows your feet to slide out — a crucial safety feature in the event of a spill. When you climb into the shell, adjust the position of the foot stretcher. Many instructors suggest that, in correct position, your thumbs will touch the bottom of your ribcage when you sit in the finish position holding the oars. The height and pitch of the oarlocks can also be adjusted, along with their distance from the sides of the shell.

Canoeing and Kayaking

Some exercise authorities recommend canoeing and kayaking as good alternatives to rowing. These two sports provide aerobic benefits, and many people find them easier than rowing. Some newly designed canoes and kayaks slip through the water with barely a ripple. Choose models with a comfortable seat and use bent-shaft paddles to minimize shoulder stress when paddling. Investigate options in your area. Always wear a life vest.

RESOURCES

Organizations

▶ American Canoe Association (P.O. Box 248, Lorton, VA 22079). Organization for canoeists and kayakers of all skill levels. Member of U.S. Olympic Committee.
▶ U.S. Canoe Association (617 S. 94th St., Milwaukee, WI 53214).
▶ U.S. Rowing Association (251 N. Illinois St., Indianapolis, IN 46020). National governing body for rowing sports and an information clearinghouse. The group can put you in touch with the nearest rowing club, equipment suppliers, and instructors.

Publications

▶ *Canoe Magazine* (P.O. Box 10748, Des Moines, IA 50340). Devoted to all forms of canoeing and kayaking.
▶ *Row for Your Life* by Barbara Kirch, Reed W. Hoyt, Ph.D., and Janet Fithian (Fireside Books, 1985). Includes a review of basic rowing techniques, guidelines and instruction groups for disabled rowers, and a national listing of rowing clubs and organizations.
▶ *Rowing: Power and Endurance* by Susan Lezotte (Contemporary Books, 1987). Endorsed by the U.S. Rowing Association.

▶ *Sea Kayaker Magazine* (6327 Seaview Ave., N.W., Seattle, WA 98107).

▶ *Small Boat Journal* (P.O. Box 400, Bennington, VT 05201). Reviews rowing shells of all kinds.

Ice and Roller Skating

Gliding on skates captures the very essence of the joy of movement. Ice skating and roller skating are now endorsed by the American Heart Association as safe, effective ways to achieve cardiorespiratory fitness. A recent UCLA study reported that skating burns fat, increases aerobic capacity, and reduces stress as effectively as cycling and running.[116] Research suggests that roller skating at a speed of 10 miles an hour is the aerobic equivalent of jogging at 5 miles per hour.[117]

It is important to keep skating continuously so that your legs and arms are constantly in motion and you stay in your target heart rate zone. If you spend too much time coasting along, the aerobic benefits start to disappear.

During winter trips to Switzerland and Austria, I've marveled at the ice rinks filled with families, school classes, and office staffs skating for half-hour sessions during mealtime breaks. At the same time, local cross-country ski trails, walking paths, and fitness centers are brimming with people enjoying active, pleasant camaraderie.

Skating provides several unique exercise benefits. First, it's a particularly good form of exercise for the pelvis and legs. Skating tones the buttocks and the outer muscles of the thighs. The smooth, pumping stride is relatively trauma-free and, unless you fall frequently, there's less chance for overuse or impact injuries common in running.

Skating sports have also hit the quiet paved roads, bicycle paths, and vacant parking lots of America. With some practice, they are sheer exhilaration for exercisers of all ages. One such sport is roller skiing, which uses ski boots and bindings with short graphite-carbon skis with rollers attached to the base to simulate cross-country skiing (ski poles optional). Another new sport, one of my favorites, is Rollerblading, using special ski-skates (with a single row of roller wheels attached to the base of high-tech hockey skate uppers) that simulate ice skating. Go where traffic is light and the weather fair.

Equipment and Facilities

Ice skating can really be one of four different sports — recreational skating, figure skating, speed skating, and hockey — any of which requires an indoor or outdoor rink with well-maintained ice. Roller skating may be done at an indoor rink or outside (as in roller skiing and Rollerblading) on paved pathways, empty parking lots, or smooth roadways where skating is permitted.

Select skates that fit your chosen type of skating, and look for good boots that are high enough to support the ankle without enclosing the calf. They should have a well-padded tongue and good cushioned support at the toes, arch, and ankles. Be certain that the boots fit well at the ankle bones, arch, toes, heel, and Achilles tendon — the major pressure points when skating. Get good-quality rollers or blades, expertly sharpened.

RESOURCES

Publications

▶ *Power Skating: A Pro Coach's Secrets* by Laura Stamm (Sterling, 1982).
▶ *Recreational Ice Skating* magazine (1000 Skokie Blvd., Wilmette, IL 60091).
▶ *Roller Skating: Fundamentals and Techniques* by Sharon Kay Stoll (Human Kinetics, 1983). A self-instruction book on traditional roller skating.
▶ *Skating Magazine* (U.S. Figure Skating Association, 20 First St., Colorado Springs, CO 80906).

Suppliers

▶ Eagle River Nordic (P.O. Box 936, Eagle River, WI 54521; 800-423-9730). Mail order source for roller skis and Rollerblades.
▶ New Moon Ski-Shop (P.O. Box 132, Hayward, WI 54843; 715-643-8685). Mail order source for roller skis and Rollerblades.
▶ Rollerblades are available from North American Sports Training (9700 W. 76th St., Suite T, Minneapolis, MN 55344; 800-328-0171).

Other Outdoor Aerobic Activities

The less steady and rhythmic an exercise, the less beneficial it is aerobically. Popular sports such as tennis, handball, racquetball, squash, basketball, and soccer involve a great deal of stopping and starting. These sports are great fun and certainly provide fitness benefits, but unless you can ensure the *aerobic* quality of each game, don't let them take the place of other outdoor or indoor aerobic activities.

17 Aerobic Exercise: Indoor Options

WHEN WE HAVE DECIDED to get into shape, most of us think of doing it at home or in a fitness club, and indoor exercise is an essential part of the fitness equation. Statistics indicate that between 60 and 80 percent of all the Americans who exercise do it at home.

Indoor aerobic activities cost money — from $10 for a jump rope to $400 or more for a cross-country ski simulator, stationary cycle, or rowing machine. To cut costs, equipment can be shared with family members or close friends. Under the right conditions, some outdoor aerobic sports can be performed indoors. Enclosed swimming pools and indoor roller rinks, ice skating arenas, and running tracks are examples. Similarly, some of the aerobic exercises listed in this book as indoor can be performed outdoors by moving equipment outside onto the patio, lawn, or deck.

Once you've decided to exercise regularly at home, *where* you do it in your home becomes a factor. Working out in a dusty garage or dreary basement undercuts enthusiasm in all but the most dedicated exercisers. Pick an enjoyable, well-lighted space to be your personal exercise center. See that temperature is controlled and the area is well ventilated. If space is limited, you can reserve a room part-time for your exercise and select a fold-up ski machine, rower, or cycle.

Most people love their fitness sessions far more when they include variety, distraction, and excitement. Find various ways to spice up your indoor exercise: listen to music, talk on the phone, watch the news or a favorite television show, learn a foreign language, or listen to books or educational lectures on audiotapes.

Cross-Country Skiing Machines

Cross-country skiing provides a smooth, superb aerobic workout. That's because the legs, hips, abdomen, shoulders, back, chest, and arms all contribute to the gliding Nordic movements.

For decades, cross-country skiers wondered how to bring their favorite skiing indoors for those long months without snow. Finally, inventors designed Nordic machines that let us glide our way to aerobic fitness year-round in the comfort of health club or home.

The best Nordic ski machines combine two basic principles: gliding along a special pair of tracks with your feet and pulling with your arms using a resistance mechanism. They have a fully adjustable pelvic cushion to push against when you ski, keeping your body aligned and relaxed with good posture. The best ski machines are designed for an easy, natural stride that simulates skiing using a one-way clutch mechanism for more resistance on the rearward rather than the forward leg motion and feature foot cups so your feet don't slip as you glide forward and back.

Leg resistance is also adjustable — from a gentle glide that simulates crossing a meadow to the powerful leg drive you need to move uphill. Arm cords provide an adjustable, variable mechanism to give greatest resistance at the beginning of the arm motion on each stride just the way real Nordic skiing does. And they're strongly constructed to remain stable and secure when you exercise vigorously.

At the time of this writing, the two finest cross-country ski machines are the Precor 515E (Precor Inc., 20001 North Creek Pkwy., Box 3004, Bothell, WA 98041; 800-662-0606) and the NordicTrack (NordicTrack, Inc., 141 Jonathan Blvd. N., Chaska, MN 55318; 800-328-5888).

Stationary Cycling

When most people think of home exercise, they think of stationary bicycling. It's one of the safest, simplest ways to build strong legs and get a good aerobic workout. Several cycles even have handlebars that move back and forth as you pedal. This involves the arm, shoulder, and back muscles in the cycling exercise.

The quality of stationary bicycles varies tremendously. Most inexpensive models are poorly designed and uncomfortable. They fail to provide accurate readings of workload during exercise, give a shaky ride, make noise, and fall apart easily.

The better-quality indoor cycles come in two basic types: mechanical bikes and more expensive models laden with electronic monitors. Both can have built-in ergometers (derived from the Greek words *ergon* for power or energy and *metron* meaning measure), which calibrate your exact workload (speed/resistance/time) while you're riding the bike. This can help you duplicate workout intensities.

Well-designed stationary bicycles have some key features:

The frame is rigid for efficient pedaling action. The seat is wide, comfortable, well padded, stable, and adjustable, with a secure locking mechanism for each height increment. The pedals have a slip-resistant rubber or metal surface. Straps can help you work on both upstroke and downstroke.

The handlebars are easily adjustable to a comfortable height where your shoulders, neck, back, and arms are not imbalanced or tense. They have grips covered with a cushioned material that helps prevent your hands from slipping when you perspire. Resistance control is calibrated for easy resetting each time you cycle. The resistance mechanism is durable; caliper models and belt-around-flywheel devices are often used. In general, the bigger and heavier the flywheel, the smoother the ride.

Gauges are accessible and easy to read. A timer and odometer are helpful to record how long and how far you have ridden. A speedometer makes it easier to maintain a steady speed and stay within your target heart rate zone.

As stated in the outdoor cycling section, it's important to be able to adjust the seat so that your leg is almost fully extended (leave 10–15 degrees of flexion in the knee) — but not locked — at the lowest point of the pedaling circle. This helps balance leg muscles and prevent injury. A common mistake is to cycle at too high a level of resistance, which can cause knee and leg pain. A reasonable goal for most indoor cyclists is to keep your legs spinning between 50 and 100 rpm as you pedal in smooth circles.

Electronic Wizardry: Efficiency or Entertainment?

Electronic bikes are simply too expensive for most of us as home exercise units, but they're increasingly popular in many health clubs. Some super-high-tech models, like the Perceptronics LaserTour, cost as much as $20,000. Others are in the $1,200–$4,000 range. Electronic bikes offer computer-programmed workouts, pulse meters, caloric metabolism estimates, and even small television screens to help you avoid boredom. The fancy gadgetry and space age appearance make them entertaining, but most of us can achieve an effective, satisfying cycling workout for far less expense.

Choices in Stationary Bicycles

When it comes to top-quality stationary bicycles that most of us can afford, there are three basic categories: upright legs-only cycles, upright integrated cycles, and semirecumbent cycles.

Upright legs-only cycles. At the time of this writing, top moderately priced cycles in this category include the Tunturi Executive Ergometer W2 (Tunturi, Inc., P.O. Box 3825, Bellevue, WA 98009; 800-426-0858), the Precor 825e (Precor Inc., 20001 North Creek Pkwy., Box 3004, Bothell, WA 98041; 800-662-0606), and Monark Mark II Ergometer 865 (Monark-Universal Fitness, 50 Commercial St., Plainview, NY 11803).

Upright integrated cycles. The Schwinn Air-Dyne (Excelsior Fitness Equipment Co., 615 Landwehr Rd., Northbrook, IL 60062) is an example of a new cycling technology. While you pedal, a special set of alternating arm levers moves forward and backward. An air-displacement wheel provides automatic increases and decreases in resistance according to how fast you move the pedals or arm levers. You may cycle in a seated position using the legs alone, the arms alone, or any arm-leg combination.

Semirecumbent cycles. Semirecumbent exercise cycles are ridden in a reclining position on a special seat that resembles a chair, with your legs extended in front of you.

On upright bicycles, the full torso weight is placed on your buttocks. On semirecumbent bikes, your weight is distributed through the back, lower back, and buttocks, making the ride more comfortable.

At the time of this writing, the best value in top-quality semirecumbent cycles is the Precor 815e (Precor Inc., 20001 North Creek Pkwy., Box 3004, Bothell, WA 98041; 800-662-0606). Other, more expensive options include The Chair (Paramount Fitness Corp., 6450 E. Bandini Blvd., Los Angeles, CA 90040) and the Pro Tec PTS Turbo 10000 (Pro Tec Sports, Inc., 1965 E. Blair, Santa Ana, CA 92075).

Rowing Machines

Rowing machine sales have skyrocketed in recent years, partly because rowers provide aerobic benefits while strengthening both the upper and lower body. All this happens smoothly, without impact or strain to muscles and joints. Rowing machines for home and gym have sliding seats and, in some cases, ergometers to measure the energy or power being produced.

Many good rowing machines are available. Some expensive models — such as the Adams Ergometer from France and the Gjessing Ergo-Row Ergometer from Norway — feature electronic wizardry and computerized components and cost up to $5,000. In contrast, the least expensive rowers (some under $100) tend to be poorly made, unstable, and unsafe.

There are two main types of indoor rowing machines on the market: hydraulic cylinder units where the resistance comes from pulling against a hydraulic cylinder, which acts like a shock absorber; and straight-pull machines where a flywheel braked by a belt, fan, or electric motor provides the resistance load.

Like rowing shells, machines use a sliding seat that moves along a rail or track, so you can use your legs and arms together during each rowing stroke. And like racing shells, the best indoor rowers have seats that are contoured to your buttocks so you don't slip around and have tracks that decline slightly toward the feet, letting you recover more easily at the end of each rowing stroke.

The most popular rowing machines for at-home use are hydraulic. You pull the oarlike handles against pressure from hydraulic cylinders. These machines are compact, quiet during operation, easy to store between workouts, and generally less expensive than straight-pull rowers. The amount of resistance depends on where the hydraulic cylinder is clamped on to the pivoting arm of the machine. Good-quality rowers need at least five different adjustment settings; ten or more are best.

At the time of this writing, two of the best hydraulic rowing machines are the Precor M 6.2 (Precor Inc., 20001 North Creek Pkwy., Box 3004, Bothell, WA 98041; 800-662-0606) and Tunturi R203 (Tunturi, Inc., P.O. Box 3825, Bothell, WA 98009; 800-426-0858). Other options include the Monarch 633 (Universal Fitness Products, 20 Terminal Dr. So., Plainview, NY 11803) and Avita 970 (M & R Industries, 7140 180th Ave., N.E., Redmond, WA 98052).

Several experts suggest that hydraulic rowers place more stress on the back and arms than straight-pull flywheel machines do.[118] In some cases this may be due to incorrect exercise form rather than the rowing machine design itself. Other authorities believe that straight-pull flywheel rowing machines better simulate real rowing out on the water.[119]

Currently one of the top machines in this category is the Concept II (Concept II, Inc., RR1 Box 1100, Morrisville, VT 05661; 802-888-7971). It provides varied resistance from a wheel system with air flaps and chain ring. You can use a full range of body movements and choose from different resistance settings. Other excellent choices are the Coffey Indoor Rower and Sculling Simulator (Coffey Racing Shells, 48 E. 5th St., Corning, NY 14830; 607-962-1982), which simulate real water rowing.

The most common rowing machine error is overworking the back and upper-body muscles while underworking the legs. Remember, the primary action in seated rowing machines is leg-powered movements.

Aerobic Dance–Exercise

One of the most popular forms of cardiorespiratory exercise in recent years is aerobic dancing. "Until the advent of aerobic dancing, it seemed that nothing could bridge the gap between enjoyment and results," says Bryant Stamford, director of the Health Promotion and Wellness Center at the University of Louisville School of Medicine. "Putting movement patterns to music provides an opportunity for variety and creativity. Because aerobic dance is usually performed by a group of people, the camaraderie that develops adds to the fun. It is a safe bet that many people now engaged in aerobic dance would not be exercising at all if jogging were their only alternative."[120]

Researchers report that, if done properly, aerobic dancing is very effective in improving cardiovascular fitness.[121]

Reducing Injury Rates

Without careful instruction, the right environment, proper shoes, and good technique, the injury rate among aerobic dance instructors and students is high. One California study reported that 75 percent of the instructors and 43 percent of the students had been injured while dancing,[122] although subsequent reviews of the data indicate that actual injury rates were closer to 10 percent of instructors and 20 percent of students.[123] Another study reported the rate of injury was 26 percent for instructors and 29 percent for students, based on 100 hours of aerobic dance activity.[124] Overall, the area most vulnerable to injury was the shins, followed by the feet, back, knees, calves, and hips.

Most aerobic dance injuries result from four factors: poorly designed shoes, improper floor surface, ill-advised routines, and overtraining. All can be controlled.

Proper Shoes: A Major Issue

Aerobic dancing shoes must stabilize the foot, absorb shock, and minimize foot twisting (torquing). Dr. Jean Rosenbaum, director of the American Aerobics Association, heads an independent research group that conducts regular evaluations of aerobic dance footwear. (For current recommendations, write to Task Group for Aerobic Footwear, P.O. Box 401, Durango, CO 80301.)

Heel support, in which the foot is cupped firmly with good ankle and arch support, is critical. So is a padded Achilles tendon collar. Aerobic dance shoes must give support in two directions — along the anterior-posterior axis (front to back) and the medial-lateral axis (side to side).

According to sports medicine podiatrist Glenn Ocker, aerobic dance shoes should meet strict standards in the following areas:[125]

Forefoot shock absorbency: "A lot of aerobic-dance movements involve landing on the front of the foot, with considerable weight placed on the ball of the foot. Shoes [require] extra cushioning beneath the forefoot to reduce the shock impact between the foot and the floor."

Lateral foot stability: "Aerobic-dance movements include twisting and turning while the exerciser is on his/her toes. Shoes [should] hold the foot in place inside the shoe during these movements. Greater stress, which can lead to injury, is placed on the ankle and knee joints if the foot is able to roll outward or inward during these movements."

Rear foot stability: "Shoes [should] hold the heel in place during common aerobic-dance movements. If the rear of the foot slips up and down or side to side, the shoe is not giving enough support to the ankle and knee joints. Shoes with a rigid heel counter will usually hold the rear foot in place."

Floor Surface

The ideal floor for aerobic dancing is hardwood suspended on springs over an air space. Wood on beams is also all right, say researchers, as are several synthetic floors, now marketed in quick-fit pieces to accommodate any size room (Sentinel Fitness, 130 North St., Hyannis, MA 02601). Knowing to avoid concrete and similarly unyielding surfaces is fairly obvious, but the problems with thick carpet are not.

"As there are so many side-to-side motions in aerobics, peculiar to this form of exercise, . . . thick carpet is out," says Dr. Rosenbaum. "Side-to-side movements on high nap carpet cause the foot to grab and the ankle to snap rather than roll. Thin, high density industrial carpet . . . is acceptable."[126]

Warm Up, Cool Down, and Don't Overtrain

As with other aerobic exercises, warm-up and cool-down periods are essential to prevent injuries. It's also important not to overtrain — limit aerobic dance sessions to a maximum of 1 hour two to four times a week and choose other aerobic activities for nondance days.

Dance Routines

Aerobic dance routines must match the fitness level and abilities of each individual participant. Instructors need to allow time for accurate pulse taking during and after every workout to ensure that dancers stay within their personal target heart rate zones. Evidence suggests that with good shoes, an ideal floor surface, and a well-designed routine, many dancers can safely perform so-called high-impact aerobics.[127] But there are certain advantages to the style of aerobic dancing now referred to as low-impact aerobics.[128]

Low-impact aerobics, a softer form of aerobic dance, takes the jarring, jumping, and lunging moves out of the dance routines, replacing them with steps that don't force the joints and with nonballistic stretches that aren't bouncy. This makes it easier for many people to stay within their target heart rate zone. In low-impact aerobics, hops, jumps, and jogs are being replaced by sidesteps, marches, and simple dance/walk combinations in which one foot remains on the floor and the dancer uses rhythmic, continuous motion without forced effort.[129]

Hand Weights

Since the intensity level of traditional aerobic dance is difficult to maintain with low-impact routines, instructors often suggest that participants use their arms more — keeping them above heart level, moving them through a variety of full-range motions, and adding one-half-pound to two-pound hand or wrist weights.[130] Ankle weights are unnecessary and may be dangerous, contributing to strains and even dislocations.[131]

Aerobic Music

Music is an integral part of aerobic dancing. But music must be matched to the length of your desired aerobic session and, most important, to *your* target heart rate zone. If the music is too slow, you don't get a vigorous enough workout; if it's too fast, you overtrain. Computer technology has enabled music scientists to match the beats per minute of various popular music selections to approximate target heart rates for aerobic dancers. The Aerobic Music Service (Box 2688, Alameda, CA 94501; 415-521-1224) is a good source for aerobic exercise music tapes.

Power Aerobics and Martial Arts Aerobics

Power aerobics refers to aerobic dance routines to which light to moderate hand weights have been added. Some aerobic dance studios and videotapes offer this as an option. Stringent guidelines are necessary to prevent injuries. Avoid too much speed and momentum, emphasize right and left sides of the body equally, and keep elbows and knees at least slightly bent for shock absorption. Maintain good posture and select music that ensures a safe workout tempo.

Martial arts aerobics, another modification of aerobic dance, is becoming popular in America. It blends martial arts techniques with aerobic dance routines and provides aerobic exercise benefits and helps build useful self-defense skills.

There are many reasons for people to learn martial arts, and in recent years self-defense classes have become very popular. Some martial arts schools now offer aerobics classes. Be certain to select a program that emphasizes smooth, flowing, balanced movements.

Aerobic Dance Videotapes

Aerobic dance routines can be performed in the privacy of your own home using videotaped routines. A great array of workout tapes is available. Many promote poorly designed, high-impact routines and dangerous stretches and lack accurate or consistent heart rate monitoring. For current recommendations about aerobic exercise videotapes, contact the professional organizations listed below.

Certified Instructors   It takes up-to-date knowledge and advanced skills to be an outstanding aerobic dance–exercise instructor. The following organizations (listed alphabetically) are involved with setting new standards.

▶ American College of Sports Medicine (P.O. Box 1440, Indianapolis, IN 46206). Sponsors professional training programs and certification examinations.

▶ IDEA: International Dance-Exercise Association, Inc. (6190 Cornerstone Court East, Suite 204, San Diego, CA 92121). A leading professional organization that sponsors conferences and seminars and publishes *Dance-Exercise Today* magazine. The IDEA Foundation (6190 Cornerstone Court East, Suite 202, San Diego, CA 92121) develops new dance-exercise certification standards and publishes the excellent *Aerobic Dance-Exercise Instructor Manual*.

▶ The Institute for Aerobics Research (12330 Preston Rd., Dallas, TX 75230). Offers a series of training and certification programs for fitness specialists and group exercise leaders.

▶ Jazzercise (2808 Roosevelt St., Carlsbad, CA 92008). One of the largest aerobic dance programs in the world.

A note about social dance aerobics: There is a new name being given to the kind of fun dancing that many of us thought didn't contribute much to physical fitness. Research directed by Betty Rose Griffith, professor of education at California State University at Long Beach, indicates that a well-designed social dance routine — her test version used a 5-minute cha-cha warm-up, 4 minutes each of waltz, samba, polka, and swing, followed by a 5-minute cool-down — can produce aerobic benefits for many people.[132] For more information, contact Sodanceabit (1401 Anaheim Pl., Long Beach, CA 90804).

Jumping Rope

It's cheap, it's portable, it's strenuous, and it's fun. In addition, jumping rope, when properly performed, can be an excellent aerobic exercise.[133] U.S. Olympic Committee researchers report that skipping rope can be as effective for aerobic conditioning as running and subjects the bones and joints to less trauma since shock is distributed through the whole leg more efficiently than most running strides allow.[134]

The American Heart Association sponsors a "Jump Rope for Heart" program across America, stating that jumping rope "can be an enjoyable way to maintain cardiovascular fitness; can provide vigorous exercise in a minimum amount of space; can be used as an individual or team activity; is simple enough for a six year old to master, while complicated enough to challenge a well-coordinated athlete; can encourage vigorous lifelong activity through development of rhythm, agility and coordination."[135]

Proper Posture, Shoes, and Floor Surface

For jumping rope, good athletic shoes are a must, and women should always wear a jogging bra (see running/jogging section earlier). The best floor surface is one that few of us have access to: the hardwood, spring-suspended floor mentioned under aerobic dancing. Carpeted and padded exercise surfaces or a level grassy lawn are good choices, far superior to concrete.

Maintaining good posture is a must when jumping rope. Keep your head up, neck long and relaxed, shoulders broad and loose, back straight, knees bent, arms relaxed, and elbows bent about 45 degrees. Use your wrists to control the rope, and keep your vision straight ahead to avoid the tendency to watch your shoetops while skipping. Jumping in front of a full-length mirror can help you monitor proper technique.

Selecting a Jump Rope

Choose a jump rope that fits your height and body structure. Generally, the correct length is such that the handles reach your armpits when you stand with both feet on the center of the rope and pull it straight up.

There are many rope designs in the American fitness marketplace. The clothesline rope is the old standby. The handles should be large enough to be held relaxed in your hands, and the rope material should be one that minimizes tangling. The beaded jump rope is a colorful, lightweight option for beginning jumpers that adds a rhythmic whooshing sound on each revolution. Avoid sloppy techniques, however, since they can result in stinging contact to the ankles or shins.

The Gyro-Jump (Gyro-Jump, P.O. Box 4500, Laguna Beach, CA 92652) features longer handles that permit a variety of jumping styles and improve upper-body fitness. Ball bearing handles give smooth, easy rotations. Intermediate and advanced jumpers can perform a rhythmic rowing-type action with the upper body. The Heavyrope (Heavyrope, Inc., 1638 Leonard, N.W., Grand Rapids, MI 49504) is a unique, weighted jump rope made from a stretchy rubber tube filled with sand-like silica beads. Heavyropes are available in 1-to-5-pound weights. Each revolution of the rope provides a dynamic strengthening action for the upper body combined with an aerobic workout. This can be a pleasant change-of-pace in your workout routine and is popular with many athletes.

Technique

Jump high enough for your feet to barely clear the rope as it passes beneath them just above the floor surface. You don't need to jump high to achieve benefits; in fact, skilled rope jumpers who can skip at high speeds scarcely leave the ground with their feet on each revolution of the rope. Don't grip the handles too tightly or tense your shoulders, neck, arms, or back. When first jumping, your goal should be to make single jumps with both legs on each arm turn (one complete circular revolution of the rope). To learn more, see *Jump! The New Jump Rope Book* by Susan Kalbfteisch (William Morrow, 1985), a good basic book by the coach of the Canadian Heart Association skipping team.

Other Indoor Aerobic Options

Other indoor aerobic fitness options include the following.

▶ Climbers. Two good ones are the very affordable legs-only Precor 718e Fitness Climber (Precor, Inc., Box 3004, Bothell, WA 98041; 800-662-0606) and the elite hand/arm/leg VersaClimber (Heart Rate, 3186-G Airway Ave., Costa Mesa, CA 92626; 800-237-2271).
▶ Motorized treadmills and stairs.
▶ Slideboards. One of my favorite lateral-motion training devices lets me perform aerobic skating techniques in heavy socks on a flat, compact, foldable device with adjustable end stops. A patented roll-up version is also on the market. (Amskate, P.O. Box 255, Syosset, NY 11791.)
▶ No-cost options, such as indoor walking programs, running in place, and stair stepping.

18 Strength and Endurance Exercises

Strengthening, Firming, Toning, Shaping

Whatever your body type, is there a difference between the physique you want and the one that faces you in the mirror every morning? It's easier than you may think to change that body shape, and one of the keys is strengthening your muscles.

More than four hundred muscles keep your body firm — or let it sag. If those muscles aren't made strong and balanced in relationship to each other — and kept that way through a weekly fitness program — they slowly wither as time goes by. Muscular strength and endurance exercises are the focus of this chapter. Contrary to popular myth, research shows they are as important for women as for men.

Abdominal exercises (Chapter 13) and posture exercises (Chapters 14 and 15) strengthen certain key muscles. Aerobic fitness programs (Chapters 16 and 17) build strength and endurance, too, sometimes in isolated body areas (such as the legs in cycling, running, skating, or walking) and at other times in several areas (such as the arms, shoulders, back, and legs in cross-country skiing or rowing). But we each need to take additional steps to guarantee that we're shaping and toning all four hundred skeletal muscles, not just a handful. And this chapter is about doing just that, as quickly and enjoyably as possible.

The dividends are many. With healthy, well-toned muscles, your body is balanced, better coordinated, and more vibrant. You can do more of what you want wherever you want to do it. You will be better able to resist fatigue, and your joints will become protected against common strains and pains that debilitate millions of Americans and turn millions more into chronic grumps and grouches. Most of these aches and injuries, scientists say, are caused by weak, imbalanced muscles and can be corrected by simple exercises suitable for men and women of all ages.

In this chapter, you'll learn how to design your own bare-minimum muscle-toning program that takes not a single extra minute of exercise time; or to go through a full-body workout where all you need are some ankle weights, light dumbbells, a flat bench, and two chairs; or to select the best values in strength-building home gyms; or to choose a health club with equipment and staff to help you achieve fast, safe results.

Muscular Strength and Endurance

Muscular strength is defined as the greatest force your muscles can produce in a complete single effort. Strength exercises are sometimes called "progressive resistance training." Muscular endurance is a muscle's ability to perform continued repetitions of the same movement. This shouldn't be confused with cardiovascular endurance, which is generally thought of as aerobic fitness.

When most Americans think of muscular strength and endurance training today, their image is of bodybuilding or weight training. They picture sweaty gyms; "no-pain, no-gain" posters; long lines of disciples crammed into big pieces of equipment and under heavy weights; burly instructors standing over them telling them how great it all is — and blocking thoughts of cheating or escape; and stiff, sore muscles in bed the next morning and probably all of next week. An accurate picture? In most cases, not any longer.

By definition, bodybuilding involves the use of progressive resistance training to create a balanced, muscular physique, usually with free weights and special machines. Weight training and strength training also utilize resistance techniques and are undertaken to build maximized strength in certain areas of the body or for a specialized sport or activity. The popularity of bodybuilding and weight training has soared in America in recent years, and a wave of new fitness centers and home gyms brings muscular strength and endurance exercise within easy reach of us all.

The List of Benefits Keeps Growing

In addition to benefits in muscle tone and shape, strength exercises build stronger, healthier bones[136] and more. The *Journal of the American Medi-*

cal Association recently published the results of a 16-week study on strength training for men and women conducted at the Oregon Health Sciences University.[137] The researchers reported that "the findings were more impressive than had been suspected"; they discovered that, for both men and women, regular strength training of sufficient intensity (described later in this section) generally led to modest improvements in blood cholesterol profiles (see cholesterol discussion in Chapter 22) and increased lean body mass and exercise ability (improving a dramatic 100 percent for both men and women), even though the participants did not change dietary habits during the study. Other recent studies report health benefits and attest to the safety of progressive resistance training.[138]

Synergistic Approach

Synergy, one of the guiding principles for *Health & Fitness Excellence,* is also the master plan for your muscles. Synergy means that the results of a concerted, unified effort can be far greater than the simple sum of the individual parts of that effort.

Throughout the twentieth century, some exercise scientists and equipment designers have claimed that the way to develop the greatest strength was to totally isolate big single muscles. While potentially valuable for rehabilitative medicine, this theory went far beyond that. It ushered in our present era whose philosophy is that it takes dozens of different specialized weight machines to strengthen the whole body. Don't believe it.

When it comes to muscles, size isn't directly proportional to importance. Some of the smallest muscles play the biggest roles. If knotted with tension or pain, the tiniest spinal rotator muscle or the little popliteus at the back of the knee can immobilize you just as quickly as a tight hamstring or shoulder muscle. Your muscles are a team — with more than four hundred members. The smaller structural muscles must be strengthened along with the larger, more dominant muscles if synergy is to be respected and balanced strength and endurance achieved.

"Isolation is not only impossible, but undesirable," says Frederick C. Hatfield, exercise scientist, world power-lifting champion, and editor of *Sports Fitness* magazine. "Synergy is the goal. Synergistic action from surrounding muscles allows for greater overload, fewer injuries, more controlled movement, fuller bodypart development and greater overall . . . strength."[139]

In any given exercise movement, muscles called *prime movers* perform the predominant motion, assisted by dozens of helper muscles called *synergists*. Still other muscles have an indispensable role as *stabilizers,* securing a limb or joint while the prime mover and synergist muscles carry out the motion. *Antagonists* are opposing muscles that can reverse the movement on command and, in some cases, provide assistance as synergists, neutralizers, or stabilizers.

Let's look at an example: the bicep curl exercise, a familiar movement in which the arm is flexed at the elbow and the palm side of the hand is brought up toward the front of the shoulder. This "most simple of all bodybuilding exercises . . . provides a classic example of synergism," says Dr. Hatfield. "No fewer than eight different muscles are involved in this exercise, with a score more acting as stabilizers of the shoulder girdle, trunk and lower body. The eight biceps 'movers' that act synergistically are the biceps brachii, brachialis, brachioradialis, pronator teres, flexor carpi longus, flexor carpi ulnaris, palmaris longus and flexor digitorum superficialis." Even the simplest strengthening exercises must utilize synergy for best results.

An understanding of such synergistic effects is important in planning a weekly program that tones the entire body, not just a few favored areas.

To achieve balanced results, without any weak points, first take a look at what strength and endurance benefits you're already receiving from other parts of your fitness program and then choose the fastest, easiest ways to take care of those muscles not yet being toned.

Option 1: The Bare Minimum

If you feel especially pressed for time, this is the option to consider first. As with aerobic exercises, when speaking of strength and endurance, the question How much do I need to do? is often a polite way of saying, How little can I get away with?

If you step back and survey your weekly fitness schedule, you can build in strength and endurance benefits without spending any extra time by combining the following groups of exercises:

1 *Aerobic exercises* (Chapters 16 and 17) that build strength and endurance in the greatest number of body areas. Cross training — selecting several different aerobic activities every week — is even better than sticking with one type of exercise. Some combined upper-body/lower-body aerobic sports are (alphabetically) aerobic dance with hand or wrist weights; cross-country skiing or ski machines; jumping rope with a weighted rope; outdoor rowing or indoor rowing machines; integrated stationary cycling; swimming; walking, jogging, running, or skating with light hand or wrist weights.

2 *Basic abdominal exercises* (Chapter 13) and *posture exercises* (Chapters 14 and 15) following the sample schedules given in those chapters.

It's also valuable to choose recreational sports (on weekends, vacations, and family outings) that strengthen some of the major muscle areas you don't catch with numbers 1 and 2 above. For example, if your favorite aerobic choices are legs-only cycling and walking without hand weights, select recreational activities like canoeing or kayaking (on peaceful waters), tennis, racquetball, squash, handball, softball, or basketball (using both hands and both arms to paddle, hit, catch, or throw). In other words, choose fun activities where you use your muscles to reach, lift, rotate, push, and pull in different ways from your regular aerobics routines.

Option 2: More Comprehensive Strength and Endurance Training

For best overall fitness, at some point you'll want to take strength and endurance training at least one step further. That means scheduling some weekly time — a lot less than most people think — for specific exercises. These may be performed without equipment (body weight resistance or dynamic isometrics) or with equipment (rubber tubing, dumbbells, barbells, or machine weights).

The rest of this chapter discusses more intensive strength and endurance training, beginning with several scientific principles and followed by methods without equipment and with equipment. Next is an example of what I call a streamlined home routine, designed with minimal equipment (ankle weights, a set of dumbbells, a flat bench, and two chairs) for people on a tight budget. And finally, I'll help you sort through the confusing choices in equipment and home gyms, ranging from garage sale bargains on dumbbells and barbells through compact home gyms that take up a few feet of floor space but let you perform dozens of different exercises and including ideas on top-of-the-line equipment for your business or neighborhood fitness center.

Once you get past the beginning and early-intermediate levels of strength training, you'll benefit from an encyclopedic, illustrated resource guide that gives a wide variety of safe exercise options for every part of the body. One book is particularly noteworthy: *Getting Stronger: Weight Training for Men and Women* by Bill Pearl and Gary T. Moran, Ph.D. (Shelter Publications/HP Books, 1986; available from Bill Pearl Enterprises, P.O. Box 1080, Phoenix, OR 97535; 503-535-3363). Another highly regarded book is *Getting Built* by Dr. Lynne Pirie (Warner Books, 1984), which focuses on bodybuilding for women.

Basic Scientific Principles and Guidelines for Strength and Endurance Training

To get the most out of strength and endurance exercises, it pays to first become familiar with some scientific guidelines. Muscular strength and endurance are increased by forcing muscles to make "specific adaptation to imposed demands" (sometimes called the SAID principle). In other words, you must regularly exercise each part of your body with enough intensity (resistance) to elicit what is known as an "adaptation response," stimulating your muscle cells to become stronger and healthier.

Progressive resistance exercise (PRE) is the safe, proven way to develop strength and endurance. Resistance in this sense can come from body weight, rubber tubing, machine weights, barbells, dumbbells, variable resistance devices, or other measures. In essence, PRE is the introduction of a specific level of resistance into a series of exercises; the level is then increased in small increments from week to week. This safely stimulates your muscles to adapt to the workload, leading to increased strength and stamina.

Isometric exercises cause tension in a stationary position with no motion of the body limbs. There's some shortening of the muscle fibers but no true movement. An example of isometrics is pushing hard against an immovable object such as a wall.

In *isotonic exercise,* a body part is moved and the muscle shortens or lengthens. Although sit-ups, push-ups, and pull-ups are isotonic, lifting free weights (dumbbells and barbells) is considered the classic form of isotonic exercise.

Isokinetic exercise is a specialized type of isotonics in which a device provides accommodating resistance, that is, resistance that can be varied by special cams and rolling levers in a machine to theoretically help you maximize effort throughout a full range of motion. Some expensive weight machines provide this type of resistance.

Breathing patterns vary somewhat with each exercise but the normal recommendation is to exhale during the increase of resistance and inhale during the lowering of resistance. Some authorities suggest a short, quick inhalation (usually through the mouth) just prior to the most difficult part of the exercise followed by a smooth, fast exhalation as the repetition is completed. Above all, don't hold your breath.

In most cases, a resistance representing 60 to 85 percent of a muscle's force-generating capacity is sufficient intensity to produce significant strength gains. Lower resistance, in the 60–70 percent range, makes it easier to perform higher numbers of repetitions for muscular endurance, whereas more maximal efforts, toward the 80–85 percent intensity level, lower the number of repetitions needed for strength development.

Reps and Sets

A *repetition* ("rep") is an individual full cycle of an exercise; for example, a traditional bicep curling exercise requires that the weight in your hands (palms out, arms down at a level below the waist) is raised (bending the arms at the elbows) from about mid-thigh level up to the front of the shoulder and back down to the starting position. The whole motion is a single repetition.

As a general guideline for beginners, between 6 and 15 repetitions of any exercise is recommended; 6–10 reps build muscular strength and 10–15 reps emphasize muscular endurance. Some fitness specialists suggest that two body areas particularly dense in muscle fibers — the forearms and calves (lower legs) — may require extra repetitions (12–25) for maximum benefits.[140]

A *set* is a group of repetitions performed in sequence. A good starting point for beginners is one to two sets. For example, let's say you decide to do two different strength and endurance exercises each for the chest, back, shoulders, and arms — eight exercises in all. Each is to be performed for 6 to 10 repetitions. Starting with the first chest exercise, select the resistance level or poundage to perform between 6 and 10 smooth, controlled repetitions (the weight is correct if the last rep is fairly hard to perform — you feel tired in a positive way, you're temporarily expended but will recover once you get a quick rest). Pause briefly (not more than 5–10 seconds in most cases) and then do 6 to 10 reps of the second chest exercise. This completes the *first set* for the chest.

After another brief rest interval (usually 60–90 seconds), go on to do one set of exercises for the other body parts. Then, if you decide to do two sets, begin with chest exercises again. Some trainers suggest performing both sets for one body part before going on. To do this, you would finish the first set of chest exercises, rest briefly, and then repeat the chest exercises for set two. Then proceed through the other body parts, doing two sets for each.

In general, don't stop to rest between exercise repetitions *within* a set. Between sets, a rest interval of 60–90 seconds may be taken. It's important that your breathing return to normal before beginning the next set of exercises. This will be challenging to your mind, since your body won't fully recover in this brief minute. Your muscles will feel like they've worked hard, but safely. It's a good, confidence-boosting feeling. The short rest intervals also give you an opportunity to focus your mind on the next exercise.

It's important not to rest longer than necessary since "if you rest more than ninety seconds before starting the next set, . . . you risk allowing your body to cool down, which makes your muscles and joints more susceptible to injury," says women's bodybuilding champion and sports medicine specialist Dr. Lynne Pirie.[141]

Overtraining — exercising too much or too often — can be avoided by keeping workouts well organized and brief. In general, beginning-level strength and endurance exercise routines can be completed in 15–30 minutes per session (see the examples later in the chapter).

Training Frequency and Routines

You need adequate rest time between workouts. Exercise physiologists have determined that, after being intensively exercised, a muscle needs about 48 hours — sometimes 72 hours — of rest to make maximal fitness gains.

Consistent, safe improvements can be accomplished using a split routine with a 72-hour rest interval between exercise sessions. In the beginning, you may elect to do strength and endurance exercises just once a week. That's fine, but soon you'll probably want to consider twice a week, which will produce greater results.

If you decide on two strength and endurance workouts per week, here's an example of a common routine, called a four-day split. The strength and endurance exercise sets are divided into two basic sections: For example, perform all of the upper body part exercises in one workout — say on Monday and Thursday — and all of the lower body part (leg) sets in another — Tuesday and Friday. (Sample weekly schedules are given in Chapter 11.)

Safety Factors and Preparations

Your mind and muscles are closely connected. Take several minutes before each session to relax, become aware of the present moment, clear your mind, and visualize your upcoming exercises. Studies report that these factors significantly influence results.[142] Specific positive-on-positive thoughts (Chapter 44) and focused concentration (Chapter 45) may be used to increase the neuromuscular excitation of the muscle fibers for greater involvement in exercise movements, creating safer, more rapid improvements.

Most safety tips are obvious: comfortable clothes that hug the body enough not to get snagged on equipment; good-fitting athletic shoes with nonskid soles; bright lighting; safe, sturdy equipment; training gloves for a firm grip and a training belt for abdominal and lower-back support if you are lifting near-maximal weights; and perhaps an exercise partner to boost motivation and act as a "spotter" for an extra safety margin on some exercises. Warm-up and cool-down periods are essential.

Finally, and most important of all, listen to your body. Begin slowly. Choose resistance levels and numbers of reps and sets with care so you stay within reasonable limits. No coach or trainer can know how you feel inside — personal energy varies from day to day, hour to hour. The right exercises will never leave you wrapped in pain or fatigue. Instead, they'll refresh and stimulate you toward better health and performance. Pay attention — and have fun.

Strength and Endurance Exercise Methods Without Equipment

Isometrics

While beneficial in certain rehabilitative and sports training situations, static isometric exercises are of limited value in a time-effective general fitness program. That's because this kind of strength development is highly specific, that is, the strength gained during isometric exercises is limited to the precise angle at which you hold your joint. For example, if you perform an isometric contraction by lifting up against an immovable countertop with bent elbows, your muscles will be stronger in that precise bent-elbow position but not when the arm is more flexed or extended.

Dynamic tension contractions (sometimes called dynamic isometrics or iso-tension exercises) use very slow movement. They offer the advantage of developing strength throughout the full range of movement for each muscle group being trained.

Once you have learned a strengthening routine and know the feeling of using weight resistance, you can perform dynamic tension exercises effectively. Soviet exercise scientists report that using mental imagery while performing weight training exercise movements *without* weights increases not only strength but also speed of movement and coordination.[143]

Dynamic isometric techniques are slow, smooth movements with contractive tension levels of 60 to 85 percent. They can be "imagery copies" of virtually any weight resistance exercise. The movement through a full range of motion gives dynamic tension a decided advantage over traditional frozen-position isometrics.

You may want to study the following streamlined at-home routine and go through it using body weight resistance, ankle weights, or dumbbells as directed. Then try the whole routine without weight resistance, providing your own imaginary resistance — tensing your muscles pretending you are still lifting the same body weight, ankle weight, or dumbbell.

Body Weight Resistance

It is also possible to create a strength and endurance routine using body weight as resistance. Push-ups, sit-ups, and dips are examples of this type of exercise.

Strength and Endurance Exercise Methods with Equipment

Rubber Tubing

Although exercises using rubber bands and surgical tubing have been around for years, the American Academy of Family Practitioners (AAFP) recently designed an exercise program called The Bodyband Workout (Feeling Fine Programs, Inc., 3575 Cahuenga Blvd. West, Los Angeles, CA 90068), complete with rubber bands and safety-conscious instruction. This form of resistance training involves holding the ends of a stretchy rubber band or tube with your hands or your feet while you perform a variety of exercises using the band or tube as resistance throughout each movement. While it won't produce the complete results possible with free weights or machines (or the streamlined at-home program presented in this chapter), it can be a good first step for some people. Similar rubber bands are available from SPRI Products, Inc. (962 N. Northwest Hwy., Park Ridge, IL 60068; 800-222-7774).

The premier rubber tubing system is the Lifeline Gym (Lifeline International Inc., 325 118th Ave., S.E., Suite 115, Seattle, WA 98009; 800-553-6633). Used by professional and Olympic athletes for special conditioning and when traveling, the Lifeline Gym is well designed and fun to use. It comes in a compact bag and includes cables, several handles, a bar, and basic instructions. Cable resistance is adjustable over a range of settings from number 1 (very light tension for injury rehabilitation) through 10 (advanced strength training enthusiasts), and more than twenty exercises can be performed. It is a good way to start strength and endurance training and, if you move up to a home gym or join a fitness club, the Lifeline can be used when you travel.

Free Weights and Associated Equipment

Most free weight exercise programs utilize barbells and dumbbells along with basic associated equipment such as leg flexion-extension benches, incline-decline benches, wrist rollers, cable pulleys, and rowing devices. Free weights have been used effectively in strength training programs for many years.

Machines

Unlike free weights, machines limit the plane of motion for each exercise and can restrict the development of synergistic and stabilizer muscles vital to balanced fitness. In some cases, machines don't provide for size adjustments (height, leg length, and arm reach) and force some users into stressful positions with higher risk of injury. And then there's expense: advanced machines are often beyond the financial reach of small home gyms and many health clubs.

Resistive exercise machines do offer several advantages over free weights. They allow you to train alone (a partner or spotter is important in some free weight exercises), may take up less space, and are usually somewhat faster to use (since they cut down on the time it takes to change barbell and dumbbell weight plates).

Constant-resistance devices are basic weight machines that employ a similar principle to barbells and dumbbells: as muscles contract through the range of movement at a particular joint, the weight feels relatively lighter or heavier at each degree of the motion even though the weight itself doesn't change. This is called constant resistance and has produced solid results over the years.

Variable-resistance devices are high-technology weight resistance machines that use special cams, rolling levers, and other devices to vary the amount of resistance, supposedly to match leverage and strength curves, thereby helping (at least in theory) the muscles carry a steady resistance through each entire movement. Newer, very expensive "accommodating resistance devices" (also called isokinetic machines) take the process a step further.

The bottom line: "Space age appearances of many machines lull users into believing that high technology equals maximum efficiency in achieving fitness goals — a sentiment that is definitely not true," says Dr. Hatfield. "Nothing beats hard work in promoting fitness. . . . I'd like to point out that all champion body builders use free weights as well as machines. While the majority of their workouts are performed with free weights, it has long been understood that in some instances machines are more effective than barbells and dumbbells. It is impossible to be more explicit in pinpointing the actual exercises that are best performed with machines. Each body builder and athlete has his or her own particular needs, anatomical structure and temperament. When you go to your spa or gym, experiment with both. Discover which method yields the best results."[144]

Streamlined, At-Home Starting Routine

Here is one example of a simple, balanced at-home strength and endurance routine suitable for beginners and early intermediates, both men and women. Equipment needed: a set of dumbbells, several pairs of ankle weights (you'll need to experiment to find the right safe but challenging poundages), a flat, stable bench, and two sturdy chairs.

Remember the guidelines presented earlier in this chapter and the fact that abdominal, lower-back, and posture exercises are given separately in Chapters 13–15. I have arranged the exercises in upper body and lower body categories because I recommend splitting the routine into separate days. Exercises listed under one body part — for example, chest — may actually benefit muscles in several areas — chest, shoulders, arms, and back. To keep things simple, I have listed the muscles by general area only, with the exception of the arms (front of the upper arms are listed as biceps, rear of upper arms as triceps). Instead of writing which specific parts of the shoulder muscle group (front, lateral, or rear) are emphasized in a given exercise, I've simply written "shoulders."

For fastest, safest results, keep all movements slow and smooth — under your complete control.

Upper-Body Routine Total time required (twice through these nine exercises, 6–10 repetitions of each): Maximum 30 minutes.

Warm-up

Standing in place, slowly move your arms in all directions without straining — up over your head, across in front of your chest, toward the back on both sides, pushing and pulling in front of you, and so on. Move the neck, shoulders, arms, and spine in the same way the dynamic flexibility exercises were described in Chapter 14. Take several minutes.

Before you begin, take another minute to lightly jog in place on a padded floor surface or lawn, moving your arms comfortably but vigorously to increase blood flow to upper-body muscles.

Chest

1. Push-ups

For chest, shoulders, and triceps. Choose one of three options below.

Wall Push-up

Starting position: Stand about arm's length away from a wall, feet about shoulder width apart, knees slightly bent, arms extended at mid-chest height, palms against the wall (see Figure 18.1).

Movement performance: Keeping your posture aligned (head and neck on line with a straight back), slowly lean forward at the ankles and hips by bending your elbows until your forehead and nose lightly touch

Figure 18.1   **Figure 18.2**

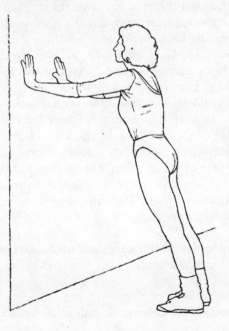
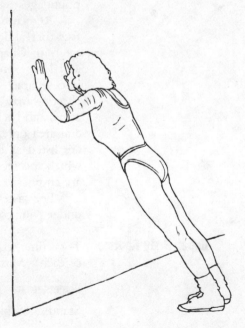

the wall (Figure 18.2). Pause for a second and then use your arm, chest, and shoulder muscles to push back to starting position. With practice, you'll be able to switch to the next two push-up options.

Beginning Push-up

Starting position: As shown in Figure 18.3, kneel on all fours on a padded floor surface, hands about shoulder width apart and positioned slightly ahead of your shoulders, feet facing straight back with toes pointing down, torso in a straight line (if this is too difficult, then slide your knees forward a bit, buttocks above them, back parallel to the floor).

Figure 18.3

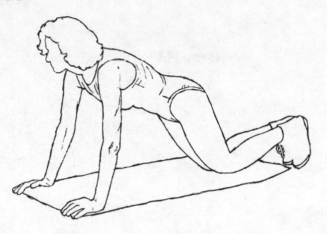

Movement performance: Slowly bend your elbows and lower your body as a unit, chest and chin moving down to nearly touch the floor (Figure 18.4), and then push back up. Don't lock the elbows. Repeat the desired number of repetitions.

Standard Push-up

Starting position: As shown in Figure 18.5, kneel on all fours on a padded floor surface, hands about shoulder width apart and positioned directly beneath your shoulders. Extend the legs straight back, supported by the balls of your feet. Keep your torso in a straight line.

Movement performance: Slowly, smoothly bend your elbows and lower your body as a unit, chest and chin moving down to nearly touch the floor (Figure 18.6), and then push back up. Don't lock the elbows. Repeat the desired number of repetitions.

Figure 18.4

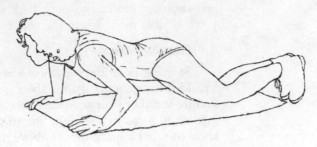

Figure 18.5

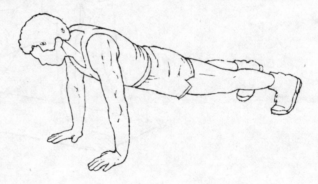

Figure 18.6

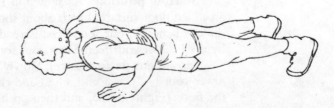

Note on the beginning and standard push-up variations: To increase the work for the chest muscles, move your hands out a little wider than shoulder width. For extra work on the triceps (muscles at the back of the upper arms) move your hands closer together, making an inverted *V* with your index fingers close to each other, palms farther apart.

2. Modified Dip 1

For chest, shoulders, triceps, and back.

Starting position: Place two sturdy, stable chairs about 24 inches apart, as shown in Figure 18.7. Bend your knees and position yourself with your feet on the floor directly beneath your buttocks between the two chairs, as shown in Figure 18.7. Use your legs to help raise and lower you, assisting your shoulders, chest, and arms. (Over time, use your legs less and less, eventually extending them in front of you as shown in Figure 18.9.)

Movement performance: Slowly lower yourself, bending your arms — with elbows moving out to the sides, not behind your back — until you feel a gentle stretch on your chest muscles (Figure 18.8), then

Figure 18.7

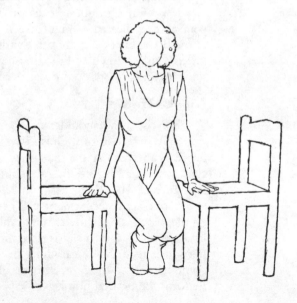

Figure 18.8

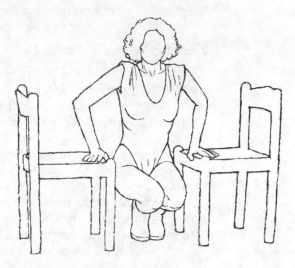

slowly extend your arms to push yourself back up to the starting position with your chest up. Keep the tops of your shoulders down — don't let them rise up toward your ears — as you lower yourself. Don't lock your elbows. Perform the desired number of repetitions.

Note: Once the basic exercise becomes very easy for you, position yourself as indicated in Figure 18.9, with legs extended toward the front of the body, knees slightly bent, and heels on the floor. Smoothly, slowly lower yourself down and then raise yourself back up to this starting position. Perform the desired number of repetitions.

3. Dumbbell Flyes

For chest and shoulders.

Starting position: Grasp two light dumbbells and lie back on a flat bench with feet flat on the floor, arms extended straight up from the chest with dumbbells lightly touching and elbows slightly bent, as shown in Figure 18.10.

Movement performance: Keeping your elbows bent and back flat on the bench, slowly lower the dumbbells out to the sides in a semicircular arc until you feel a slight stretching sensation in the chest muscles. Do not lower them below shoulder height (Figure 18.11). Then return the dumbbells along the same semicircular arcs back to the starting position. Perform the desired number of repetitions.

Figure 18.9

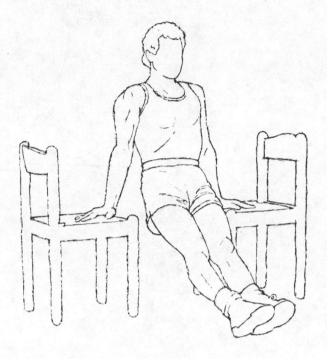

Upper Back

4. Bent-Over Rowing

For the back.

Starting position: Stand to the left of a flat bench or stable chair with a dumbbell in your left hand. Extend your left leg back about 18 inches to the rear and keep both knees bent. Bend over from the hips, place your right palm on the bench or chair seat for support and to brace your torso, keeping your right elbow slightly bent (Figure 18.12).

Movement performance: With your left hand held so the palm is facing your body's midline, slowly pull the dumbbell up until it lightly touches the side of your ribcage, rotating the left shoulder slightly upward at the top of the movement (Figure 18.13). Slowly lower the dumbbell back down to the starting position. Perform the desired number of repetitions with the left hand, then switch positions and put the dumbbell in your right hand. Perform the desired number of repetitions.

Figure 18.10

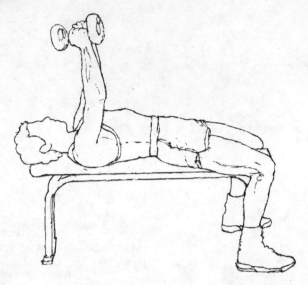

Figure 18.11

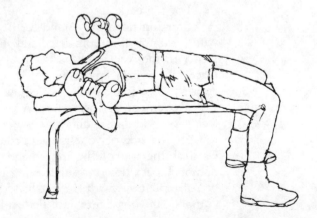

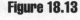

Figure 18.12   Figure 18.13

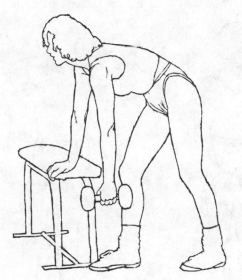

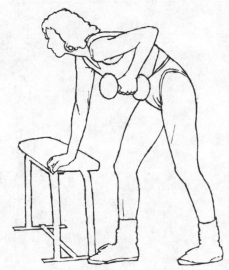

Shoulders

5. Side Lateral Raises

For the shoulders.

Starting position: Grasp two light dumbbells and stand with your feet about shoulder width apart. Stand with erect posture, knees slightly bent, and upper body leaning slightly forward from the hips. With palms facing each other, arms bent slightly, bring the dumbbells lightly together several inches in front of your hips (Figure 18.14).

Movement performance: With the elbows remaining bent throughout the entire movement, slowly raise the dumbbells in semicircular arcs out to the side and upward until they are approximately shoulder height (Figure 18.15). As you raise the dumbbells, pretend you have pitchers of water in each hand and are going to water some plants hanging about shoulder level. As you reach the top of the movement, rotate your shoulders (not wrists or arms) forward slightly so that the front weight of the dumbbell moves a bit lower than the rear, as if you were pouring water onto the imaginary plants. Slowly lower your arms back in the same semicircular arcs to the starting position. Perform the desired number of repetitions.

Figure 18.14   **Figure 18.15**

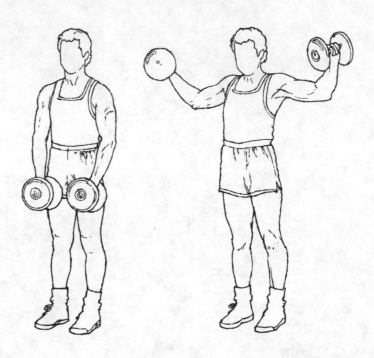

6. Upright Rowing

For shoulders and back.

Starting position: Grasp two light dumbbells and stand with your feet about shoulder width apart, elbows slightly bent, dumbbells resting just in front of your upper thighs (Figure 18.16). Lean the upper body slightly forward (bending at the hips) to avoid arching your back during the movement.

Movement performance: Keeping your elbows bent and the dumbbells about 10 inches apart and close to the body, slowly pull the dumbbells straight up until they reach collarbone height (Figure 18.17). The elbows will end up above your hands and about shoulder height at the top of the movement, shoulders rotated slightly to the rear. Slowly lower the dumbbells back to the starting position. Perform the desired number of repetitions.

Figure 18.16

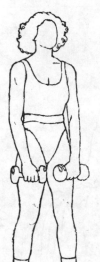

Figure 18.17

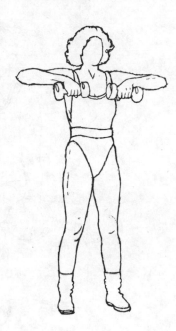

Arms

7. Bicep Curls

For the front of upper arms.

Starting position: Grasp two dumbbells and sit on a stable chair or bench, with good erect posture, arms extended downward with elbows slightly bent, palms facing the sides of your legs (Figure 18.18).

Movement performance: Alternately curl the right and left arms up in front of the body to the shoulder (Figure 18.19), rotating the hands so your palms are facing your shoulders at the top of the movement. Lightly press the insides of your upper arms against the sides of your torso and keep them in this position throughout the upper part of the movement. Slowly lower your hand to the starting position as the other hand comes up. Perform the desired number of repetitions.

8. Modified Dip 2

For the triceps — back of upper arms, chest, shoulders, and back.

Starting position: This is similar to Modified Dip 1, but it shifts

Figure 18.18   **Figure 18.19**

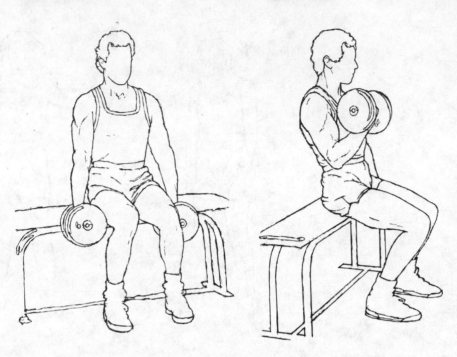

the emphasis from the chest to the triceps. Place two sturdy, stable chairs about 24 inches apart. Position yourself as shown in Figure 18.20, with knees bent and feet on the floor directly beneath your buttocks between the two chairs. Use your legs to help raise and lower your body, assisting your shoulders, chest, and arms.

Movement performance: Slowly, smoothly lower yourself by bending your arms — with elbows pointing behind you — until you feel a gentle stretch on your chest muscles (Figure 18.21), then smoothly extend your arms to push yourself back up to the starting position. Keep the tops of your shoulders down — don't let them rise up toward your ears — as you lower yourself. Don't lock your elbows. Perform the desired number of repetitions.

Note: Over time, you may be able to use your legs less and less, eventually extending them in front of you as shown in Figures 18.22 and 18.23.

Figure 18.20

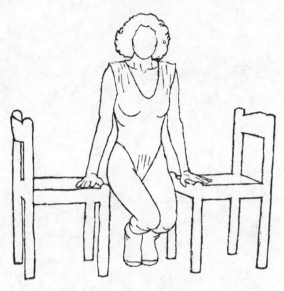

Figure 18.21

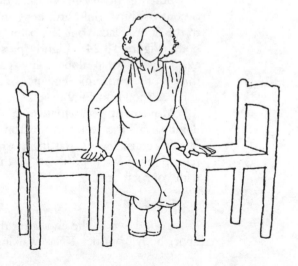

Figure 18.22

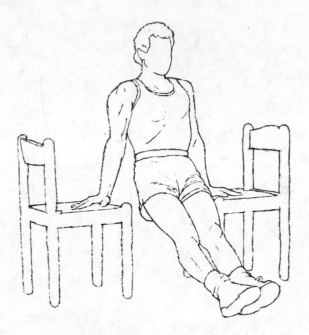

9. Bent-Over Arm Extensions

For the triceps — back of upper arms.

Starting position: Grasp a dumbbell in your right hand and bend over at the hips, right arm bent at the elbow, until your torso is parallel to the floor. Place your left palm on a flat bench or chair to brace your body (Figure 18.24). Lightly press the inside of your upper right arm against your torso along a line parallel to the floor (and keep it there through the entire movement). Begin with your arm bent at a 90-degree angle as shown in Figure 18.24.

Movement performance: Slowly straighten your arm, bringing the dumbbell to the rear and up from its starting position (Figure 18.25). Slowly return to the starting position. Perform the desired number of repetitions. Switch positions to the other side and perform repetitions with your left arm.

Cool-down

Cool down at the end, after the second time through this complete upper-body routine. Keep walking for several minutes, moving your

Figure 18.23

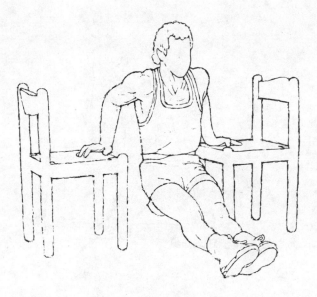

arms, shoulders, and torso. Allow your breathing and heart rate to gradually return to normal.

Lower-Body Routine   Total time required (twice through these six exercises, 6–15 repetitions of each): Maximum 15 minutes.

Warm-up

Before you begin, take a minute or two to walk around, smoothly lifting your knees up high and lightly jogging in place on a padded floor surface or grassy lawn. Slowly perform simple dynamic flexibility exercises like those given for the hips, legs, knees, ankles, and feet in Chapter 14.

Thighs

1. Modified Knee Bends

For upper thighs.
Starting position: This exercise is the same as the modified knee bend recommended in Chapter 16. By adding resistance, you can expand the benefits. Assume a comfortable standing position with your feet

Figure 18.24   **Figure 18.25**

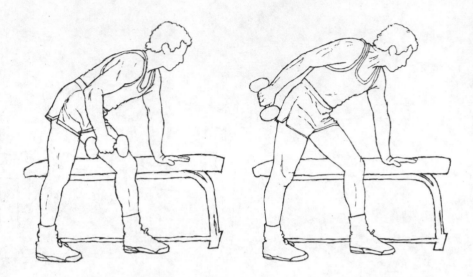

spread shoulder width apart. To increase resistance, hold the dumbbells in your hands with arms down at your sides (Figure 18.26). Your weight should be evenly distributed on both feet.

Movement performance: Slowly bend your knees and lower your body into a squat position (Figure 18.27), being certain that the knees do not extend in front of the toes during the movement. As you move downward, your knees will come forward several inches, your buttocks will move to the rear and your trunk-torso line will incline slightly forward (your back is straight — the slight bend comes from the hips). This lets you maintain solid balance over both feet. When you reach your lowest squatting position (not lower than sitting in a chair at first), gently reverse the movement and, keeping your chest and head up, raise your body back to the original standing position. Perform the desired number of repetitions.

2. Outer-Thigh Lifts

For outer thighs, buttocks, and lower back.

Starting position: Try this exercise first without ankle weights; then add weight if desired. Lie on a padded floor surface on your right side in a straight line with your right arm comfortably supporting your head and your left arm helping to balance your body. Assume a pelvic-balanced (aligned) position (Figure 18.28).

Figure 18.26   **Figure 18.27**

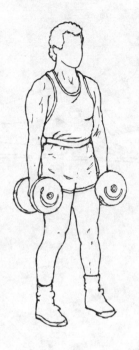

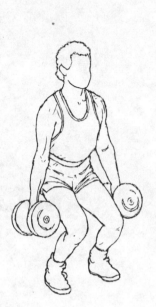

Movement performance: Raise your left leg smoothly and slowly upward about 12 to 16 inches, as shown in Figure 18.29. Do *not* twist your body out of position. Slowly return to the starting point. Perform the desired number of repetitions and then switch to the left side and repeat the exercise.

3. Inner-Thigh Lifts

For inner thighs and groin area.

Starting position: Try this exercise first without ankle weights; then add weight if desired. Lie on your right side on a padded floor as pictured in Figure 18.30. Support yourself with your right elbow and forearm and left hand. Rotate the hips slightly back to about 45 degrees. Place the sole of your left foot securely on the floor so that your right leg can move upward freely. Rotate your right (bottom) leg out so that the heel and toes are parallel to the floor.

Movement performance: Slowly, keeping your right foot flexed and your right leg straight, lift your right leg as high as you comfortably can (Figure 18.31) without rolling your hip back. Then slowly lower

Figure 18.28

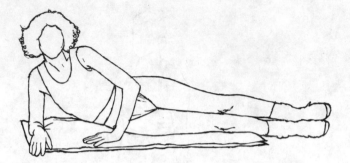

Figure 18.29

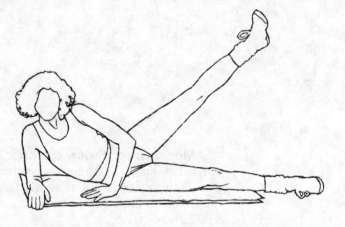

your leg back to the floor. Perform the desired number of repetitions and then change sides and repeat with the left leg.

4. Leg Extensions

For thighs.

Starting position: Try this exercise first without ankle weights; then add weight if desired. Sit on the edge of a bench or chair, with pos-

Figure 18.30

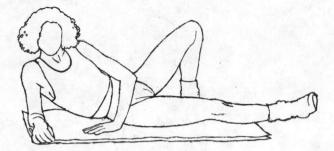

Figure 18.31

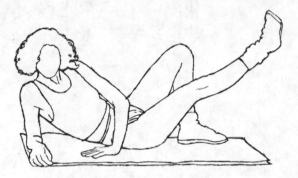

ture erect, both feet firmly on the ground, and hands supporting you by gripping the edge of the seat (Figure 18.32).

Movement performance: Lift your right leg off the ground and slowly extend it fully to the front, no higher than the height of the bench (Figure 18.33). Then slowly return to the starting position, keeping your foot flexed (don't point your toes). Avoid tilting or turning your pelvis or shoulders or tensing your upper body. Perform the desired number of repetitions and then change to the left leg and repeat the exercise.

Note: If you are wondering why I don't recommend the traditional leg curl exercise, it's because of the advice of rehabilitative medicine expert Dr. Rene Cailliet, who thinks the leg curl is useless in a general fitness program and may be dangerous because it strains the lower back.[145]

Figure 18.32   **Figure 18.33**

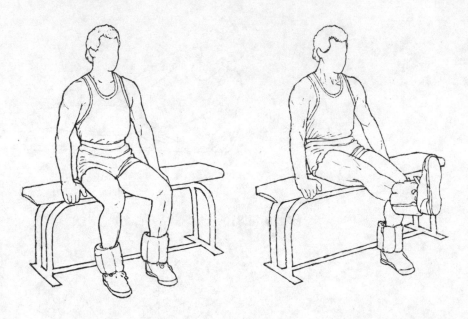

Calves

5. Toe Raises

For the calves and feet.

Starting position: As shown in Figure 18.34, place the toes and balls of your feet on a block of wood (a 2-by-4 or 2-by-6 will be fine), toes pointed straight ahead, and grasp a sturdy object with your hands to maintain balance. Sag your heels as far below the toes as comfortably possible (the heels may or may not touch the floor).

Movement performance: Slowly rise up as high as you can on the balls of your feet (Figure 18.35) and then slowly return to the starting position with your heels lowered as close to the floor as possible. Be certain that the ankles do not roll outward. Perform as many repetitions as desired.

Note: You may wish to try a more advanced version of this exercise using one leg at a time instead of two. Another option is to hold a dumbbell in the hand corresponding to the leg being exercised. For greater overall muscular development in the lower legs and feet, add the varia-

Figure 18.34   **Figure 18.35**

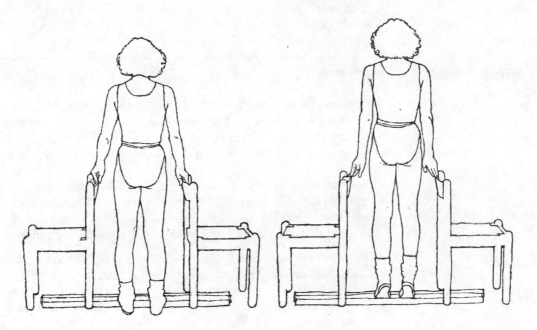

tions of (a) raising up more on the "inside ball" of your foot and then
returning to the ground and (b) raising up more on the "outside ball" of
your foot and then returning to the ground.

6. Toe Taps

For the calves and feet.

Starting position: Sitting in a chair with both feet about 6 inches
apart and flat on the floor.

Movement performance: Leaving your heel on the floor, slowly
lift the front of your right foot as high as you can, starting a kind of
slow-motion up and down movement like tapping your toes. This exercise helps balance the toe raise exercises and prevent some of the shin
splints that are common to runners, walkers, and aerobic dancers.

Note: For greater overall muscular development, add this variation:
(a) lift the front of your foot higher on the "inside ball" area (your big
toe will end up higher than your little toe) and return to the starting position, and (b) lift the front of your foot higher on the "outside ball" area
(your little toe will end up higher than your big toe) and return to the
starting position.

Cool-down

Cool down when you finish the second set of the six exercises in this lower-body routine.

Equipping a Home Fitness Center

Home exercise centers, often called home gyms, have become very popular. For many families, having a home exercise area promotes family fitness, saves time spent commuting to and from an exercise facility, and, over several years, may cost considerably less than belonging to a health club.

However, it's often advisable to first join a local fitness club to familiarize yourself with various types of equipment and exercise routine options before making any long-term home gym decisions. If you're convinced that a home gym is right for you, consider the following:

If finances or space for a home gym are especially limited or if you are inexperienced in strength and endurance exercise, consider the portable Lifeline Gym (mentioned previously under "Rubber tubing"), or think about making a cooperative purchase with close relatives or neighbors.

If you have available space and the finances to make a moderate investment, the more expensive strength and endurance equipment and machine options will probably better match your improving fitness levels in the years ahead.

Compare designs and features: What form of resistance is used? What is the unit's adjustability to different-sized people? Does it have multistation features? How many different exercises can be safely and optimally performed (it varies greatly, from a single exercise to dozens)? Contact a variety of companies, including those listed in bodybuilding and sports publications and those recommended by fitness professionals in your area. Compare prices, service, and warranties.

High-Quality, Cost-Effective Options

Under $500: free weights and associated equipment. Home fitness centers can make very effective use of free weights (dumbbells and barbells) and some simple pieces of associated equipment. For the best value in free weights, buy them secondhand. Watch the classified advertisements in your local paper. Look for solid iron barbells and dumbbells rather than plastic filled with sand budget versions. A straight, strong, knurled barbell bar and a pair of dumbbell bars are essential. Between 120 and 170 pounds of weight plates is a good starting point. Choose pairs of plates in the following weights to permit greatest safety and small-increment adjustments in poundage: 25 pounds, 10 pounds, 5 pounds, 2½ pounds, and 1¼ pounds. A set of four "wrenchless collars" will safely secure the plates to the bars during exercise.

Several accessories and pieces of no-frills equipment expand the setup: a pair of training gloves and waist belt for lower-back support; an adjustable incline-decline bench; a flat bench; a leg flexion-extension bench; a pull-up bar; a dip bar; and perhaps several simple cable setups for pressdowns, crosses, rowing, and other exercises. Some of these pieces of equipment can be obtained in combination benches designed for home use. Once again, look for options in your local health clubs, and shop the classified ads for bargains.

$500 to $800 range: machines. There is a staggering array of home exercise machines available in America. Resistance can be provided by body weight, weight stacks, elasticized cables, springs, shock absorbers, and other designs. Machines have the advantage of generally taking up less space than a collection of barbells, dumbbells, and benches. But many machines are poorly designed and poorly manufactured.

The Consumer Products Safety Commission has reported a dramatic increase in injuries from home exercise machines. Avoid discount merchandise, advises Phil Rosenthal, assistant director of the Institute of Sports Medicine and Athletic Trauma in New York. "Nothing good is really cheap. . . . Most of the equipment is not harmful — if you buy a decent machine."[146]

The following home exercise machines are well designed, durable, and cost-effective. While there are many reliable products — and new ones are being introduced to the marketplace regularly — these should give you a basis for comparison:

▶ Bow-Flex 2000X (Bow-Flex of America, Inc., 1151 Triton Dr., Suite B, Foster City, CA 94404; 800-654-3539). A cable-and-pulley system, it can provide the user with more than fifty different exercise options. The Bow-Flex features high-tech plastic power rods that feel superior to surgical tubing or stretch cord. The operation is smooth and quiet, and resistance is easily adjusted.

▶ Mega-Gym (Healthstyles, Inc., 3049 Alta Vista, Sarasota, FL 33577). A home unit for beginning and early-intermediate strength and endurance training. It's ideal when you have virtually no free space, since it takes up less than 1½ square feet of floor space when the bench is folded up and it has a beautiful wooden frame (it looks good enough to mount on the wall in your office, bedroom, or den). Designed by a French exercise physiologist and built in Sweden, the Mega-Gym features a vertical, wall-mounted chassis and an adjustable incline-decline bench with fixed position and sliding seat options. It uses an adjustable pulley-and-cable system that lifts two independent stacks of variable weights.

Over $800. Hundreds of companies now manufacture commercial-quality strength and endurance machines for sale to individuals, clubs, and gyms. Outfitting your home exercise center with this equipment may end up being a bit like financing a trip around the world or buying a small vacation home — plan to spend $2,000 to over $40,000 for a new equipment collection. Used equipment with warranties may be available for considerably less.

For current comparison information, contact the following companies.

▶ David Fitness Equipment Inc. (Carriage Four, 1086 Teaneck Rd., Teaneck, NJ 07666; 800-843-8577).
▶ Eagle Fitness Systems (Cybex, 2100 Smithtown, Ronkonkoma, NY 11779; 800-645-5392).
▶ Hydra-Fitness Industries, Inc. (2121 Industrial Blvd., Belton, TX 76513; 800-433-3111).
▶ Muscle Dynamics, Inc. (17022 Montanero St., Suite 5, Carson, CA 90746; 213-637-9500).
▶ Nautilus Sports/Medical Industries, Inc. (P.O. Box 1783, Deland, FL 32721; 800-874-8941).
▶ Paramount Fitness Equipment Corp. (6450 E. Bandini Blvd., Los Angeles, CA 90040; 800-421-6242).
▶ Polaris (P.O. Box 1458, Spring Valley, CA 92077; 800-858-0300).
▶ Universal Gym Equipment, Inc. (930 27th Ave., S.W., Cedar Rapids, IA 52404; 800-553-7901).

19 Balance, Agility, and Coordination Exercises

WHY, YOU MAY BE WONDERING, are separate exercises needed to develop balance, agility, and coordination? Don't aerobics, stretching, and strengthening exercises take care of that?

There's no doubt that all activities — *every* motion we ever make — influences our fitness. But to most of us, good balance, agility, and coordination seem "good" mostly because of how everyone else moves around. Elegantly coordinated people — elite dancers, gymnasts, yogis, martial artists, and others — are rare in the Western world. And this rarity makes their kind of natural gracefulness seem, well, unnatural. Yet brain scientists[147] now realize that we could all develop a far greater sense of physical mastery — balance, agility, and coordination — than most of us have ever imagined.

Good, you may be thinking, but that takes years of intense training, doesn't it? Surprisingly, it doesn't; it requires as little as 6 minutes a week. How? By progressively developing your mind, senses, and muscles in some new ways, little by little, day by day. That's the focus of this chapter.

A central theme reappears here: the golden circle of *Health & Fitness Excellence*. As martial arts masters have observed for centuries, once you start to expand your balance, agility, and coordination beyond normal limits, you experience a cascade of secondary benefits. New levels of physical balance have a way of turning into greater life balance — in emotions, attitudes, and actions.

Several definitions:

Balance is the dynamic ability to control shifts in the body's center of gravity, maintaining equilibrium in a full range of stationary and moving positions. Balance depends upon the ability to integrate visual input with inner-ear equilibrium centers and accurate kinesthetic (muscle movement sensing) perception. Dynamic balance isn't a gift, it's *learned*.

Agility is the competence to smoothly and precisely change position and direction without loss of balance. Agility, like balance, is integral to work, sport, and recreation. It enhances performance, increases our adaptability and resilience, and prevents injuries. Agility is developed only through practice.

Coordination is the ability to integrate all fitness factors (including perception, flexibility, strength, endurance, speed, balance, and agility) into a synergistic, productive whole. Coordination is "a harmonious relationship of movements, a smooth union or flow of motion in the execution of a task," writes exercise physiologist Brian Sharkey. "Coordination . . . *is achieved by practice* [emphasis added]."[148]

2-Minute Program

Here's a simple basic program to increase your balance, agility, and coordination. The time required is as little as 2 minutes three days a week (see sample daily exercise schedules in Chapter 11). If you'd like to devote more time to it, that's great — but not essential. I have listed some popular options that require more time later in this chapter.

Tibetan Balance and Agility Exercises

These simple exercises — developed by martial arts masters — have been used successfully for many centuries in the East. They are taught to young children and practiced by men and women throughout their lives. Each exercise is performed slowly, smoothly, and with total control. In the beginning, use a handrail or other solid object for support.

The central principle is omnilateral movement. Tibetan martial artists use the image of a sphere, understanding that the flexible, centered human body can move gracefully in any direction within an imaginary sphere — in this case, one circumscribed around your body a little more than an arm's length away — made up of millions of tiny points of light. Wherever possible with comfort and safety, movements to the left should be balanced with complementing movements to the right; motions up with motions down; inside to outside; front to back; circles moving up and to the right with circles moving down and to the left; and so on.

Choose buoyant posture — with your head floating, neck long, shoulders broad and relaxed, chest open, back straight, and pelvis level. In an alert, relaxed way, preplan your movements so that your *whole body* takes on a kind of fluid integration and unity — feet guiding legs, legs guiding waist, waist guiding torso, torso guiding shoulders, shoulders guiding arms, arms guiding hands. Avoid the random leg-here, hip-there, where-are-my-hands-supposed-to-be-anyway kind of motions.

1. Double-leg Moving Balance Exercise

Time required: 1½ minutes.

Starting position: Stand comfortably with feet about shoulder width apart, knees slightly bent, elbows flexed 30 to 60 degrees, arms held in a relaxed and balanced position (grasp a solid object with one hand for support if necessary).

Movement performance: Keeping both feet on the ground, slowly and smoothly raise and lower your vertical torso, bending at the knees. Your upper body moves as a whole — up and down, left and right, forward and back — with your head properly extended on a straight neck. Next, bending at the knees and hips (not the waist or lower back), smoothly lean your torso in an oblique (diagonal) angle halfway between straight ahead and left, then return to center. Now lean halfway between straight ahead and right, then back again, and so on. Be creative, moving in as many different directions as capture your interest today, while leaving the feet on the ground. Imagine standing on footprints painted on the ground. You may come up on the balls of your feet or heels or pivot your stance, but don't twist or slide completely off the footprints.

Then change your foot positions, standing wider or narrower than shoulder width or with one foot farther in front of the other, with toes pointing straight ahead or off to the left or right, and so on. Begin a new series of movements. If you find a certain position is uncomfortable or painful, work gently around it. Stop after a minute and a half if this is the time you have allocated today.

2. "Touch the Universe" Exercise

Time required: 30 seconds.

This is a pleasantly challenging, smooth but fast exercise in which you add hand and upper-body movements to the double-leg moving balance exercise.

Starting position: The image: You are standing inside a beautiful sphere of soft, sparkling lights, all about the size of a silver dollar. Keep your knees bent, moving from unlocked straight legs to very bent knees. Your posture is aligned from your hips to your neck, and your whole body moves fluidly with each arm motion. At first, you may want to hold on to a solid object with one hand for support. Create this exercise in your own way.

Movement performance: It is a flowing, silken movement, nothing abrupt, nothing tense. As smoothly as you can — maintaining complete control of your balance and getting a little faster each time you practice — reach to touch different points of light with one hand, then the other, again and again; up high, down low; forward, backward; left, right; in straight lines, inside circles, outside circles. Reach to touch sparkling little lights in all parts of the imaginary sphere surrounding you. Gradually develop the ability to put your moving balance leg exercise beneath you as you touch dozens of points with your hands in 30 seconds. Each time you do this exercise, encourage yourself to be a little smoother, a little more relaxed, a little faster, reaching a few new points of light in the sphere.

3. Option: Advanced Single-leg Moving Balance Exercise

This is a more advanced technique to be performed only after the double-leg moving balance drill feels comfortable. The movement orientation is the same, but only one leg is in contact with the ground. Once again, grasp a solid object for support whenever necessary.

Begin by elevating one foot only an inch or two off the ground, which allows a quick, safe recovery if you should momentarily lose your balance. In a relaxed and controlled way, move slowly within the imaginary sphere of directional possibilities, reaching high, low, forward, backward, left, and right with the whole body; bend the knee of the support leg smoothly up and down while moving the free leg in complementing directions to preserve and enhance balance. Then rest for a moment and switch legs. Begin again.

These exercises feel wonderful whenever you can find an extra half minute here or there during the day. They quickly clear the mind and open the senses.

Other Exercises for Balance, Agility, and Coordination

The following exercise options can be added to your fitness program as desired.

Mini-Trampolining

Also called rebounding, mini-trampolining is an enjoyable, productive exercise for developing balance and agility.[149] It is used by thousands of families across America and in a number of athletic training routines.

A mini-trampoline can be placed in a convenient spot at home near the television or telephone, at work in the lunch room or hallway, or even right outside the bathroom door — anyplace where you can catch an extra few seconds, or even a minute or two, of balanced, agile movement.

"[Rebounding exercise builds] coordination, stamina, agility, balance [and] rhythm . . . without the usual trauma associated with other forms of exercise," says learning abilities expert Alfhild Akselsen, from

Norway.[150] Research at the University of California at San Diego confirms this.[151]

Mini-trampolines come in a variety of shapes and sizes. Quality in construction varies considerably. Investigate options in your area and by mail order, and compare features and costs.

Rebounding is fun — but be aware of safety factors. It is advisable for beginners or those with balancing problems to purchase a rebounding handrail or put the mini-trampoline next to a secure object that you can hold on to for stability. Maintain balanced posture and avoid the tendency to look at your feet when bouncing. Use your arms for balance, bending them at the elbow and moving them in a relaxed manner. Here are several beginning exercises:

Basic bouncing exercise. Stand on the mini-trampoline with your feet comfortably spaced about shoulder width apart, knees slightly bent. Bounce lightly and rhythmically without letting your feet lose contact with the mat surface of the rebounder. The total up and down motion is only a few inches. This is an easy, energizing exercise.

Jogging. When jogging on a mini-trampoline, alternately raise and lower your legs in a smooth motion. For most people, striking the mat on the down motion with simultaneous contact from both the ball of the foot and heel is best. Don't raise your knees too high on the upward leg movements — remain in full control of your balance. The arms can give you stability throughout the jogging motion. Use heterolateral movements: raising your right arm as you lift your left leg, your left arm as you lift your right leg, and so on.

High-knee jogging. This exercise is basically the same as jogging, but with the knees being lifted higher on the upstroke of the jogging motion.

Other rebounder exercises. Once you are comfortable with the mini-trampoline, you can add a variety of dancelike footwork and creative arm movements, but keep safety in mind. Acrobatic tricks, abrupt twisting motions, and other high-risk movements have no place in a health and fitness program.

Jumping Rope

As described in Chapter 17, jumping rope improves balance, agility, and coordination. It has been used as a training technique by tennis players, boxers, martial artists, gymnasts, dancers, and professional sports champions for many years. Jump ropes are convenient to use and handy to take along with you in purse, briefcase, or backpack.

Develop your skills slowly. For extra foot dexterity and hand-foot coordination, practice skipping rope with both feet together; then one foot at a time; alternating your feet; high stepping; and crisscrossing.

Aerobic Dancing

Aerobic dancing (Chapter 17) can be a fun-filled exercise activity with significant benefits to balance, agility, and coordination. The key is to choose an integrated variety of dance routines — different movements that use the upper and lower body in safe but challenging new ways — reaching, bending, turning, weight shifting, and so on.

Martial Arts Routines

A number of martial arts systems feature graceful, flowing exercise movements that involve the entire body and improve balance, agility, and coordination in a pleasant, relaxed way. Many people know of tai chi chuan. With some basic instruction by a qualified teacher, it's easy to learn and practice on a daily basis.

"Although its roots are in ancient China, T'ai Chi Ch'uan is very suitable for tense Westerners," says Da Liu, former member of the United Nations, author of *T'ai Chi Ch'uan,* and the man many credit with introducing tai chi chuan to the United States. "It has the advantages of regular exercise combined with a definite emphasis on the gracefulness and slowness of pace that Western society so conspicuously lacks. . . . The relaxed, gentle movements of T'ai Chi Ch'uan keep the body from being tense and awkward. . . . Each form requires balance. . . . Coordination of body, mind, and breathing is essential. . . . T'ai Chi Ch'uan should be performed slowly and carefully so that the utmost quiet will be achieved . . . to enhance . . . concentration, energy, breath control, and patience. . . . T'ai Chi Ch'uan is based on effortlessness. Its movements are free and smooth. All unnecessary exertion is avoided. . . . Moving smoothly and gracefully, the student achieves his art as naturally as a child in playing."[152]

"[Tai chi chuan] can be performed at any speed for any length of time," reported Dr. Allan Ryan, editor of *The Physician and Sports Medicine,* after a recent trip to China. "It exercises every part of the body, if a complete set of exercises is carried out, and it develops coordination and balance."[153]

Springing, Bounding, Lunging, Leaping, and Sprinting

If you are already at an intermediate fitness level or are serious about developing advanced sports skills, read this section now. If not, earmark it for future reading after the rest of your *Health & Fitness Excellence* program is well under way.

Balance, agility, and coordination can also be enhanced by quick-reflex movements that combine strength with speed. Research in the United States, Europe, and the Soviet Union document the value of speed training (short sprints and rapid arm movements) and plyometric exercises (jumping, springing, and leaping; bounding, hopping, and skipping; lunging; swinging and throwing; and other direction-change movements).

The term *plyometrics* is thought to have originated from the Greek word *Pleythyein,* which means to augment or increase. In sports science, plyometrics refers to "exercises characterized by powerful muscular contractions in response to rapid, dynamic loading or stretching of the involved muscles."[154] Add the sports title of "explosive-reactive power" to these exercises and it really sounds as if they should be reserved for secret Olympic training camps. But let's stop to think about it for a moment.

Even if you don't compete in sports, simplified versions of these exercises are worth considering at some point as a way to add variety to your fitness sessions and positive stimuli to keep your brain and senses developing in new ways. How much time are we talking about? Not hours of wind sprints or leaps and lunges that risk life and limb. But as little as 5 minutes once or twice a week doing reasonably paced short sprints and some skipping, bounding, jumping, or other drills that are fun. There isn't space in this book to detail specific exercises, but the resources indicate where you can learn more.

RESOURCES

▶ *Plyometric Training* by Michael Yessis, Ph.D., and Frederick C. Hatfield, Ph.D. (Fitness Systems, P.O. Box 222, Canoga Park, CA 91305; 1986; 800-544-5485). An upper- and lower-body program for speed-strength development. Includes specific applications to many sports.

▶ *Plyometrics* by James C. Radcliffe and Robert C. Farentinos, Ph.D., 2nd Ed. (Human Kinetics Publishers, P.O. Box 5076, Champaign, IL 61820; 1985; 800-DIAL-HKP). Well-illustrated program. A corresponding videotape is available.

▶ *Secrets of Soviet Sports Fitness and Training* by Michael Yessis, Ph.D. (Arbor House, 1987). Practical ideas on integrating advanced Soviet sports science techniques into your fitness regimen.

▶ *Tai Chi Chuan* by Marshall Ho'o (Karl-Lorimar Video, 17942 Cowan, Irvine, CA 92714; 1987; 800-328-TAPE). A good step-by-step video lesson and basic book by the chairman of the National Tai Chi Chuan Association.

▶ *Tai Chi* by Chia Siew Pang and Goh Ewe Hock (CRCS Publications, 1985). A book teaching 44 Chinese tai chi positions with correct posture.

Step 3

NUTRITIONAL WELLNESS

20 Introduction

MYTH: Good nutrition simply means a modern diet from "the four major food groups."

FACT: According to leading nutritional scientists, the modern American diet is far from ideal. For best health and fitness we need to eat an *extraordinarily varied diet* from many different food groups. An optimal diet is high in carbohydrates and fiber, moderate in protein, and low in fat, cholesterol, salt, alcohol, and caffeine. (*See Chapter 21.*)

MYTH: Don't eat between meals. Snacks make you fat.

FACT: If you overeat high-fat foods, you'll gain body fat — no matter when you eat. But if you want to burn excess fat — and think, feel, and perform at your best — it's a priority to eat small amounts of fresh, wholesome, low-fat, high-fiber food five or six times a day. (*See Chapters 21, 22, and 27.*)

MYTH: Food choices have little or nothing to do with how you think, feel, and perform.

FACT: There is compelling new evidence about a mind-mood-food connection. Learn how *your* best food choices may give you greater control of your emotions, energy, mental sharpness, and performance. (*See Chapter 27.*)

MYTH: Your thirst tells you when you need more water. And during warm weather it's best to drink extra fluids with meals.

FACT: Thirst can be an unreliable indicator of your body's true need for water, and dehydration contributes to fatigue and poor performance. We each lose about 10 cups of water a day, without taking into account fluids lost during exercise or from hot weather, physical work, stuffy offices, or airline travel (where you can lose up to 2 pounds of water in a three-hour flight). Coffee, tea, stress, alcohol, and other factors make the dehydration even worse. And mealtime is usually the wrong time to drink extra fluids. (*See Chapter 22.*)

MYTH: Food allergies are the biggest nutritional issue of the century. They're the leading cause of fatigue, headaches, grouchiness, anxiety, depression, and illness.

FACT: While many individuals may be sensitive to a few isolated foods, bona fide food allergies are very rare for people who eat a widely varied diet and follow a balanced, fitness-oriented lifestyle.

MYTH: Vitamin-mineral supplements are the key to good health and are a smart form of nutritional insurance in place of a good diet.

FACT: These claims are false. A widely varied optimal diet of wholesome, fresh foods — backed by the other six steps of *Health & Fitness Excellence* — is vastly more important than any vitamin or mineral supplement. (*See Chapter 28.*)

Food is more than a source of nutrients. It's a social phenomenon. We are in the midst of a nutritional revolution in America, and we're paying a terrible price for misinformation. Contradicting experts with isolated facts and inexperts with no facts vie for media attention. Food industry advertisements pound away at our subconscious minds. Fad diets leave millions disillusioned and well experienced at dietary failure.

As consumers, we are faced with perplexing decisions — nutritional choices with immediate and lasting influences on our entire life. Our diets can *cause, contribute to,* or help *prevent* a variety of diseases, and science has made one point especially clear: Dietary apathy isn't a safe haven anymore. To ignore the responsibility for personal nutrition is to invite disaster.

The Changing American Diet

The American diet has been changing steadily since the early 1900s under the influence of new technologies, affluence, government programs, working parents, health concerns, and more. In addition, the nation's $200 billion per year food industry plays a major role in influencing food habits, capitalizing on the public's desire for certain tastes and convenience.[1]

Aren't Americans the best nourished people on earth? Unfortunately, we are not. "Although poor nutrition has traditionally been thought of in terms of vitamin, mineral, and protein deficiencies," says Michael F. Jacobson, executive director of the Center for Science in the Public Interest, "millions of Americans suffer another kind of malnutrition: too rich a diet — too many calories, too much fat, too much salt (sodium), too much cholesterol, too much alcohol. It is somewhat ironic that after centuries of worrying about starvation, much of humankind finally overcame deprivation only to suffer the ravages of food excesses."[2]

Environmental factors such as diet and smoking are thought to contribute to 80 to 90 percent of all human cancers in America,[3] with dietary factors alone contributing to an estimated 60 percent of cancers in women and 40 percent of cancers in men.[4] A recent report in the *Journal of the National Cancer Institute* estimated that 90 percent of deaths from colon cancer (the leading cause of cancer death) in the United States might be prevented by dietary modifications.[5] The American Heart Association has identified strong links between diet and heart disease.[6]

Caution: Don't Lose Sight of the Golden Circle

While nutrition *is* very important, it isn't the panacea that one-sided enthusiasts would have us believe. Science has shown that all health and fitness factors are interrelated. For instance, exercise (which improves circulation, tones muscles, and helps control excess body fat), relaxation skills (which release tension), and even mental imagery (which can reduce anxieties and boost self-esteem) can help the body better digest and assimilate nutrients from the foods you eat. In turn, this nutritional improvement helps every part of your body and can also enhance your ability to control your thoughts and emotions. This is another example of the golden circle of *Health & Fitness Excellence*.

Is Nutritional Wellness Expensive?

Is best-quality nutrition more expensive than poor nutrition? With rare exceptions, no. In fact, *those who fail to change their diet in light of new health facts will probably do so in the future simply because of the rising cost of foods*. "People concerned about nutrition spend about one-third less money on their food bills than those people whose shopping carts are overflowing with soda pop and hot dogs," reports Michael Jacobson.[7]

Beyond the Old "Balanced Diet"

For a quarter of a century, physicians, dietitians, and nutritionists have recommended the U.S. Department of Agriculture's "Basic Four" food guide. The four food groups — milk, meat, fruit-vegetable, and grain — are the basis for virtually all traditional nutrition programs taught in America.

The original intent of the Basic Four was to provide a simple approach to nutritional adequacy. But in light of today's knowledge, it inadvertently condones or ignores certain disease-promoting dietary problems, such as high fat, cholesterol, and sodium. Despite its obvious flaws, the Basic Four still prevails because of powerful political allies in the food industry and traditional nutrition circles.

So even though there is little scientific doubt that it's time to modify the Basic Four, change has been slow. Thanks to years of practice at the encouragement of dietary authorities and food-industry advertising, Americans en masse feel stuck. Either we plead ignorance to the evidence and just keep right on eating the way we have learned to eat, or we're forced to struggle with letting go of some deeply set bad habits — such as meal skipping, overeating, and a lingering passion for the high-fat, high-sugar, low-fiber, magically adulterated cuisine that is still being sold all around us.

The answer? A variety of proposals have been made. The "food exchange" systems formulated by the American Diabetic and Dietetic Associations are very helpful for many people who are beginning to improve their diets. Some software programs developed by nutritional scientists for home computers also offer valuable guidance.

From a balanced perspective, nutritional wellness comes down to some simple but often overlooked principles. We'll examine each of them in the next chapter.

21 Eight Scientific Nutrition Principles

By SCIENTIFIC STANDARDS, the average American diet still falls short of ideal nutrition. But contrary to popular opinion, a superior day-to-day diet costs no more — in time or money — than a mediocre one. And best nutrition doesn't depend on exotic fresh produce, rare condiments, a cupboard full of vitamin and mineral supplements, or prepackaged "all-natural" foods. It's far simpler than that. An optimal diet is founded on eight basic principles.

1. An Exceptionally Varied Diet

Eat an exceptionally varied semi-vegetarian or vegetarian diet. The central theme of nutritional wellness comes down to eating a widely varied diet of fresh, wholesome foods that, overall, are unrefined and high in complex carbohydrates and fiber, adequate but not excessive in protein, and low in fat, cholesterol, and salt.

While many Americans assume they eat an adequately varied diet, research proves otherwise. In fact, experts now know that an extraordinarily varied diet — that means *real* variety, biological variety, not a dozen different snack foods — can improve digestion, increase nutrient availability, reduce toxin and food allergy risks, and help fight excess body fat.

An exceptionally diversified diet also gives pleasure in eating. We humans have what scientists call "sensory-specific satiety" — we love variety in foods. This is an inborn and universal need and one reason why strict, monotonous diets are difficult for most of us to follow.

Take a quick inventory right now of how many *different* foods you consumed last week in your meals and snacks: whole grains (a dozen different grains are readily available in America), legumes (more than twenty-five varieties of beans, peas, and lentils are marketed nationwide), vegetables and fruits (more than seventy-five varieties are sold in some produce stands), and other foods.

Semi-Vegetarianism and Vegetarianism

For many years, most Americans were openly critical of vegetarians, but scientific findings have begun to change that attitude. "We tend to scoff at vegetarians, call them the nuts among the berries," says Dr. William Castelli, director of the federal government's respected Framingham Heart Study in Massachusetts, "but the fact is, they're doing much better [healthwise] than we [nonvegetarians] are."[8]

Vegetarianism falls into several categories. *Vegans* eat vegetables, whole grains, legumes, fruits, nuts, and seeds, but no animal products — not even milk or eggs. *Lacto-vegetarians* include dairy products in their diet. *Lacto-ovo-vegetarians* include both dairy products and eggs. *Semi-vegetarians* may include dairy products, eggs, and occasional fish, poultry, or meat in their diet.

Medical researchers have carefully studied tens of thousands of vegetarians (in most cases lacto-vegetarians or lacto-ovo-vegetarians) over decades and have found that they are generally well nourished and have significantly less chronic, degenerative diseases than the rest of the U.S. population.[9] As a group, vegetarians have been found to have lower blood pressure and more ideal blood cholesterol levels; less incidence of heart disease, osteoporosis, obesity, arthritis, diabetes, and kidney disease; a lowered risk of certain cancers; and a generally stronger immune system.[10]

A lacto-vegetarian or lacto-ovo-vegetarian diet is also now considered a positive part of many prevention and treatment programs for obesity, constipation, diverticular disease, coronary artery disease, diabetes, hypertension, and, to some degree, breast cancer, colon cancer, and gallstones.[11]

Researchers have discovered that vegetarians and semi-vegetarians don't just eat less meat — they also tend to eat more whole grains, legumes, vegetables, and fruits than do nonvegetarians. The fiber, vitamins, minerals, and other substances in these foods may help prevent vegetarians from developing cancers. And millions of Americans are discovering that vegetarian and semi-vegetarian diets not only are nutritious but are relatively inexpensive and offer a tremendous variety of delicious meal and snack options.

When statistically compared with Americans, the Japanese — whose traditional diets tend to be vegetarian-oriented and very low in fat — experience only about one-fifth as much breast and colon cancer.[12] "Our working hypothesis is that mutagens in fried and broiled meat initiate and high-fat diets *promote* cancers of the breast, prostate and colon," say scientists at the American Health Foundation in Valhalla, New York. "Fried potatoes and similar foods contain some mutagens, but meats contain one thousand times more."[13]

The more meat in the diet, the more likely too is consumption of agricultural and industrial chemical carcinogens. One particular class of insecticides, chlorinated hydrocarbons, is known to accumulate in the body fat of animals and humans.

But, you may be wondering, aren't vegetarians deficient in iron and vitamin B_{12}? There is no doubt that beef is richer in iron than most other foods, but new research reports that many plant foods, such as lentils, beans, and green leafy vegetables are also excellent sources.[14] While some cases of anemia have been reported in vegetarians,[15] this may have been due to a lack of variety in their diets.

Recent discoveries show that iron absorption from grains and legumes can be significantly enhanced when vitamin C is present — in the form of tomatoes, green peppers, potatoes, chilis, turmeric, and lemons. One international group of experts reports: "The effect of ascorbic acid [vitamin C] on [non–meat source] iron absorption has been tested in a number of dietary settings and in every case has been shown to be profound. It plays a particularly critical role in diets in which little or no meat is present."[16] One recent study showed that iron absorption was quadrupled in meals that contained enough vegetables to provide 65 milligrams of vitamin C.[17] Lactic acid (contained in yogurt and other cultured dairy products) is also thought to perform a role similar to that of ascorbic acid in increasing assimilation of iron.[18]

It was also thought for many years that vegetarians were deficient in vitamin B_{12}. But by the early 1980s, these conclusions were judged premature or based on scientific oversights.[19] Sophisticated research techniques have revealed that vitamin B_{12} is made by bacteria high enough in the human intestinal tract that it can be absorbed into the body.[20] And the absorption of vitamin B_{12} is reportedly as high as 70 percent for vegans, compared with 16 percent in meat eaters.[21] Excess fat and protein in the diet — commonly seen in meat eaters — increases the need for B_{12}. Although the American Dietetic Association still recommends that vegans include a reliable B_{12} source (either supplements or fortified foods) in their diets, vegetarians with widely varied diets high in complex carbohydrates and fiber, moderate in protein, and low in fat appear to run little risk of vitamin B_{12} deficiency.[22]

A growing number of athletes are becoming vegetarians and report improvements in strength, performance, and endurance. In one study, athletes placed on a high-fat, high-protein diet promptly found that their endurance had been cut in half, according to U. D. Register, professor of biochemistry and nutrition at Loma Linda University and one of America's leading authorities on vegetarianism. In contrast, with a high-carbohydrate vegetarian diet, the athletes' endurance levels doubled over their normal levels.[23]

Some people have become vegetarians for religious reasons, others for moral or ethical rationale: meat not only contributes to health problems but also represents an extravagant style of life in a world of shortages and poverty.[24] According to the Worldwatch Institute, the average 1-pound feedlot steak costs the world 5 pounds of grain, 2,500 gallons of water, 1 gallon of gasoline, and at least 35 pounds of eroded topsoil.[25]

2. Small Meals and Snacks

Eat frequent small meals and light snacks. "Millions of Americans have fallen into a pattern of too-late-for-breakfast, grab-something-for-lunch, eat-a-big-dinner, and nibble-nonstop-until-bedtime," writes *New York Times* health columnist Jane Brody. "They starve their bodies when they most need fuel and stuff them when they'll be doing nothing more strenuous than flipping the TV dial or pages of a book. When you think about it, the pattern makes no biological sense."[26]

Large meals swamp your digestive system and interfere with absorption of nutrients. It's easier for the gastrointestinal tract to absorb nutrients from small amounts of food every two to three hours during the day.

When you eat too much at a sitting, you experience a postprandial dumping syndrome — lots of blood is drawn to the digestive tract. When this happens after a large meal, there is not enough blood flowing to the brain or muscles to supply energy and you experience a kind of after-meal stupor. Before long, this lethargy becomes the norm. Worse, when the meal is high in fat and refined foods, it can cause additional fatigue and can sabotage thoughts, feelings, and performance.[27]

Breakfast and Lunch Matter!

Regularly skipping meals — such as breakfast or lunch — hurts health and productivity. In fact, making a habit of missing one or both of these meals can help guarantee a lasting struggle with excess body fat. Skipped or delayed meals may cause blood-sugar levels to drop below normal, resulting in fatigue, loss of concentration, headaches, weakness, hunger, and more stress.[28]

Yet here's the current situation: Over half of American families have at least one member who regularly skips breakfast. Half of all school children have little or no breakfast. Recent large-scale national surveys indicate that the number of people skipping breakfast has increased by one-third in less than five years[29] and includes two out of every three people aged twenty to thirty-four.[30] In addition, the number of Americans skipping lunch nine days out of ten has increased 63 percent in the past decade.[31]

A nutritious breakfast improves physical and mental performance. Benefits include faster reaction time, higher productivity during the late morning hours, and less muscle fatigue. Breakfast-skipping children are more likely to be listless and have difficulty concentrating and solving problems in school.[32] And after missing a meal like breakfast or lunch, the body has difficulty in replacing the missing nutrients.[33]

Between-Meal Snacks

Do you know one of the fastest ways to eliminate midmorning and midafternoon performance slumps while improving your health? Between-meal snacks. That's right. Of course, this doesn't mean junk food treats or eating large main meals and then *adding* snacks. Rather, we're talking about improving the quality — and cutting back on the size — of breakfast, lunch, and dinner and *then* adding some light between-meal snacks.

With this plan, the body's digestion, absorption, and metabolism function more efficiently, contributing to a steady supply of energy and improved mind power, emotional control, and physical effectiveness. In addition, those who eat five or more small daily meals generally have lower serum cholesterol levels, less heart disease, and an improved ability to process blood sugar.[34]

Overall, daily caloric intake should be adequate to maintain your desired body weight (discussed in Chapters 29–32). For a rough estimate of daily calorie needs for a generally healthy adult, multiply body weight in pounds times 12 for sedentary people, between 12 and 15 for low-to-moderate-activity people, between 15 and 18 for moderately to very active people, and 18 or more for extremely active people. Compare this figure to your normal daily calorie intake. For a more accurate estimate, consult your physician or a qualified nutritionist such as a registered dietitian.

The Golden Circle — Again

Just as your diet affects all the other aspects of *Health & Fitness Excellence,* the other six steps in this program influence your nutritional state. Here is an example to think about: Sustained negative stress and a problem-focused view of life force the adrenal glands to release steroid hormones called glucocorticoids.[35] These stress hormones block the entry of glucose into many types of cells to preserve the glucose for "emergency" muscle movements and physical actions. This restricts glucose to brain cells and they can die.[36] Solution? As you can see, to achieve your best health and fitness it takes more than just good nutrition. It takes an integrated program that includes stress management, exercise, balanced posture, and mental development.

Sensible Meal/Snack Plan

Here is an example of how to schedule meals and snacks throughout the day:

6:00 A.M.	Arise
7:00 A.M.	Small breakfast
9:45 A.M.	Light snack
12 noon	Small lunch
3:00 P.M.	Light snack
6:00 P.M.	Moderate supper
8:30 P.M.	Very light snack
11:00 P.M.	Bedtime

3. Drinking Water and Minimizing Alcohol and Caffeine

Drink plenty of water between meals and eliminate or limit intake of alcohol and caffeine. As we'll see in the next chapter, water isn't a source of calories — it's an essential nutrient. Most of us drink far too little of it, and this negatively influences our health and performance. Make it a priority to drink at least six to eight glasses of water every day. And limit caffeine intake to a maximum of 300 mg per day. (Caffeine is found in coffee, tea, chocolate, and cola drinks.) That's zero to four 6-ounce cups of caffeine beverages per day (and drink none if you are pregnant or breastfeeding). Limit alcohol consumption as your doctor directs. The maximum is generally one to two drinks a day (a drink is usually defined as 1.5 ounces of hard liquor, 4 to 5 ounces of dry table wine, 3 ounces of sherry or port wine, or 12 ounces of beer).[37]

4. Awareness of Nutritional Needs and Preferences

Respect your body's unique nutritional needs and preferences. "Readiness to ignore individual differences," says medical researcher Andrew Weil, ". . . accounts for a great deal of the contradictory dogma that characterizes the health professions, a problem glaringly visible in disputes over nutrition and diet."[38] We are each unique — genetically, physically, psychologically, biochemically. While certain food choices and combinations may promote *your* best energy and performance levels, the same dietary choices may be less pleasant or more stressful for others.[39] Moreover, food taste preferences are deepset habits, so it is important to let them change slowly as you introduce new foods into your daily menus.

Keeping a Diet Record

The first step to changing your diet is getting your eating habits out in the open. It's surprising how many of us don't remember from day to day — sometimes hour to hour — what we eat and drink. An accurate, written diet record is a valuable aid in charting *what, how much, when,* and *in what order*. Such a journal also helps pinpoint recipes and meal plans that not only please your personal tastes but give you a nutritional advantage in terms of energy and productivity.

To begin a diet record, use a small notebook and label a page for each day over the next two to four weeks. (Remember, this written record is a short-term awareness tool, not a lifelong task.) Take this notebook with you throughout the day and enter every food and beverage you consume, along with the time and approximate quantity. Take several minutes at the end of the day to look back over your meal/snack/beverage pattern. What simple improvements can you make tomorrow or next week? *Change* depends on *awareness*.

It's What You Eat Most of the Time . . .

Dietary fanatics ultimately fail. Besides being intolerable to live with, they will probably collapse in the end from stress. Dietary "cheating" — eating not-great foods — is usually acceptable on occasion (unless it violates your religious or spiritual beliefs or the treatment advice of your physician).

By all means, choose high day-to-day dietary standards, but build in some flexibility. Don't abandon social contacts just because meals or snacks offered at friendly gatherings are not ideal. Calmly change whatever you can whenever you can. Holiday recipes aren't always made from exemplary ingredients, but the love and camaraderie surrounding them provide vital nourishment of their own. Family bonds, friendship, laughter, recreation, and other benefits of social get-togethers contribute joy and health to life.

There is usually something you can do in a kind, gentle way to improve food choices when you're away from home. You might offer to bring a dish or two to a family dinner or to help your friend or neighbor with the chef's hat if the meal is prepared in a home kitchen. When dining out, pick the restaurant whenever you can and choose the most health-promoting (or least health-stressing) recipes on the menu. When traveling by air, order special meals and snacks in advance. On a train, bus, or car trip, pack your own meals or snacks when possible.

Be certain to modify your dietary habits slowly. "You cannot change your eating patterns overnight," explains Dr. Ruth Kunz-Bircher, longtime director of Switzerland's Bircher-Benner Medical Clinic. "To do that would almost certainly result in failure. Never try to give up your old ways all at once."[40]

---

5. Regular Mealtimes

Establish regular daily times for meals and snacks. Scheduling your meals and snacks at the same times each day may improve digestion and metabolism.[41] For nearly a century, the Bircher-Benner Clinic (a private medical center and nationally licensed hospital in Switzerland that has treated thousands of people since the late 1800s) has endorsed an "order of life" therapy as part of its health and fitness programs. Meals and snacks are taken at the same time every day in a relaxed, positive environment. Staff members at the clinic believe this benefits people of all ages and conditions.[42]

We live in accordance with so many other scheduling priorities — work, appointments, television viewing, recreational events, dates — that it's high time we placed when we eat our meals and snacks at the top of that list.

6. A Positive Mealtime Environment

Create a positive mealtime environment. How pleasant are your mealtimes? Do you discuss family affairs, personal problems, financial decisions, or world events? Do you listen to television or radio news while eating? Debate or argue? Choose crowded, noisy restaurants or grab a quick bite on the run?

A positive mealtime environment helps the body properly and completely digest foods and absorb nutrients. It makes little sense to carefully select high-quality foods and organize balanced, delicious meals if environmental chaos reigns — if each bite is barely chewed and hurriedly swallowed or if your abdomen and neck are tense from bad news or heated discussions. Stress encroaches on digestion.

Set some house rules and guidelines. Enforce them. For a period lasting from 15 minutes *before* to 15 minutes *after* each meal and snack, ban intense discussions, negative comments, and complaints. Turn off the television set and turn the stereo to soft, positive background music. We are overinformed about problems we can do little, if anything, to solve. The national and local news can contribute to feelings of helplessness and hopelessness that are known to depress the immune system.[43]

Create a relaxed, unhurried atmosphere. Have all household members help in some way with meals — planning, preparation, serving, or cleaning up. If necessary, take the phone off the hook. Put a vase of fresh flowers, a favorite small plant, or centerpiece on the table. Have everyone sit with comfortably erect posture (this improves attitudes and digestion, as noted in Chapters 33 and 34). Slow down the eating pace.

Focus the meal on positive conversation and happy thoughts. Take a moment, if appropriate, to join hands and say a positive affirmation or mealtime prayer. Don't just count your blessings; *imagine* them clearly in your mind.

During mealtimes, the Bircher-Benner Clinic forbids all talk of the past and insists on a positive present and future orientation. If past problems dominate you in the present, you are interfering with more than digestion — you are blocking your own path to best health and fitness.

7. Relaxing at Mealtimes

Relax before, during, and after eating. Do you hold tension in your "stomach"? Millions of us do. This muscular tightness restricts circulation and can contribute to digestive disorders, fatigue, cramping, lower-back pain, headaches, and other conditions.

"The glands in your mouth can produce two kinds of saliva," say stress researchers Dr. Jeffrey A. Migdow and James E. Loehr. "When the diner is relaxed and ready to eat, the parotid glands produce saliva that contains digestive enzymes and is watery; it easily dissolves food being chewed. Under stress, however, the sublingual glands exude a thick saliva that is devoid of digestive enzymes. Clearly, relaxing before a meal is the first step toward ease of digestion."[44]

Relaxation is one of the missing ingredients in otherwise well-designed nutritional programs. Here's a simple method for relaxing before every meal and snack: Sit comfortably with good posture. Place your left palm on your abdomen. Over the next 10–30 seconds, take several deep breaths, clearly imagining your stomach area releasing *all* tension, feeling your abdominal muscles letting go. Take another moment to focus your mind on this new relaxed feeling.

The first few times you use this exercise, you might not notice a dramatic difference. But persevere. Your sense of touch is establishing a biofeedback path through your nervous system, promoting increased circulation and decreased muscular tension. Maintain this relaxed, aware state before, during, and after each meal and snack.

8. Eating Slowly and Enjoying It

Eat slowly, limit extra fluids with meals, chew thoroughly, and enjoy. "Slow down! You're eating too fast" is the often-heard parental admonition. Unfortunately, this good advice is rarely followed. Millions of us "eat on the run" at almost every meal. Even when our schedule doesn't demand it, we hurry.

In response to stress, the entire digestive tract experiences a type of shutdown, explains stress researcher Dr. Peter G. Hanson. "People who eat on the run under stress do themselves a lot of harm by forcing food at high speed into their inactive stomachs. Stomach bloating, nausea, discomfort, cramps, and even diarrhea can result."[45]

Eating too quickly also contributes to overeating and excess body fat. Part of the food in each meal is converted to glucose, and blood-sugar levels begin to rise. This prompts a release of insulin from the pancreas. Within approximately 20 minutes of the first bite of a meal or snack, receptors in the cerebrospinal fluid signal the brain to let the digestive tract know that you are full.[46] But when you rush your meals, it's easy to keep right on eating until the 20-minute mark, and then when the signal finally comes, it's too late.

Of course, few of us have the time for leisurely two-hour meals. But with some practice, we *can* take control of our mealtime/snacktime attitude and environment.

And remember, digestion begins in your mouth with each bite of food. Poorly chewed, quickly swallowed foods interfere with digestion. So chew well.

It also pays to keep an eye on extra fluids at mealtime. Many people have made it a habit to drink several glasses of water, milk, juice, soft drinks, tea, or coffee with each meal. This extra fluid, when combined with solid foods in your stomach, can dilute the concentration of enzymes and interfere with digestion.[47] Relaxing, eating more slowly, and chewing each bite of food thoroughly makes it easier to cut back on extra fluids with meals. A small glass of water or low-fat or nonfat milk (which becomes a semisolid in the stomach), sipped slowly with a meal, is fine. But drink most fluids *between* meals.

A Basic Nutritional Supplement

A raging debate surrounds the issue of nutritional supplements — taking extra vitamins and minerals beyond those you obtain from your diet. Is it necessary or advisable? Is it safe? For a straightforward, referenced look at this subject, see Chapter 28.

RESOURCES

Nutrition is a complex subject. No single book covers it all. Throughout the following chapters, I recommend publications that I feel are especially valuable. And in the Resource list at the end of this book, I list some of the best magazines, journals, and newsletters. In addition to *Health & Fitness Excellence,* the following books are a good starting point for a home library on nutrition.

▶ *The Complete Eater's Digest and Nutrition Scoreboard* by Michael F. Jacobson, Ph.D. (Anchor/Doubleday, 1985). This revised and updated guide examines the food industry and government research on nutrition. It describes common food additives, stating which are recognized as probably safe, which are dangerous, and which have not received adequate testing. The nutrition scoreboard rates the basic nutritive value of a wide range of common foods.

▶ *Guess What's Coming to Dinner: Contaminants in Our Food* by the staff of Americans for Safe Food (ASF, 1501 16th St., N.W., Washington, DC 20036; 202-332-9110; 1987). This booklet gives an overview of food contaminant problems in America, including pesticides, animal drugs (hormones, antibiotics, and others), microbial contamination, molds, and chemicals. Presents sensible precautions and proposes short-term and long-term solutions.

▶ *The Health & Fitness Excellence Cookbook* by Leslie L. Cooper (Advanced Excellence Systems, P.O. Box 1085, Bemidji, MN 56601; 218-854-7300; 1989). Complements and expands on the dietary recommendations in *Health & Fitness Excellence* and offers practical suggestions for meal planning and food preparation. Features unique 14-day cool weather and 14-day warm weather meal/snack menus and gives a complete nutritional analysis (including percentages and grams of fat, cholesterol, protein, carbohydrate, fiber, calcium, and sodium) for each recipe, meal, snack, and complete day's menu. Preparation times are listed for each recipe and an index notes the recipes that can be prepared in 5 to 30 minutes.

▶ *Jane Brody's Nutrition Book* by Jane E. Brody, updated edition (Bantam, 1987). This nutrition fact book by the award-winning *New York Times* health columnist is filled with good, sensible information.

▶ *Jean Carper's Total Nutrition Guide* by Jean Carper (Bantam, 1987). Based on the U.S. Department of Agriculture's scientific analysis of the nutrients in more than 2,500 foods.

▶ *Nutrition Wizard* (Center for Science in the Public Interest, 1501 16th St., N.W., Washington, DC 20036; 202-332-9110; 1987). Computer software designed by Michael F. Jacobson, Ph.D., who received his doctoral degree in microbiology from MIT. *Nutrition Wizard* is intended as a comprehensive program to help people eat a more healthful diet. The first part gives a standard analysis of dietary needs based on age, body size, and activity level. The second part uses a databank with more than 1,700 food items (which can be expanded by the user) to analyze recipes, meals, and an entire day's diet for twenty-five nutritional components, including protein, carbohydrate, soluble/insoluble fiber, fat (polyunsaturates, monounsaturates, and saturates), cholesterol, sodium, and many other minerals and vitamins. Easy to use. Good, clear instructions.

▶ *Nutritional Analysis System: The Food Processor II* (EHSA Research, P.O. Box 13028, Salem, OR 97309; 503-585-6242). Sophisticated, professional-level computer software used by a number of leading government organizations, hospitals, research centers, and universities.

22 Essential Nutrients: A Painless Primer

YOU DON'T HAVE TO BECOME a nutritional biochemist or registered dietitian to select food wisely for yourself and your family. Nonetheless, it's important to understand the basic principles of nutritional science, especially in light of recent discoveries. This chapter shares some highlights.

Oxygen

Oxygen is necessary for energy production and brain function and in prevention of disease and premature aging. Although some nutritional authorities overlook it, oxygen cannot be taken for granted.

Studies show that most adults and many children are oxygen-deficient because of lack of exercise, an unfit heart, poor posture, shallow breathing, nutritional (including iron) deficiencies, stagnant air at home or work, muscle tension, and other factors. While you can remain technically "alive" with very little oxygen reaching your body's cells, you are far from being at your best.

How do you train the body to take in an ideal amount of oxygen, circulate it to every cell, and use it to produce energy and burn excess fat? The only sure way is an integrated program like *Health & Fitness Excellence*. Good nutrition is part of the answer; so are breathing exercises

(Chapter 12), aerobics (Chapters 16 and 17), stress management (Chapters 3–10), balanced posture (Chapters 33 and 34), and mental development (Chapters 43–48).

Pure Water

Water is a forgotten nutrient. It is crucial to every function in the body — temperature regulation, nerve impulse conduction, circulation, metabolism, immune system, eliminative processes, and all the rest.

Dehydration occurs when you don't take in enough water to replace all that's lost through perspiration, respiration, urination, and other body processes. Dehydration reduces blood volume, creating thicker, more concentrated blood, which may stress the heart and is less capable of providing muscles with oxygen and nutrients and eliminating accumulated wastes.[48]

It takes surprisingly little fluid loss — 1 percent — for your body to become dehydrated, and you can't depend on thirst to tell you that it's happening.[49] "Even a tiny shortage of water disrupts your biochemistry," says Michael Colgan, nutritional researcher and recent visiting scholar at Rockefeller University. "Dehydrate a muscle by only 3% and you lose 10% of contractile strength and 8% of speed. Water balance is the single most important variable in top performance."[50]

You don't have to be perspiring profusely or urinating frequently to lose water. You are losing it all the time. If you work in a stuffy building or live in a dry home, you lose large amounts of fluid by invisible evaporation from the skin and lungs. If you're a frequent business traveler, the rapid circulation of dry airplane air can cause your body to lose as much as *2 pounds* of water in a three-to-four-hour flight.[51] And alcohol and caffeine, both diuretics, *increase* the body's fluid loss. So does stress.

Drinking plenty of water prevents dehydration and helps regulate body temperature, promote smoother skin, keep bowel movements more regular and soft, increase resistance to infections by hydrating the mucous lining of the respiratory tract, maintain a higher volume of urine production (which decreases fatigue), and help prevent kidney stones, urinary infections, edema (fluid retention), and elevated blood pressure.[52]

Water also plays a critical role in keeping the brain adequately hydrated, say sports medicine authorities Dr. Bob Goldman and Robert M. Hackman. "Even a slightly dehydrated body can produce a small but critical shrinkage of the brain, thereby impairing neuromuscular coordination, concentration, and thinking."[53]

How much water do you need to drink? It depends on many variables, including the foods in your diet, metabolic rate, weather, temperature, climate, physical activity level, and stress factors. In general, *we each need to drink more water than our thirst calls for.*

Each day the average person loses at least 2 cups of water through breathing, another 2 cups through invisible perspiration, and 6 cups through urination and bowel movements. That's *10 cups a day* without taking into account fluids lost through perspiration in exercise or hard physical work.[54]

Next let's consider where your body gets — or should get — its fluids. "Because most food contains a large amount of water," says public health researcher Philip Collins, "you obtain approximately three and a half cups from what is eaten over the course of a day. Interestingly, the body's metabolism itself is another source; as it makes and uses energy, one of its daily byproducts is about half a cup of water. Therefore, taking into account the approximately four cups provided by food and metabolism, and the ten cups lost, *the average person needs to drink six to eight cups of water daily just to keep functioning well* [emphasis added]. This requirement changes, of course, according to the environment and the type and quantity of food you eat."[55]

Dehydration is a common cause of poor athletic performance,[56] in part because muscles have a very limited ability to store water. Traditional athletic diets, high in protein and low in carbohydrates, result in ketosis, a condition in which incomplete metabolism causes the formation of toxic compounds called ketones, which dehydrate muscles. Drinking plenty of water helps prevent this, and so does a diet rich in complex carbohydrates.[57]

Here are several recommendations: (1) In general, drink between 6 and 8 cups of pure water every day, preferably between, rather than with, meals. (2) Develop new water-drinking habits. Keep water accessible during the day and keep track of how much you consume. Put a glass or cup of water next to you at work. (3) Sip beverages slowly. *Cool water* (40–50°F) is more quickly absorbed than warm and, contrary to popular opinion, won't cause cramping.[58] (4) *Precede* exercise sessions with extra water, generally 1 to 2 cups taken in the hour or so preceding training. Drink another 1/2 to 1 cup of water 15 to 20 minutes before the workout. If pure water isn't available where you exercise, bring your own. (5) Take short breaks to drink small amounts (1/4 to 1/2 cup) of water every 20 to 30 minutes *during* intensive exercise or athletic sessions. (6) Consume more water (1/2 to 3 cups) immediately *following* exercise sessions and sports activities.

If you're like most of us who've spent years underhydrated, all this may have you wondering why you haven't dried up and blown away before now. But like suboptimal breathing habits (from which it's easy to grow accustomed to being tired) and chronic tension (from which the slightest easing of muscle tightness can trick you into thinking you're relaxed), persistent dehydration, however slight it may be, covertly cuts your quality of life. The solution takes some getting used to, but it's well worth the effort.

Pure Water

Until recently, most Americans took water quality for granted. But recent studies report that a great percentage of water supplies are laden with toxic chemicals, poisons capable of causing cancer, heart disease, birth defects, neurological disorders, organ damage, and other illnesses.

First, an antiparanoia statement: Every drop of water that passes over your lips doesn't have to be perfect. Nonetheless, it's essential to know the facts about pure water, know how to have your water supply tested, and know your options if you find a contamination problem.

"The Environmental Protection Agency (EPA) reports that more than 700 potentially hazardous chemicals have been found in U.S. drinking water," states Jonathan King, staff member of the Center for Investigative Reporting in Washington, DC.[59]

Twenty percent of all community water supplies don't meet standards of the Safe Water Drinking Act of 1974, according to the EPA, because of harmful levels of bacteria or mineral contaminants (such as lead or arsenic). In addition, the EPA estimates that nearly two-thirds of rural Americans drink water that is potentially unsafe.

Lakes, streams, and rivers hold only about 4 percent of the fresh water in the United States. The remaining 96 percent is contained in vast underground reservoirs in porous layers of sand, gravel, or rocks. This groundwater supplies the drinking water for 90 percent of all rural residents and over half the total U.S. population.

Small amounts of groundwater pollution can have a devastating effect. A single gallon of gasoline can make the well water for a community of fifty thousand people unfit to drink for years.[60] Until recently, some people thought groundwater was magically "self-purifying" and protected from pollution because it seemed so distant from the toxic industrial chemicals and by-products, sewage, pesticides, herbicides, heavy metals, and other contaminants on the surface. We now know that this protection doesn't exist.

Drinking-water supplies across the United States have been shown to contain toxic heavy metals (lead, cadmium, mercury, cobalt, copper, and others), cancer-causing organic chemicals, sodium, nitrates, asbestos, arsenic, radioactive substances, and a wide range of toxic industrial chemicals. Everything that we inject into our environment — chemical, biological, or physical — ultimately finds its way into the earth's water.

Chlorine and Other Chemicals

Chlorination of surface water was first introduced in 1908 as part of improved public sanitation, and epidemics of cholera, dysentery, typhoid, and other water-borne bacterial diseases became rare in the United States.

But some authorities contend that, while the addition of chlorine to our drinking water undoubtedly reduced infectious illnesses, it may have contributed to other diseases, including cancer. More than a dozen studies suggest an association between cancer and chemicals in drinking water,[61] and municipal water supplies have been found to be laced with chemicals that are known or suspected to cause cancer.

In their well-intentioned attempts to clean up the drinking water, municipal water companies are currently using more than fifty different chemicals. A single chemical, perhaps harmless when isolated, can be added to the water, react with other chemicals, and form new toxic chemical compounds.

Fluoridation

As a means to prevent tooth decay, water fluoridation is endorsed by the American Dental Association (ADA), World Health Organization, Centers for Disease Control, U.S. Department of Health and Human Services, U.S. Public Health Service, American Cancer Society, and dozens of other organizations. As a public health measure, there is no doubt it has been successful in protecting millions of people against serious tooth decay. The ADA reports that fluoridation of drinking water provides a twentyfold return in dollars saved in repairing decayed teeth.

Although water fluoridation has become an emotion-charged political issue in some parts of the country, dozens of controlled studies report no link between fluoridation of community water supplies and increases in disease rates.[62]

But with fluoride now present in many water supplies, toothpastes, and mouthwashes, one growing concern is how much fluoride is too much, especially for young children. Research projects by the ADA and other organizations are under way to find the answer.

Check with your city water supply officials. If your water contains more than 0.7 to 1.2 parts per million (ppm) of fluoride (or in excess of about 1.2 mg fluoride per liter) and you choose to drink it without filtering or purifying it (by distillation or reverse osmosis methods) and you use a fluoridated toothpaste, do not have your family members use a fluoridated mouth rinse or have children take vitamins with fluoride unless prescribed by your dentist.[63] For the most up-to-date guidelines, write the ADA (Bureau of Health Education, 211 E. Chicago Ave., Chicago, IL 60611).

Bacterial Contamination: Still the Biggest Problem?

Despite the publicity surrounding chemical pollution, the number one water quality problem is still bacterial contamination. Nearly one-third of all rural American drinking water contains more than the federal limit of 1 coliform bacteria per 100 milliliters.[64] Other bacteria — many of them pathogenic — are turning up in water supplies nationwide. As noted, chlorine and other chemicals kill bacteria but create other concerns. For many of us, home water purification methods offer the best overall answer.

Soft Water

Studies in the United States, Canada, Great Britain, the Netherlands, and Sweden suggest that softened water is actually worse for drinking and cooking than straight tap water.

All pollutants from raw tap water remain in soft water with the exception of calcium and magnesium salts, which are replaced by sodium salts. This can add up to 100 milligrams of extra sodium per quart of water.[65] Worse still, softened water tends to leach lead, cadmium, and other metals from pipes, adding these toxins to your water. Don't use softened water for drinking or cooking.

In contrast, hard water contains relatively high amounts of dissolved mineral salts, which may in some way help prevent heart disease.[66] In areas where hard water is consumed there is lower incidence of heart disease and heart attacks, according to studies sponsored by Dartmouth Medical College and the University of Missouri.[67]

Lead and Other Dangers

Even if it were possible to have 100 percent pure water as it leaves the reservoir, there would still remain the serious question of whether it is fit to drink by the time it reaches the faucet. Many Americans live with an extensive network of underground pipes made from materials such as copper and lead, which can poison body tissues. Other plumbing materials, such as plastic polyvinyl chloride (PVC), have unknown health effects. These facts underscore the need to consider home water purification.

Several Solutions

It may take many years and billions of dollars to stop pollution and devise effective government methods of purifying enough water to meet our growing population needs. Fortunately, we don't have to await government action to obtain pure water for drinking and cooking. North Americans now spend nearly $2 billion each year for bottled water and almost that much for water filters.[68]

Before you decide to drink bottled water or invest in a home water purifier, it is a good idea to have your tap water tested. Pollution danger signs include brown, cloudy or murky-looking water; smelly or bad-tasting water; foam; and sudden changes in appearance or taste. However, many toxic chemicals are invisible, odorless, and tasteless. Laboratory analysis is the only certain means of identifying safe drinking water.

The U.S. Environmental Protection Agency (EPA, Water Division, Washington, DC 20460; 800-426-4791) now provides a toll-free hotline for general and technical information about the quality of drinking water. If you cannot find a reputable analysis lab locally (check with your community health department), contact WaterTest (P.O. Box 186, New London, NH 03257; 800-426-8378). To find out more about what you can do about water pollution, write for "Safe Drinking Water For All" (League of Women Voters Educational Fund, 1730 M St., N.W., Washington, DC 20036) and "Manual for Evaluating Public Drinking Water Supplies" (Water Supply Division, Environmental Protection Agency, Washington, DC 20460).

If yours is among the 13 million American homes that rely on well water, some health department officials recommend that you have your water checked annually for coliform bacteria and nitrates. And every five years, arrange for a more extensive test.

Water Purification Methods

Let's assume you have tested your water and decided to purify it or buy bottled water. What are the options?

Short-term expedient methods. Letting the water run from the faucet at full force for 2 or 3 minutes each morning before use can help clear copper, cobalt, lead, or cadmium that may have dissolved out of your water pipes overnight. Boiling your water for 20 to 30 minutes (uncovered) will help eliminate bacterial problems and aid in the removal of volatile chemicals that may be present. Even whipping the water in a blender for 15 minutes with the top off may help to remove chlorine, chlorinated hydrocarbons, and chlorinated pesticides. None of these options, however, provides a long-term solution to pure water needs.

Bottled water. You can buy bottled water prepackaged or bottle your own directly from a nearby spring in a nonindustrial area where few pollutants reach the water. If you buy it, look for water labeled something like "natural spring water bottled directly from the source."

Contact bottled water manufacturers to ask where the water comes from, if and how it's processed, the kind and amount of chemicals and minerals in it, results of recent bacterial tests, and how often such tests are made.

Bottled water comes in a bewildering variety of forms. Still water, spring water, natural water, distilled water, mineral water, purified water, seltzer, and naturally sparkling water have joined the parade of options.

Because of widespread groundwater contamination, some of these bottled waters are actually less pure than tap water. In fact, bottled water with a name like "spring type," "spring pure," "spring-like," or "spring fresh" isn't spring water at all but simply processed tap or well water. The New York State Health Department recently reported that traces of chemical solvents and other substances — including petroleum derivatives — exist in 48 of the 93 bottled water brands sold in New York state.[69]

With the cost of bottled water approaching a dollar per gallon, and a year's supply exceeding two hundred dollars per person, many people are investing in home water filtration or purification systems. Consider a group purchase — with friends or neighbors — to reduce the initial expense.

Home water treatment systems. Different home water treatment technologies deal with different types of contamination.

Activated-carbon filters remove most volatile chemicals, such as chlorine (and chlorine by-products like trihalomethanes), industrial solvents, and pesticides. But activated carbon generally cannot eliminate bacteria, viruses, nitrates, dissolved solids, particulates, or heavy metals such as mercury and lead.

Carbon filters must be changed regularly (by using a test kit and following manufacturer's instructions) since their effectiveness lessens with use, and, if unchanged, they can become breeding grounds for bacteria. For a comparison of various designs and efficiency ratings, see test results published in *Consumer Reports* (256 Washington St., Mt. Vernon, NY 10553).

Reverse osmosis (RO) filtration involves the passage of water through a semipermeable membrane that permits the movement of water but prevents passage of organic and inorganic contaminants because of their larger molecular size. Although they can remove virtually all particulates, most pesticides, volatile organic chemicals, bacteria, and heavy metals, RO units filter out only about 50 to 70 percent of nitrates and cannot block some small trihalomethane chemicals such as chloroform — a known carcinogen. "Combination RO purifiers" — containing a prefilter, an RO membrane, and an activated carbon filter — are currently the best RO option.

Steam distillation generally removes most contaminants, but reliability depends on the design of the distiller and how well it is maintained. Not all units effectively remove pesticides or certain volatile chemicals. Because of this, some companies are manufacturing purifiers that combine distillation, activated carbon filtration, and multistage RO filtration.

Test your water supply to determine which contaminants need to be removed, and then choose your home water treatment method accordingly. For help in choosing a reliable water treatment device, the EPA recommends contacting the National Sanitation Foundation (P.O. Box 1468, Ann Arbor, MI 48106). This organization establishes industry standards and conducts certification tests on home water treatment systems.

Protein

Next to water, protein is the most plentiful substance in the human body, used for tissue growth and repair and a host of other biochemical purposes. Compelling research indicates that *most Americans eat at least twice as much protein as they need,* and this excess leads to health problems.

During digestion, protein is broken down into its smaller components, called amino acids. Some twenty-two amino acids are known to be vital for humans. Of these, nine are labeled essential amino acids because the body cannot manufacture them from other amino acids. They must come from your diet and, since protein cannot be stored by the body, you must provide a new supply each day.

Most animal proteins, including eggs, meats, fish, and dairy products, contain reasonable amounts of all nine essential amino acids and are therefore called *complete proteins.*

Proteins in grains, legumes, and vegetables lack ideal amounts of one or more essential amino acids, typically lysine, tryptophan, or methionine. If a single grain, legume, or vegetable is eaten by itself, the body cannot take advantage of its protein; therefore these foods are called *incomplete proteins.* However, by eating two or more of these vegetarian foods that make up for each other's essential amino acid deficiencies, you create complete proteins. Such food combinations are called *complementary proteins.*

The proteins we eat most in the Western world — in meats, eggs, and nuts — are too high in fat to be included often in a health-promoting diet. Nearly all vegetables, including green, yellow, and starchy ones, contain some protein that, over the course of the day in varied small meals and snacks, can make a solid contribution to your protein requirements. For example, if you combine corn, which is low in the essential amino acids lysine and tryptophan, with beans, which are high in lysine and tryptophan but low in methionine, you end up with protein that is as complete as that found in eggs or steak, but without the fat.

Legumes (soybeans, lentils, kidney beans, black-eyed peas, chickpeas, navy beans, pinto beans, split peas, lima beans, and others) can be combined with grains (barley, corn, buckwheat, rice, oats, wheat, and so on) to make delicious, inexpensive recipes with plenty of complete protein. Or meals with vegetables, legumes, and grains can include small amounts of animal proteins, such as low-fat or skim milk or small amounts of fish or poultry. In essence, the animal proteins act as condiments, adding extra complete protein to meals based primarily on vegetarian ingredients.

The myth that we need huge amounts of dietary protein has been soundly destroyed by science. While athletes do need more daily protein than sedentary people,[70] some athletes consume 5 to 15 times the amount of daily protein they actually need and can use![71] According to government statistics, on average, even infants and children in the United States consume about twice the Recommended Daily Allowance (RDA) of protein.[72]

Here's another fact that few people know: You can get fat eating too much protein.[73] Your body cannot store excess protein and must eliminate it as toxic wastes or convert it to glucose or fat for storage. This wastes energy, cuts performance and endurance, increases blood acidity, dehydrates, causes mineral loss (especially calcium) and deficiency of certain vitamins (notably B_6), encourages intestinal putrefaction, burdens the liver, kidneys, and other eliminative organs, and contributes — over time — to chronic fatigue, constipation, excess body fat, and lowered resistance to degenerative diseases such as osteoporosis, heart disease, certain cancers, and premature aging.[74] What a list!

Recommendations for protein consumption: How much protein do you need every day? The exact amount varies, based on age, weight, sex, biochemical individuality, digestion and absorption rates, health condition, levels of stress and physical activity, and other factors.[75] For healthy adults, the U.S. Senate Select Committee on Nutrition and Human Needs recommends that 12 percent of total daily calories should come from protein (at 4 calories per gram).

One calculation formula for adults, based on World Health Organization guidelines, is 0.8 gram of protein per day per kilogram of ideal body weight.[76] To estimate, divide your weight in pounds by 2.2 and multiply that number by 0.8. Another way to calculate daily protein needs in grams for an average healthy person is to multiply body weight in pounds by: 1.0 for newborns (0–½ year); 0.9 for infants (½–1 year); 0.8 for young children (1–3 years); 0.5 for children (4–10 years); 0.45 for early teens (11–14 years); 0.4 for later teens (15–18 years); and 0.36 for adults (19 and up). Older adults, pregnant and nursing women, and some serious athletes may require an additional 20 grams or more of protein per day — consult your physician and qualified nutritionist.

Most normal healthy adults require between 40 and 70 grams of protein per day. The body uses dietary protein most efficiently when it is consumed in small amounts (as part of light meals and snacks) five or six times a day.

Fats

Most American diets are overloaded with fat. This is not only unnecessary for good nutrition and delicious dining, it's harmful to health. From 1910 to 1980, average per capita fat consumption in the United States rose from 125 to 156 grams per day.[77] Today, the average American diet still includes more than 40 percent of its total calories from fat — nearly twice the amount recommended by many experts. Even if you are cutting back on salad dressings, butter, and margarine, you probably still eat far more fat than you realize because it is hidden in so many foods.

Where is most of the fat in the average American diet? Margarine, butter, mayonnaise, salad oils, frying oils, and shortening make up about 10 to 20 percent of it. Fats in red meat, poultry, and fish account for about 30 to 40 percent of average dietary fat. Real and imitation dairy products constitute another 15 to 25 percent, and the remainder of fat comes from eggs, nuts, seeds, and other sources.

High-fat diets are linked to cancers of the breast, colon, prostate, endometrium (uterus lining), ovary, pancreas, and lung;[78] autoimmune disorders;[79] cardiovascular diseases including atherosclerosis (plaquing of the arteries), beginning soon after infancy, and hypertension.[80] High-fat diets have also been associated with poor calcium absorption from the intestines.[81]

A regular, small amount of dietary fat is vital to good health. Polyunsaturated fats — found in grains, seeds, nuts, soy foods (like tofu), and some vegetables — provide linoleic acid, known as an essential fatty acid since, without it, the body cannot utilize fats properly. Linoleic acid is readily converted in the body to arachidonic acid, an important membrane constituent. Together, linoleic acid and arachidonic acid make up a sequence of fatty acids collectively called the omega-6s. These days, with such a wide variety of whole foods available, a dietary deficiency of linoleic acid is nearly impossible. We rarely need to obtain it from extra vegetable oil in the diet.

Another important fat is eicosapentaenoic acid (EPA). It is a polyunsaturated fat made from the essential fatty acid linolenic acid (lino*lenic* acid has a very different metabolic role from lino*leic* acid). EPA belongs to a series of fatty acids called omega-3s (discussed in more detail later).

Dietary fats help transport fat-soluble vitamins A, D, E, and K so that they can be absorbed and utilized. Fats are used in the cells of the body to help with membrane formation, nerve impulse conduction, hormone production, brain functions, aerobic metabolism, cholesterol metabolism, blood platelet adhesion control, immune roles, reproductive function (and sexual wellness), skin and hair health, and more.

For all of us who are weight conscious, here's a key fact: The body is exquisitely well equipped to convert excess dietary fats into excess body fat. That means unequivocally that *excess dietary fat is fattening* — much more fattening than carbohydrates, even refined sugar. (For details, see Chapter 31.)

The wonderful news is that most whole grains and legumes are very low in fat or are virtually fat-free, as are nearly all garden vegetables and fruits. It pays to become very aware of the fat in the foods you eat. For ideas on reducing the fat content of your diet, see Chapters 25 and 26.

More than 90 percent of dietary fat is composed of complex molecules consisting of three fatty acids — saturated, monounsaturated, and polyunsaturated. Animal fats usually contain a high percentage of saturated fatty acids, while most vegetable fats (which include many vegetables, grains, legumes, nuts, and seeds) contain mainly unsaturated (mono- or polyunsaturated) fatty acids. The significance of these various forms of fat to our health and the role that fats play in our diet are discussed in the following sections.

What is the percentage of fats in oils? Here are several examples (the percentage of saturated [S], monounsaturated [M], and polyunsaturated [P] fats are given in parentheses following each oil):[82] butter (68%S, 28%M, 4%P); coconut (86%S, 6%M, 2%P); corn (13%S, 24%M, 59%P); olive (14%S, 72%M, 9%P); peanut (19%S, 46%M, 30%P); safflower (99%S, 12%M, 74%P); sesame seed (15%S, 40%M, 40%P); soybean (15%S, 23%M, 58%P); and sunflower (11%S, 21%M, 68%P).

Note: Beware of snacks and other packaged foods listing "pure vegetable oil" as an ingredient. Coconut, palm kernel, and palm oils are 86, 81, and 49 percent saturated, respectively.[83] The first two are even more saturated than beef fat and lard. And don't be misled by the "cholesterol-free" claim. While these three vegetable oils don't *contain* cholesterol, they do *raise* cholesterol levels in the blood.

Cholesterol

Cholesterol is a waxlike substance with a complex, unusual molecular structure that resembles some of the hormones that are manufactured from it. When we hear the term cholesterol, it usually represents total cholesterol — the full amount of cholesterol in the blood, measured in milligrams per deciliter (mg/dL).

The cholesterol in the blood is characterized by three different types of lipoproteins, the compounds that transport the cholesterol around the body: high-density lipoproteins (HDLs), low-density lipoproteins (LDLs), and very-low-density lipoproteins (VLDLs). The total cholesterol content in the blood — referred to as total serum cholesterol — is the sum of all three types of lipoproteins found in the blood.

LDL cholesterol is generally regarded as the predominant culprit in heart disease.[84] Some LDLs are of great benefit to the body, delivered via receptors to the cells for productive work in cell growth. But other LDLs, teamed with a villainous chemical called apolipoprotein B, adhere to the artery walls specifically in the coronary arteries next to the heart, as part of the formation of a complex substance called plaque. The higher the LDL level in the blood, the greater the risk of heart disease.

VLDL cholesterol is manufactured by the liver and transports various fatty substances such as triglycerides and LDLs. The higher the VLDL level, the more LDL the liver can produce.

HDL cholesterol, often referred to as "good cholesterol," is the protective type. It actually draws cholesterol away from the coronary arteries. In general, therefore, the higher the HDL level, the greater the protection against heart disease.

As an ideal total serum cholesterol reading, 200 mg/dL has been the target advised by both the American Heart Association and National Institutes of Health in recent years.[85] However, the results of a major new study, published in the *Journal of the American Medical Association,* suggest that a lower level is better.[86] The best total cholesterol level for the average adult may be in the range of 180 to 190 mg/dL or even lower, and recommended total cholesterol-to-HDL ratio (which many health organizations now consider the most important cholesterol number) should generally be below 4.6 for males and below 4.0 for females.[87] In addition to providing protection against coronary heart disease, reducing elevated levels of serum cholesterol also reportedly reduces the risks of colorectal cancer.[88]

When you have your blood tested, be certain that your doctor or laboratory is using the reference standard established by the Centers for Disease Control. That is the most stringent standard for accuracy. To be assured that you are receiving a true reading, you may also want to have your cholesterol checked two or three times, at least one month apart, and then average the results.[89]

Is there a formula for controlling cholesterol levels? According to researchers, LDL production is *decreased* by regular aerobic exercise (which, as noted in Chapters 16 and 17, provides the additional benefit of *raising* protective HDL levels), stress management, and a widely varied vegetarian or semi-vegetarian diet that is low in fat and refined sugar[90] and includes soluble-fiber-rich foods such as vegetables, legumes, certain grains and fruits, and oat bran.[91] For further details about the important issue of cholesterol, the best book to date is Dr. Kenneth H. Cooper's *Controlling Cholesterol* (Bantam, 1988).

There is also another aspect of the disease prevention picture to consider: reducing dietary fats that create free radicals.

The Dangers of Free Radicals

One widely supported theory of degenerative disease and premature aging is the *free radical theory*. Among the most prevalent and destructive mutagens, free radicals are unstable, highly reactive, "pyromaniac" molecular fragments that can harm cells throughout the body. A major dietary source of free radicals is polyunsaturated fatty acids.

Polyunsaturates are especially vulnerable because of their many double bonds, which react easily with oxygen (oxidize) to form lipid peroxides and free radicals. The free radicals set off chain reactions that convert more fats to peroxides, which in turn produce more free radicals, and so on, creating a destructive effect that biochemists call a cascade. The predominant damage is caused by the effect of free radicals to mutate DNA (cellular genetic material), which can lead to cancer, heart disease, and premature aging.

While a high intake of *any* dietary fat may contribute to cancer, scientific studies of animals link polyunsaturated oils to the formation of cancerous tumors and the original damage in coronary artery disease.[92] When heated, polyunsaturates produce considerably more free radicals than butter does.[93] And thus while shifting away from saturated fat toward polyunsaturates is a proven factor in reducing serum LDL cholesterol levels, polyunsaturates may at the same time be contributing to cancer, heart disease, and other ailments.

An answer? First, most of us need to cut back on — and control — our intake of *all* kinds of fat. Then we must make the wisest decisions about the fats we do choose to eat. As we'll see in a moment, monounsaturate-rich olive oil looks promising as one choice for baking, cooking, and salad dressings.

In optimum health, the body possesses the proper nutrients to neutralize free radicals at precisely the right times, before they can do serious damage.[94] These free radical quenchers, some called antioxidants, include beta-carotene (a precursor to vitamin A found in orange and dark green vegetables), vitamins A, C, E, B_1, B_6, lecithin, cysteine (an amino acid), zinc, selenium, catechols (a class of chemicals found in potatoes and bananas), indoles (protective substances found in broccoli and cabbage-family foods), chlorophyll (found in most fresh green vegetables), and oxygen.

Epidemiological studies show that the risk of both cancer and heart disease is reduced by low-fat diets containing antioxidants in whole foods: grains, legumes, vegetables, fruits, and so on. Nutritional supplements are another consideration (see Chapter 28).

Saturated Fats Raise Disease Risks

When you consume more than about 5 percent of your total daily calories from saturated fats (in beef, veal, pork, eggs, butter, cheeses, coconut oil, and palm oil), you run the risk of elevating LDL cholesterol levels and promoting disease. Moreover, a high intake of saturated animal fats is thought to increase the need for essential fatty acids,[95] which can create a vicious cycle leading to excess body fat and other health problems.

Pros and Cons of Margarine, Problems with Hydrogenated Fats

Margarine is produced from polyunsaturated oil and, while it has been widely adopted as a cholesterol-free substitute for butter, its chemical makeup may cause it to be associated with other health problems. In biochemical terms, oils in their natural state consist of a variety of fatty acids arranged in a precise natural molecular pattern. When oils are partially hydrogenated (have hydrogen artificially pumped in to "stiffen" them and make them more spreadable — a desirable quality for margarine), their molecular architecture becomes, in the words of one biochemist, "completely disorganized."

Widespread use of hydrogenated oils in cakes, cookies, fried foods, mayonnaise, salad dressings, puddings, shortenings, crackers, snack chips, candies, bread, breadings, and frostings causes unintentional changes to occur in the fatty acids that remain unsaturated — in biochemical terms, the molecules are rearranged from a natural "cis" pattern into an unnatural "trans" position.

Researchers suggest that excessive consumption of trans fats may cause health problems. Partial hydrogenation may interfere with the production of hormone-like chemicals called prostaglandins, may raise serum cholesterol levels,[96] and may interfere with several of the body's protective mechanisms.[97] And evidence suggests that the average adult may be consuming several times the government's average per capita estimate (used to determine dietary cautions) of 8 grams per day.[98]

Another problem with margarine, mayonnaise, salad oils, and other products made from polyunsaturates is that "the unsaturated fatty acids combine with each other to form unnatural structures — chemists say the acids polymerize. This happens particularly when oils are used for deepfat frying. The longer the oil has been in the cooker, the greater the number of polymerized products that soak into the fried items."[99]

Part of the Answer: Olive Oil in Small Amounts

What are the answers to the what-fat-is-good-fat question? First, recent medical studies recommend reducing total dietary fat — *all* fat — to 20 to 30 percent of total daily calories. Second, from a health and fitness standpoint, it looks as if a predominant cooking and salad oil — used in controlled quantities — should be olive oil.[100]

Why the plaudits for olive oil? It is high in monounsaturated fatty acids (75–80 percent) that, like polyunsaturates, have been found by researchers to help lower LDL cholesterol levels. But unlike polyunsaturates, which also lower protective HDL cholesterol levels, monounsaturate-rich olive oil reportedly doesn't affect HDLs.[101]

Olive oil may offer additional protective effects against cardiac disease. In particular, Stanford University research suggests that olive oil can help lower systolic and diastolic blood pressure,[102] and other studies suggest that it helps reduce the abnormal or stressful formation of blood clots that lead to strokes and heart attacks.[103] Recent studies on breast and colon cancer report that, unlike polyunsaturated oils, olive oil apparently doesn't promote tumors.[104]

Researchers also suggest that olive oil assists the natural rhythms of the digestive tract, reduces excess bile acids, may stimulate pancreatic secretions, and provides some protection from disease and premature aging brought on by free radicals.[105]

Extra-virgin (from the first pressing) and virgin (from the second pressing) olive oils are not refined, and some authorities recommend these types of olive oil because they are well protected against oxidation (which creates free radicals).[106]

In some recipes, such as sweet-tasting baked goods that are high in complex carbohydrates and fiber and low in fat, olive oil doesn't taste good to most people (although new "light" olive oils taste better). In these cases, an acceptable choice may be the smallest possible amount of high-quality unsalted butter.

In a diet that is low in overall fat and in which beef and other flesh foods are at most rarely consumed, there is a little open space within health guidelines for a very small amount of saturated fat — and butter can be used. But in this case, it is a matter of taste, not health. As long as your serum cholesterol level is moderate and is being controlled or reduced with the help of aerobic exercise and a low-fat semi-vegetarian diet that includes monounsaturates and a wide variety of soluble-fiber-rich whole foods, very small amounts of butter may be acceptable.[107]

Butter, because of its highly saturated butyric acid, is far less prone than polyunsaturates to form free radicals when heated. In addition, butyric acid may offer some minor anticancer and antiviral effects.[108]

It is surprising how few recipes actually need butter for good taste and, when called for, how little butter is necessary in recipes flavored with other food ingredients and spices or seasonings. The amount of cooking fat can be reduced even further with nonstick or well-seasoned cookware surfaces.

Other Discoveries

Between 5 and 40 percent of the fat in seafood is omega-3 fatty acids, including eicosapentaenoic acid (EPA).[109] Recent medical research suggests that EPA helps reduce heart disease and heart attack risk by helping to streamline the blood platelets' clotting actions, reducing LDL cholesterol, and increasing HDL.[110]

EPAs are found in significant quantities in deep-water fish, notably salmon, albacore tuna, mackerel, herring, and sardines, and to a lesser extent in cod, whitefish, bonito, shad, pompano, halibut, bluefish, bass, trout, and some other varieties. Some of these fish — and fish oil capsules — are also moderately high in cholesterol.[111] So it is important not to eat big portions. Some lesser-known sources of omega-3s may be good adjuncts or alternatives: dry beans, soy tofu, seaweed, butternuts, and walnuts.[112]

Studies suggest that eating EPA-rich fish just once or twice a week may provide protection against cardiovascular disease, aid in the production of certain prostaglandins, and possibly benefit diabetics[113] and those who suffer from arthritis.[114] But always remember the whole picture: A widely varied low-fat diet high in complex carbohydrates and multifactor fiber plus exercise, stress management, positive mental images, and a host of other factors play significant roles in disease prevention.

Should all of us rush out and buy EPA supplements? Not without professional guidance, experts say.[115] In some people, fish oil supplements may actually increase the LDL cholesterol level.[116] EPA and related fats are particularly prone to rancidity when encapsulated and, if overconsumed, may suppress levels of vitamin E.[117]

Special note: Be leery of new "miracle fats." One type is known as sucrose polyester (SPE), a class of compounds formed by binding sucrose (sugar) to fatty acids. SPEs look, feel, and taste like fat, and the body absorbs them poorly, if at all. The commercial dream by SPE inventors — and scores of other food chemistry entrepreneurs — is a noncalorie fat substitute that could make billions of dollars by taking some of the junk out of junk food. But on the down side for consumers, SPEs reportedly interfere with vitamin absorption.[118] Groups of animals fed some doses of SPE developed pituitary tumors, leukemia, or abnormal liver changes[119] and others exhibited abnormalities in their offspring.[120]

To remain up to date on nutritional issues, including potential and proven risks — as well as advantages (if any) — of new "miracle fats" and fat substitutes, subscribe to *Nutrition Action Healthletter* (Center for Science in the Public Interest, 1501 16th St., N.W., Washington, DC 20036; 202-332-9110). Other recommended periodicals are given in the Resource list at the end of the book.

Recommendations for fat consumption: There are no panaceas when it comes to dietary fat — the truth is that most of us still need to cut back on fat intake in general. But "cut back" doesn't mean "cut out." *Some* dietary fat is essential, although a small but growing number of experts recommend a mere 10 to 15 percent of total daily calories from fat.

Overall, a reasonable scientific goal seems to be an average for adults of between 20 and 25 percent of average total daily calories from fat, including about one-third as polyunsaturates, one-third or less as saturates, and the balance as monounsaturates.[121] (Note: Infants and most young children need a greater percentage of total calories from fat — see your physician.)

To calculate 25 percent of total daily calories in grams of fat per day, multiply your total daily caloric intake by 0.25 and divide the result by 9. Examples: At 2,000 total calories per day, fat intake should not exceed 55.5 grams; at 2,500 total daily calories, fat should not top 69.4 grams.

Reduce dietary fat intake by reading labels, using a food scale to weigh portions and a cookbook that lists the fat content in each recipe, cooking and sautéing with vegetable broths instead of fat, using nonstick sprays and pans, adding garlic, onions, and a variety of spices to enhance the flavor of low-fat recipes, choosing low-fat or nonfat dairy products instead of whole milk, cream, or high-fat cheeses, and so on. Chapters 24–26 and 29–31 offer a number of additional suggestions for reducing dietary fat intake.

The U.S. Senate Select Committee on Nutrition and Human Needs recommends limiting dietary cholesterol intake to less than 100 milligrams (mg) per 1,000 calories, not to exceed 300 mg per day. But a number of authorities now recommend lower limits — in certain cases a total of 100 mg per day or less.[122]

A widely varied diet of whole, fresh foods including vegetables, legumes, and grains, occasional seafood (if desired), and a very small amount of fresh raw nuts and seeds will provide an ample supply of omega-6 and omega-3 fatty acids for best health.

Carbohydrates

Carbohydrates are one of the most misunderstood nutrients. There are many reasons for this, including the widespread fear that "starchy" foods are responsible for obesity. As scientists have learned in recent years, exactly the opposite is true — to lose excess body fat the most important foods to eat are complex carbohydrates (high in starches and fiber), including whole grains (prepared as cereals, side dishes, breads, pastas, muffins, bagels, and crackers and in soups, puddings, and casseroles), vegetables (including potatoes), and legumes. As noted in Chapters 29–32, two of the genuine culprits in obesity are excess dietary fat and inactivity.

At the turn of the century, North Americans ate 40 to 50 percent of daily calories in the form of complex carbohydrates. Over the past century, however, we have followed the trend of affluent nations worldwide, passing over "peasant" foods like whole grains, vegetables, and legumes in favor of what used to be banquet fare — expensive animal foods like meat and poultry, rich cheeses, and desserts.

Carbohydrates provide essential fuel — glucose — for energy production in the brain and every cell of the body. Glucose also helps maintain body temperature, digestion, movement, breathing, tissue repair, and immune system functions. There are three basic types of carbohydrates, labeled according to the complexity of their molecular structure: *monosaccharides* (simplest), *disaccharides,* and *polysaccharides* (most complex). Polysaccharides ("starches") consist of many sugar units, bonded together by nature in whole foods with associated protein, fiber, vitamins, minerals, and other nutrients, resulting in what we call *complex carbohydrates*.

Complex Carbohydrates: Essential to Good Health

Since Neolithic times, twelve thousand years ago, most human beings have survived on diets with little if any meat but lots of whole-grain carbohydrates. In fact, that long-standing diet — still eaten by peasants, farmers, and other groups of people in remote areas of the planet — provides such a good basic source of nutrients that the World Health Organization Expert Committee on Cardiovascular Disease has stated that these people are "well nourished . . . and have a good life expectancy at all ages."[123]

Complex carbohydrates are digested slowly and efficiently, providing a steady source of energy without the biochemical roller-coaster effect of concentrated sugars.

Recommendations for carbohydrate consumption: The American Heart Association recently joined other health organizations in recommending that Americans cut back on refined carbohydrates and increase their complex carbohydrate consumption to 55 percent of total daily calories.[124] Other authorities suggest 60 percent or more.[125] But, in spite of this guidance, the typical American diet remains excessively high in fat and *refined* carbohydrates such as white wheat flour and white sugar. We have already noted problems from excess dietary fat. Now let's look at those related to refined carbohydrates.

Problems with Sugar

The reason sugar and starch are both listed as carbohydrates is their chemical similarity. All carbohydrates — simple or complex — are actually made up of one or more simple sugars, the most prominent being glucose, fructose, and galactose. By themselves, each of these three is a monosaccharide. When two are joined together, they form a disaccharide. Example: Glucose plus fructose equals sucrose (table sugar). Glucose plus galactose equals lactose (milk sugar). When more than two simple sugars are linked together, a polysaccharide (complex carbohydrate) is created. Some polysaccharides contain more than one thousand glucose molecules hooked together.

The body extracts the sugars in carbohydrates — whether simple or complex — for energy. Glucose, also called blood sugar, is usually the sole source of energy for the brain and nervous system, and the liver is equipped to convert other simple sugars, such as fructose, into glucose so they can be used as fuel.

Simple sugars present health and performance problems when large amounts are regularly consumed as refined sweeteners, which are devoid of vitamins, minerals, fiber, and other features of complex carbohydrates.

Refined white sugar — sucrose — tops the list of "empty calories," along with its counterparts corn syrup, brown sugar, dextrose, maltose, and cane syrup. High intake of refined sugar has been linked to a variety of health problems, including elevated levels of blood fat and cholesterol,[126] a chromium (trace mineral) deficiency associated with heart disease and diabetes,[127] and development of breast cancer.[128] "In some cases sugar can dramatically boost the liver's production of VLDL cholesterol, an especially dangerous type, . . . [and] coronary risk factor," warns a recent report by the Stanford University Center for Research in Disease Prevention.[129]

The simple sugar molecules in sucrose require very little digestion, entering the bloodstream and quickly raising blood-sugar levels far above normal. In response, the body's insulin secretion mechanism is activated to remove the excess glucose from the blood, causing a downswing in blood-sugar levels.

Even so-called "natural sugar alternatives," such as fructose, maple syrup, maple sugar, date sugar, barley malt, honey, brown rice syrup, molasses, fruit juice, fruit concentrates, and so on, are no panacea. Many of these sweeteners contain more minerals than sucrose, and some are released into the bloodstream more slowly (fructose, date sugar, fruit juice, and fruit concentrates). But in spite of these variations, there is one underlying message: *No* sweetener used excessively is healthful.

Artificial Sweeteners

What about artificial sweeteners? Retailers sell about $8 billion worth of artificially sweetened products each year.[130] It is a lucrative, growing aspect of the food market. Because of links to cancer, saccharin is scheduled to be fully banned in the near future, just as cyclamates were banned in 1970 by the Food and Drug Administration (FDA). But the most popular artificial sweetener thus far is aspartame, called "NutraSweet" and "Equal."

Two hundred times sweeter than sucrose, aspartame is composed of two amino acids, phenylalanine and aspartic acid, leaves no unpleasant aftertaste, and is promoted in a masterful advertising campaign. Yet there is a bitter controversy surrounding aspartame, stirring strong debate among scientists, consumer groups, and the public about whether it is truly safe.[131]

"On one side," reports a recent issue of *Tufts University Diet & Nutrition Letter,* "are those who point to the more than 3,500 complaints that the Food and Drug Administration has received from consumers who claim that aspartame-containing foods have caused illnesses ranging from diarrhea and nausea to mood changes, anxiety, and seizures. On the other side are those who cite the findings of the Centers for Disease Control, an Atlanta-based government agency that gave aspartame a clean bill of health four years after evaluating more than 500 of the initial consumer complaints and finding no evidence that this sugar substitute could bring on any of the adverse health consequences blamed on it by its users."[132]

Going beyond safety, however, here's the main point: Very few people *need* to consume artificial sweeteners of any kind. There is little evidence that they help anyone lose excess body fat or keep from gaining it. Studies even report that long-term users of artificial sweeteners are more likely to *gain* weight than nonusers over the course of a year, regardless of initial body weight.[133]

Fiber

The different kinds of fiber all come from the cell walls of plants. They play a major role in keeping digestion moving smoothly and help prevent heart disease, obesity, and colon cancer.

In countries where the consumption of fiber-rich foods is low, people experience up to eight times the incidence of colon cancer as in countries where fiber intake is high.[134] Digestive and gastrointestinal tract diseases afflict nearly half of all Americans,[135] and cancer of the colon is a leading cause of cancer death. Constipation is a daily problem for an estimated 100 million U.S. citizens.

In comparison, the people of underdeveloped nations with an average of 5 or 6 times the amount of fiber and complex carbohydrates in their diets have virtually no incidence of these disorders. In recent years, the U.S. Department of Health and Human Services, the Surgeon General, the Public Health Service, the National Cancer Institute, and the National Institutes of Health all have urged Americans to eat less fat and refined carbohydrates and to consume more food high in starch and fiber.

The expression *dietary fiber* refers to all plant material resistant to digestion. It isn't actually "roughage," although fiber does help to produce a smooth, prompt transit through the digestive tract.

Fiber is divided into two categories. *Water-insoluble fibers* include celluloses (found in wheat bran), lignin, and hemicelluloses (found in whole grains and vegetables). Although they can't be dissolved in water, they absorb water, which means they swell up and add bulk, making it easier for the intestines to pass along waste products. Other dietary fibers are called *water-soluble fibers* and include pectins (found in apples, citrus fruits, legumes, and certain vegetables), gums, and mucilages (found in oats and legumes). These fibers have very different activities from the crude, water-insoluble fibers.

All fibers help slow down the absorption of glucose into the bloodstream since they are bound to digestible carbohydrates in whole foods. Pectins and gums slow sugar absorption from the intestines. Both fiber properties appear helpful to diabetics[136] and can aid us all in keeping blood-sugar levels more even.

Water-soluble fibers also bind with bile acids, which are produced by the gallbladder from cholesterol. As the body uses bile acids, it produces more, pulling cholesterol out of the bloodstream and thereby lowering serum LDL cholesterol levels.[137] High fiber intake has also been shown to aid in losing excess body fat and may even lower blood pressure by about ten percent.[138]

Recommendations for fiber consumption: Eat a widely varied diet of fresh whole foods to ensure that you get plenty of fiber in its various forms. Whole-grain breads and pasta, oat bran and oatmeal, legumes, brown rice, fruits, and vegetables are good choices.

How much total fiber should a person consume per day? The National Cancer Institute recommends 20 to 35 grams, although the average American consumes only about 10 grams. Other authorities suggest that average-sized adults should consume between 30 and 60 grams of total fiber per day,[139] and it is generally best to get your daily fiber from food rather than supplements. And remember, wheat bran is only a small part of the fiber picture.

Some of the best sources of fiber,[140] with the grams of fiber per 100 grams of that food listed in parentheses, are the following:

Water-insoluble fibers: all-bran (24.9), shredded wheat (10.2), barley (7.4), asparagus (2.8), Brussels sprouts (2.7), green beans (2.3), carrots (1.9), and broccoli (1.7).

Water-soluble fibers: dry oat bran (7.2), dried white beans (1.7), dried split peas (1.6), cooked rolled oats (0.8), strawberries (0.8), apples (0.7), and bananas (0.6).

If you aren't already accustomed to a fiber-rich diet, *gradually* increase the amount of high-fiber food in your diet in order to avoid temporary flatulence, bloating, or diarrhea.

Vitamins and Minerals

Vitamins are complex organic (carbon-containing) substances. They are essential, often in very small amounts, to support the body's normal growth, maintenance, and best health.

Often called the "spark plugs" of the cells, vitamins act as antioxidants, enzyme constituents, and catalysts for cellular metabolic reactions and immune function. Most vitamins cannot be manufactured by the body and therefore must be obtained from the diet. Because they perform so many vital functions in the body, vitamin reserves are rapidly depleted and must be consistently replaced.

An optimal diet will provide your body with a good supply of essential vitamins every day. Broad-spectrum, moderate-dosage nutritional supplements can provide added protection for those who need it. (See Chapter 28.)

Minerals are inorganic (without carbon) substances that are vital to many human structures and functions. They cannot be manufactured by the body and must be obtained from water and whole foods.

In recent years, a number of trace minerals or microminerals (manganese, zinc, selenium, chromium, molybdenum, and others) have been identified by researchers as having health and healing roles that are different than, but just as important as, the major minerals or macrominerals (calcium, magnesium, potassium, iron, sodium, and phosphorus).

Should we take isolated mineral supplements, that is, separate supplements of calcium, magnesium, iron, and so on? In most cases, probably not. Nutritional supplements containing balanced combinations of essential minerals may be helpful for some people. But it's easy to imbalance the body's mineral ratios by taking excessive amounts of individual minerals.

Salt

Except for sugar, table salt — sodium chloride — is the leading food additive in the United States. Excessive consumption has been linked to depression, bloating (edema), weight gain, obesity, headaches, hypertension (high blood pressure), and kidney disease.[141]

The body certainly needs salt, but only about a quarter teaspoon a day. The average consumption in the United States is about 20 times that amount.[142] Medical researchers in New Zealand found that consumption of common table salt can increase the amount of calcium lost through the kidneys, specifically in young women.[143] The scientists reported that adding a teaspoon of salt to the daily diets of young women can cause enough calcium loss to decrease bone mass an average of 1.5 percent annually.[144]

If you are still adding salt to your foods, it makes sense to gradually reduce the amount, beginning to enjoy the delicious variety of tastes in whole, natural foods. Salt is an acquired taste and habit. A recent national study showed that people forced to reduce their salt intake ended up liking their low-sodium diets.[145]

Because the human body has a great ability to conserve sodium, even people who work at heavy labor jobs in hot weather or who exercise intensively rarely need additional sodium beyond that found in whole, natural foods. For the estimated 20 percent of the U.S. population who are especially salt-sensitive, the Center for Science in the Public Interest (1501 16th St., N.W., Washington, DC 20036; 202-332-9110) offers a "Sodium Scoreboard" poster and a book entitled *Salt: The Brand Name Guide to Sodium Content.*

23 Contaminant-Free Food

CONVENTIONAL GOVERNMENT and industry propaganda asserts that America has the safest food supply in the world. But a surprising percentage of what is sold here isn't safe.

Food contaminated with pesticides, antibiotics, hormones, bacteria, molds, and additives, has become a concern in recent years as overuse, misuse, and abuse of these toxic chemicals and animal drugs has escalated. Ironically, the foods that health-conscious Americans are striving to eat more of — fresh vegetables and fruits — are among those most likely to be contaminated.

Our food supply can and should be made safer. Some problems can be solved by each of us as individuals, while others need to be addressed politically. One place to start is with ecologically sound farming and gardening.

Regenerative, "Organic" Growing Methods

The words *natural* and *organic* have been greatly abused in the food industry and in fad diet books. What do they really mean?

In *The Nutrition Debate: Sorting Out Some Answers*, Joan Dye Gussow, chairperson of the department of nutrition education at Columbia University and member of the Diet, Nutrition and Cancer Panel and Food and Nutrition Board of the National Academy of Sciences, says that even the food technologists and scientists who consider the word *natural* to be undefinable "were in 'reluctant agreement' that *natural* referred to treatment after the harvest and that it had something to do with 'minimal processing and the absence of artificial or synthetic ingredients or additives. . . . [And] *organic* was acknowledged, 'albeit often reluctantly,' to have a popularly agreed-upon meaning having to do with how the food was produced."[146]

Many people favor organic gardening and farming mainly because of the environmentally conserving agricultural practices it employs. It is a sustainable, biological approach to farming. "The fundamental concept of growing 'organically' is that the farmer uses practices that are in harmony with nature, and avoids the use of chemically synthesized herbicides, fungicides, pesticides or acidulted fertilizers," says organic-farming advocate Frank Ford. "For example: the grower may introduce beneficial insects to control harmful ones; apply natural mulches, mechanical cultivation, or even tolerate weeds; he may apply compost, manure, seaweed, etc. or depend on the natural fertility of the soil."[147]

There is little erosion on organic farms, since the farmer is dependent on maintaining a high humus content in the soil, and humus-rich soil does not erode. This is a critical concern because our land is disappearing. Today's chemical farmers tend to work the ground so hard that the soil is blown away or washed away at the rate of nearly 2 billion tons of American farmland every year. That means for every ton of corn produced, more than 500 tons of soil are permanently lost.[148]

Another reason more farmers are changing growing methods is economic. In a number of cases, they can increase their income by farming with fewer chemicals, or none at all, according to a recent report in *Science*.[149]

Some acreages are also being converted to intensive year-round commercial gardening using high-tech, low-cost greenhouses that produce fresh produce every month of the year, even in Minnesota.[150]

Pesticides, Herbicides, and Fungicides

Destructive health effects of toxic agricultural chemicals are well documented and include genetic mutations and cancer. It is important to determine that the foods we eat are free of these chemicals — pesticides, herbicides, fungicides, and others, which in this chapter I will collectively refer to as "pesticides." Many are so dangerous to human health that they are banned by the U.S. Food and Drug Administration (FDA) yet are still manufactured in America and sold to foreign countries where they're sprayed on crops that may then be imported and consumed in America.

Between 71 and 80 percent of all pesticides sold in the United States have not been sufficiently tested for carcinogenicity, states a recent report by the National Academy of Sciences.[151] For genetic mutations, 21 to 30 percent of all pesticides have not been adequately tested; for birth defects, 51 to 60 percent; and for adverse effects on the nervous system, 90 percent.

Understaffed, underfunded, and some say undermotivated, the FDA has far from ideal control over testing produce in the United States. Pesticides and fungicides — many known or suspected to be mutagens or carcinogens — turn up repeatedly in produce samples tested.[152] As more and more food is imported from countries with few, if any, safety standards, the problem appears to be escalating. The imported food bill in America is topping $24 billion a year.

Although some critics claim that pesticide risks are exaggerated, scientists at the Environmental Protection Agency (EPA) believe the risk is real. In a recent report, *Unfinished Business: A Comparative Assessment of Environmental Problems,* a group of seventy-five EPA experts and career managers rated pesticide residues among the top three environmental cancer risks.

During the past 30 years, pesticide use has increased more than tenfold — at least 1,100 percent[153] — yet insects are destroying more crops than ever and, in the process, are becoming more resistant to the new and increasingly expensive chemicals being created to exterminate them. More than 200 million tons of pesticides containing more than one thousand active ingredients are used annually on croplands in California alone.

There are also many unseen costs of pesticide use. For example, of the more than one billion pounds of active pesticide ingredients sprayed annually in the United States, as little as 1 percent actually reaches the target pests.[154] The rest ends up in the environment — contaminating water, land, air, and food. Private and government-funded agricultural experiment stations are developing ways to use harmless insects to control harmful ones. This is an important step in reversing the pesticide spiral — it now takes more and stronger chemicals to control insects. Why? Because an increasing number of pest species have become immune to mild, low-dosage chemicals.

Chemicals can be especially concentrated in beef, pork, and poultry and sometimes even in dairy products and eggs. "The Food and Drug Administration (FDA) now acknowledges that there may be up to 20,000 or more brands of animal drugs currently being used, of which only 2,500 have been approved for usage," reports the *Washington Post.* "According to the FDA, these drugs may pose a threat to the U.S. meat, milk, and egg supply. . . . It is also suspected that at least 3,500 of the unapproved drugs may leave residues in milk, eggs, and meat capable of causing cancer or birth defects in humans who eat the foods."[155]

Children may be especially vulnerable. Researchers at the Natural Resources Defense Council and other organizations are finding that children aged one to five, for example, may receive six to twelve times greater exposure to pesticides than adults.[156] There are two main reasons: children tend to eat more for their body weight and eat more pesticide-laden foods such as fresh fruits, vegetables, and juices.

Antibiotics

Experts are becoming increasingly alarmed over the misuse and overuse of antibiotics as a routine feed additive for commercial food animals. For more than forty years, antibiotics have been an effective medical aid in combating infectious diseases in both humans and animals. Yet today we are in danger of squandering this medical miracle. Massive overuse of antibiotics — not only in health facilities but also on the farm — is breeding strains of drug-resistant microorganisms.[157]

Thirty-five million pounds of antibiotics are produced each year in the United States; about half are prescribed for humans, and the remainder are fed to farm animals to promote growth or prevent disease. According to FDA estimates, antibiotics are administered to approximately 80 percent of all poultry raised in the United States, 75 percent of pigs and hogs, 60 percent of beef cattle, and 75 percent of the dairy cows.[158] In 1971, the British government banned the use of antibiotics as feed additives for animals. The World Health Organization supported this ban, and Holland, Germany, Czechoslovakia, and the Scandinavian countries adopted similar restrictions, but the United States did not.[159]

Microbial Contaminants

Food-borne infections strike approximately 20 to 90 million people each year in the United States and kill 9,000 of them.[160] Dr. Robert Tauxe at the Centers for Disease Control says that salmonella contaminations are increasing in incidence faster than contamination from any other food-borne microbe.[161]

The increase in salmonellosis is linked to the widespread practice in the meat industry of feeding antibiotics to cattle, pigs, and poultry.[162] New "super-salmonella" strains of bacteria are now antibiotic-resistant. High-speed mechanical methods of slaughtering and eviscerating animals, particularly poultry, increase the risk that salmonella (present in fecal material) will contaminate the meat.[163] To reduce the danger of salmonella poisoning, meat and poultry must be handled hygienically and cooked thoroughly.

Determining Your Pesticide Intake

Pesticides have infiltrated our food supply. Even if you consider only fruits and vegetables, the problem is so widespread that recent data from the Natural Resources Council show high pesticide residues in the following percentages of domestic (D) and imported (I) produce samples: apples (48%D/53%I), bell peppers (30%D/82%I), carrots (47%D/58%I), celery (72%D/75%I), cucumbers (29%D/80%I), grapefruit (60%D/48%I), lettuce (52%D/58%I), peaches (52%D/58%I), spinach (46%D/23%I), strawberries (61%D/87%I), and tomatoes (23%D/70%I).[164]

An important question, of course, is What is safe? In setting acceptable pesticide residue limits, the U.S. Department of Agriculture (USDA) and Food and Drug Administration (FDA) still use outdated, inaccurate estimates of how much fresh produce the average American eats. For example, the FDA sets its pesticide safety level assuming that an individual eats only 7½ ounces (about one-half) of a single melon *per year*. Similarly, the agency assumes that each year we eat no more than one avocado, 1½ cups of summer squash, one mango, 2½ tangerines, 1½ cups of cooked Brussels sprouts, and less than a half cup each of almonds, artichokes, blueberries, plums, nectarines, and radishes.[165]

For an optimal, varied diet, these levels are ridiculously low. Yet, according to government figures, eating more than any of these amounts in a year could theoretically expose an individual to a level of pesticide risk above that now considered safe by the government.

And beef, pork, and poultry have chemical residue problems too. The more meat in the diet, the more likely is the intake of agricultural and industrial chemical residues. For example, one class of insecticides — chlorinated hydrocarbons — can accumulate in the body fat of animals and humans. A recent report from the General Accounting Office states that 143 chemical residues are present in meat at levels above those determined safe by the government. Of these, 42 are suspected of being carcinogenic and 26 have been linked to birth defects and fetal mutations.[166]

Until effective, stringent standards are adopted and enforced, it is difficult to ascertain pesticide residue levels or verify organic growing methods once foods have left the farm or garden. What can we do about it? I list some specific recommendations later in the chapter.

The Illusion of Freshness

The availability of fresh produce year-round has to rank as one of the biggest agricultural achievements of the twentieth century. Throughout the months of late fall, winter, and early spring, Americans buy tons of produce — spending a total of almost $40 billion a year — under the illusion that it's fresh, health-promoting, and a good value for the money. It is none of these.

The "fresh" produce that millions of us buy every week during much of the year may be uncooked, even occasionally unprocessed, but it's never fresh. The costs are high and nutrients are often shockingly low — even altogether absent — because of premature harvesting, long-distance travel, and storage. Add in liberal amounts of pesticides during all phases of production, and the not-so-fresh "fresh" produce becomes worse than nutrient-deficient: it's harmful. And there is also the humanitarian issue to consider: this produce increasingly comes to American markets from distant lands, where farm workers are poisoned in working with the pesticides as well as subjected to other exploitive and inhumane labor practices.[167]

Nutritional scientists have discovered that fresh-frozen American vegetables are often a better nutritional and dollar value than the unfresh "fresh" produce mentioned above. Nutritional scientists Michael Colgan, a recent visiting scholar at Rockefeller University,[168] and David Reid of the University of California at Davis,[169] have both reported testing a variety of fresh produce and finding some of it completely void of key nutrients — for example, "fresh" oranges with no vitamin C, "fresh" carrots with no vitamin A. In a matter of a day or two after harvesting, vitamin content of produce can drop 75 percent or more.

By picking foods prematurely, or "green," growers have found that they remain hard, as if fresh, during transportation and avoid enzyme-related spoilage problems. Before shipping, some vegetables and fruits are gassed with ethylene and coated with waxes containing petroleum, animal-tallow, shellac, polyethylene, fungicides, or sprouting inhibitors. These embalming techniques are aimed at sealing in a ripe-looking color and texture.

With the dramatic increase in fresh produce consumption by Americans in recent years comes increased health risk. "The big problem in this country and Canada is that there simply isn't a strong constituency pressuring for food free of residues of widely used pesticides," says Charles M. Benbrook, executive director of the board on agriculture of the National Academy of Sciences' National Research Council. "Perhaps the day will come when people will raise such pressures, but it has not happened yet — even in the face of clear information that there are residues in the food supply."[170]

Supposedly, FDA regulations require waxed, chemical-treated produce to be labeled accordingly. Retailers are supposed to affix a label to the bins of bulk items listing waxes, fumigants, and fungicides. But the law simply isn't enforced.

Moldy Foods

Some of the most potent carcinogens are found in molds that can show up in bread, some cheeses, and peanuts.[171] Called mycotoxins, these poisons produced by molds are another category of food contaminants. In recent years, cancer researchers have expressed concern about a class of potent food-related carcinogens called aflatoxin, which is produced by molds that grow on nuts and legumes (particularly peanuts), corn, and cottonseeds, especially when they are weakened by drought or are improperly stored. Although experts claim that the actual risk to most of us may be relatively small, aflatoxins have been shown to produce cancer of the liver, and have been implicated in mental retardation of infants from women exposed to these poisons.[172]

Humans are exposed to aflatoxins primarily through consumption of peanuts and peanut products, some corn products, and milk from dairy cows fed aflatoxin-contaminated feed. Popcorn and sweet corn reportedly tend to resist aflatoxin molds and are therefore usually contaminant-free.[173]

Pickled, Barbecued, Smoked, and Burned Foods

Most commercially available salt-cured, salt-pickled, or smoked foods contain nitrites and/or nitrates added as curing agents and for coloring and flavoring. These chemicals promote the formation of cancer-causing substances called nitrosamines and should not be eaten.

In addition, "burned/brown foods are perhaps the major sources of dietary carcinogens," warns Dr. Sheldon Saul Hendler, internist and biochemist on the faculty at the University of California, San Diego School of Medicine. "There are substances in protein that when . . . browned or burned become highly mutagenic."[174]

The National Cancer Institute recommends that Americans choose grilled, barbecued, and smoked foods "less often." In barbecuing meats, the incomplete combustion of animal fat creates potent carcinogens called polycyclic hydrocarbons.[175] Studies also indicate that people who eat a lot of smoked food have a higher incidence of cancer of the stomach and other parts of the digestive tract.[176]

What You Can Do Right Now

1. *Eat a widely varied vegetarian or semi-vegetarian diet and grow your own vegetables and fruits whenever possible.* A diet made up predominantly of

plant foods — vegetables, fruits, grains, and legumes — decreases overall intake of toxic substances because you're eating foods low on the food chain. In addition, the fiber found in plant foods may help counteract or bind and eliminate a number of chemical residues and food additives that might otherwise be absorbed.[177]

If it fits your interests and schedule, take a serious look at growing some of your own food. Gardening is a great family activity and a way to save money while improving food freshness and quality. Back yard gardens, window gardens, and neighborhood cooperative gardens are among the options. In every reasonable way, avoid unnatural pesticides and other toxic agricultural chemicals. Join the National Gardening Association (180 Flynn Ave., Burlington, VT 05401), which publishes *National Gardening* magazine, and also consider subscribing to *Organic Gardening* (33 Main St., Emmaus, PA 18049).

2. *Buy the freshest, cleanest food possible.* Since imported produce generally contains more pesticide residues, try to choose domestically grown food, especially in-season, locally grown varieties. According to a National Academy of Sciences report, produce from the western United States tends to have less fungicide residue (which accounts for over half of the total estimated carcinogenic risk from pesticides) than produce from the more humid East and Southeast.[178] Be alert for freshness — don't buy or eat wilted, discolored, bad-smelling food of any kind. Pull off the outer leaves of lettuce and cabbage heads, where residues may accumulate, and trim the leaves and tops off celery.

3. *Get the most nutritional value from the produce you grow or buy.* Cut fresh foods at the last minute before eating to avoid nutrient loss related to oxidation. Use as little water as possible when preparing the foods. Cover pans when boiling or steaming to shorten cooking time and preserve nutrients.

4. *Wash fresh vegetables and fruits before eating.* Sandra Marquardt of the National Coalition Against the Misuse of Pesticides, suggests throughly scrubbing produce with vinegar or mild detergent to help break down some of the fungicide-loaded wax, although "there's no guarantee it gets rid of the residues."[179] Richard Wiles, of the National Academy of Sciences' National Research Council, is skeptical: "I'd wash, wash, wash, and hope."[180] Wayne Bidlack, a professor of nutrition and pharmacology at the University of Southern California School of Medicine and a researcher on fiber in fruits and vegetables, reports that he washes his produce in soapy water before eating it.[181]

Peeling waxed produce helps, too, although you lose nutrients by discarding the skin. Today not only apples and cucumbers tend to get waxed, but so do avocados, bell peppers, cantaloupes, eggplants, grapefruits, lemons, limes, melons, oranges, parsnips, passion fruits, peaches, pineapples, rutabagas, squash, sweet potatoes, tomatoes, and turnips. But even removing the peels of fruit and vegetables won't affect the residue concentrations of some toxic chemicals since many pesticides and fungicides can penetrate the peel.

5. *Avoid moldy foods.* Don't eat nuts or seeds that have the least suspicion of moldiness or rancidity. Use the sensitive receptors of your eyes, nose, and mouth to detect bitterness, moldiness, discoloration, or "old" appearance of foods — and then don't buy them, or discard them if you find these signs in foods you already have at home.

Some companies, such as Arrowhead Mills (Box 866, Hereford, TX 79045) and Walnut Acres (Penns Creek, PA 17862), sell peanuts, peanut butters, cornmeal, and grits that are certified aflatoxin-free.

6. *Handle and prepare animal flesh foods with great care.* If you eat beef, pork, poultry, or fish, avoid the fatty parts where most pollutants end up accumulating. Next, minimize microbial infection risks. Here are several tips: Defrost frozen foods in the refrigerator or microwave oven — not on a counter at room temperature. Rinse poultry inside and out with cold water to remove some bacteria before cooking. Use a meat thermometer and cook beef to an internal temperature of at least 160°F, other red meats to at least 170°F, and poultry to a minimum of 180°F. Cool cooked foods in the refrigerator. Keep foods at room temperature not longer than one hour before or after cooking.

Pay attention to personal hygiene. Bacteria can be transferred to utensils, dishes, and foods if you don't thoroughly wash your hands after going to the bathroom, diapering the baby, or blowing your nose. And after handling any meat products, wash your hands and utensils very carefully before handling any other foods. Wash cutting boards (don't use wood since it absorbs contaminants and can't be cleaned) and plates holding raw meat very thoroughly with soap and hot water immediately after use. Do not serve any food on the unwashed plate that held the raw meat. Reheat leftovers completely before eating.

7. *Say no to burned and most barbecued foods.* Don't eat darkly browned or burned foods and, in general, don't consume barbecued foods. If you eat barbecued foods on special occasions, here are several important guidelines. Don't use high-fat meats. Avoid basting foods with high-fat mixes — baste instead with lemon juice, wine, or tomato-based barbecue sauces to add flavor. Keep a squirter bottle of water close by in case the coals flame. If the smoke gets heavy, reduce it with water. Wrap vegetables and fish in foil to preserve flavor and protect from smoke. After cooking, scrape off any charred material on the surface of foods.

8. *Become an "American for Safe Food."* A growing demand for safe, fresh food will eventually force farmers and grocers to make changes that will benefit everyone in the long run except perhaps the chemical and drug manufacturers.

A recent campaign was launched by the Center for Science in the

Public Interest (CSPI) called Americans for Safe Food (ASF, 1501 16th St., N.W., Washington, DC 20036; 202-332-9110). I strongly encourage you to join and to start or support an ASF coalition in your community. A current listing of mail order sources of contaminant-free food is available from ASF by sending a stamped, self-addressed envelope.

One booklet to have in your home library is *Guess What's Coming to Dinner: Contaminants in Our Food* (written by the national ASF staff in 1987). Other good resource guides are *Pesticide Alert: A Guide to Pesticides in Fruits and Vegetables* by Laurie Mott and Karen Snyder (National Resources Defense Council, 122 E. 42nd St., New York, NY 10168; 1988) and *Eating Clean* by the Ralph Nader Group (P.O. Box 19367, Washington, DC 20036; 1987). To learn about misuses and abuses of chemicals in farm animals, see *Modern Meat: Antibiotics, Hormones, and the Pharmaceutical Farm* by Orville Schell (Random House, 1984).

NutriClean: Identifying Excellence in American Agriculture (149 Franklin St., Oakland, CA 94607; 415-832-1415), is an organization developing parts-per-billion measurement technologies to detect residues of pesticides and other chemicals. NutriClean uses dated silver, gold, and platinum seals to let consumers know the rating of fresh produce. The program is already being successfully used in some supermarkets in major California cities, and plans are reportedly under way to establish a national network of growers, distributors, and testing facilities.

9. *Encourage local farmers and gardeners to join the following organizations:*

▶ Americans for Safe Food (noted above).
▶ Regenerative Agriculture Association (222 Main St., Emmaus, PA 18049). The association, dedicated to a more sustainable, cost-effective food future, has more than eighty thousand members and is growing rapidly. It provides member farmers with findings of worldwide research and practical guidelines for reducing production costs and phasing out agricultural chemicals in food, water, soil, and air. Members receive *New Farm* magazine.
▶ Institute for Alternative Agriculture (9200 Edomonston Rd., Suite 117, Greenbelt, MD 20770). This organization is directed by I. Garth Youngberg, organic farming coordinator during the Carter administration. The IAA was established to pull together farmers already practicing organic agriculture with academic professionals and researchers who are willing to sidestep the political pressures of chemical-dependent agriculture to study organic methods objectively.
▶ National Coalition Against the Misuse of Pesticides (530 Seventh St., S.E., Washington, DC 20003). NCAMP has organized an effective coalition to lobby for stronger federal legislation to curb the use of dangerous agricultural chemicals.

10. *Shop at reputable, responsive stores. Demand and select the freshest vegetables, fruits, and other whole foods, locally grown whenever possible.* Put your local supermarket managers in touch with organizations like Americans for Safe Food (ASF) and NutriClean. Support regional organic farmers and farmers' markets in your community.

Have local ASF groups visit the managers of your area supermarkets and urge them to offer contaminant-free foods and to label all food that may contain potentially harmful chemical residues. Ask to see affidavits or scientific tests by independent laboratories verifying that foods are free from pesticides, herbicides, and other chemical additives. The greater the public demand for high-quality foods, the easier they will be to obtain.

11. *Write to your local newspaper and representatives in Congress* (U.S. House of Representatives, Washington, DC 20515; and U.S. Senate, Washington, DC 20510), urging a ban on chemicals known or suspected of posing a serious risk to consumers; advocating national definitions for organic foods; requiring full-disclosure labeling and dating of foods; and demanding more research by the USDA and FDA on minimizing the use of agricultural chemicals and developing safe, alternative agricultural methods.

12. *Don't become fanatical.* There is no excuse to permit food contamination to continue. But don't forget to keep things in perspective. While we work toward final solutions to this problem, most of us continue to be at considerably greater risk from factors such as tobacco smoke, alcohol, drugs, radiation, high-fat diets, inactivity, distorted thinking, chronic negative stress, and not wearing seatbelts than from pesticides.[182]

Once you have done what you can about the food contamination issue right now, schedule your future action plan. Then enjoy your meals and devote your energy to the other important aspects of *Health & Fitness Excellence.*

Caution: New "Miracles" in Food Preservation

The mammoth food industry avidly pursues new preservation and packaging methods. Every time I hear the expression "miracle" used in this commercial field, my skepticism and curiosity are aroused.

Food irradiation is one example. If you or I were exposed to 100 kilorads of radiation, we'd be dead in less time than it takes to eat a piece of fruit or small vegetable salad. Ironically, the next fruit or vegetables you eat may have been irradiated with that same 100 kilorads, the dosage recently approved by the FDA. The FDA has approved food irradiation[183] for beef, pork, poultry, seafood, vegetables, grains, fruits, herbs, and spices.

How does food irradiation work? Low levels of radiation (using cobalt-60 or cesium-137, by-products of wastes from nuclear weapons or power plants) emit radioactive rays into the food to kill insects, molds, and bacteria that may cause food spoilage or disease.

Proponents of food irradiation claim that after years of government testing, it is an environmentally safe and cost-effective alternative to chemical pesticides with known carcinogenic effects.

What an amazing process: Foods, once irradiated, can last for years, maybe centuries, on grocery store shelves without refrigerator space or any special protection. Yet little is known about the long-term safety of consuming irradiated foods (which themselves are not radioactive). The irradiation controversy centers on the chemicals that radiation produces in food. Irradiation alters a fraction of the natural chemicals found in whole foods, producing so-called radiolytic products (RPs). Many RPs appear identical to substances normally present in the food, although that doesn't make them safe. Other products of irradiation, called unique radiolytic products (URPs), have never been found in nonirradiated food and thus are of considerable concern to scientists.[184]

And there are other reasons for apprehension. Irradiation produces far more free radicals than normal cooking does. Free radicals react with chemicals in foods to produce new radiolytic products, some potentially carcinogenic.[185] A recent study identified RPs as a possible cause of precancerous conditions in the digestive tracts of animals.[186]

Britain has rejected food irradiation because of the lack of solid evidence about its safety.[187] When researchers fed a small group of malnourished Indian children irradiated wheat, they discovered abnormal chromosome numbers in their white blood cells, a change that has been associated with cancer.[188] A recent study raises other serious questions: A number of disorders, including testicular tumors, developed in animals fed irradiated chicken.[189]

Irradiation destroys vitamins — notably E, C, and B_1 — and leaves foods unprotected from rancidity and grains and nuts susceptible to carcinogenic aflatoxin molds.[190]

The FDA estimates that 10 percent of the chemicals in irradiated food are, in all probability, unique — that is, they are not found in nonirradiated foods and may be unknown to science. Although the FDA assumes that the concentrations would be too small to affect human health, irradiation energies are much higher than those involved in cooking and therefore may be more likely to produce harmful chemical reactions and possibly cell mutations that could initiate cancer in humans.[191]

FDA regulations now require that any "whole food" product treated with radiation need only be labeled with a little flower-like symbol. Apparently, everyone is supposed to know what the flower stands for.

Food products having some, but not all, ingredients treated with radiation don't have to be labeled. For example, salads with 95 percent of the ingredients irradiated would *not* have to be labeled. In addition, there is no requirement that restaurants, nursing homes, airlines, or hospitals disclose that meals contain irradiated foods. Without full-disclosure labeling, how can we choose the foods we eat away from home?

"I asked six leading medical scientists here at Rockefeller University the simple question, 'Would you eat food that had been irradiated with Cobalt 60 to preserve it?' " writes nutrition researcher Michael Colgan. "Five said 'No' and one said 'Only if there was nothing else.' "[192]

Here are several resources for more information about food irradiation.

▶ *Food Irradiation: Who Wants It?* by Tony Webb, Tim Lang, and Kathleen Tucker (Thorsons, 1987). Examines the facts about the safety and wholesomeness of irradiated food and the question of whether the technology is controllable and needed.

▶ Health and Energy Institute (Suite 506, 236 Massachusetts Ave., N.E., Washington, DC 20062). Compiles research and publishes an introductory brochure entitled "Food Irradiation: What Are the Hazards?"

▶ Coalition to Stop Food Irradiation (Box 59-0488, San Francisco, CA 94159) and the Health Research Group (2000 P St., N.W., Washington, DC 20036). Both organizations have irradiation research information available and are monitoring government and private research efforts.

One way to minimize any health risk from irradiated food is to make certain it is clearly labeled, and then don't buy it. Support local farmers who produce top-quality fresh foods sold in your area.

24 High-Quality, Fresh Whole Foods

WHAT DO I HAVE TO GIVE UP? is the first question many people ask when trying to change their diet. Most of us like the foods we are used to eating. The correct approach to making changes is quite the opposite, however: What are the hundreds of delicious *new* foods I can choose for my diet?

Vegetables and Fruits

For thousands of years, vegetables and fruits have been a basic human food. They offer a great variety of tastes and colors, and fresh, organically grown vegetables and fruits are generally low in fat, rich in carbohydrates, high in certain vitamins and minerals, and in some cases a good source of protein and fiber.

As noted in the previous chapter, it is important to find vegetables and fruits that are fresher and safer than standard produce — or grow your own. When buying, favor vegetables and fruits that grow in your area and support local farmers. Then widen your horizons. Learn about vegetables and fruits you've never eaten or perhaps haven't enjoyed in the past. Be daring enough to regularly include new varieties in your diet. *How many of these popular vegetables do you eat?* Artichokes (glove), artichokes (Jerusalem or sunchokes), arugula, asparagus, bamboo shoots, beans (green, yellow, and string), beets, beet greens, bok choy (pak choi), broccoli, Brussels sprouts, cabbage (red and white), carrots, cauliflower, celeriac, celery, chard, chicory, Chinese cabbage, cilantro, collards, corn, cucumbers, daikon, dandelion, eggplant, endive, escarole, garlic, green onions (bunching and scallions), horseradish, jicama, kale, kohlrabi, leeks, lettuce (romaine/cos, Boston, Bibb, butterhead, head, green leaf, red leaf, celtuce/stem, etc.), mushrooms (all edible varieties), mustard greens, okra, onions (all varieties), peas (all varieties), peppers (bell: red, green, yellow), peppers (chili, jalapeño, etc.), potatoes (all varieties), pumpkins, radishes, rutabagas, Savoy cabbage, sea vegetables (all edible varieties), shallots, spinach, sprouts (all fresh, edible varieties), summer squash (zucchini, yellow, etc.), sweet potatoes, tomatoes (botanically a fruit yet eaten like a vegetable; all varieties), turnips, turnip greens, water chestnuts, watercress, winter squash (acorn, banana, buttercup, butternut, Hubbard, patty pan, spaghetti, turban, etc.), and yams.

How many of these popular fruits do you eat? Apples, apricots, avocados, bananas, dates, berries (bilberries, blackberries, blueberries, boysenberries, cranberries, elderberries, gooseberries, huckleberries, loganberries, raspberries, red currants, strawberries, etc.), carob, cherries, chokecherries, figs, grapefruits, grapes, guavas, kiwi fruits, kumquats, lemons, limes, mandarin oranges, mangoes, melons (cantaloupe, casaba, cranshaw, honeydew, muskmelon, persiamelon, watermelon), nectarines, oranges, papayas, passion fruits, peaches, pears, persimmons, pineapple, plantains, plums, pomegranates, prickly pear, prunes, quince, raisins, rhubarb, tangelos, and tangerines.

Locally grown vegetables and fruits "fresh from the garden" are best. Don't wash them before storing them because excess moisture encourages rot and causes a loss of water-soluble nutrients. To maintain crispness, refrigerate most vegetables in a paper bag in the crisper bin of your refrigerator. Store fruits and vegetables separately to maximize freshness. Store hard-rind winter squashes, potatoes, and onions in separate bags or containers in a cool (45–50°F), dry, dark area instead of the refrigerator. Quick-frozen vegetables should be kept solidly frozen. Canned vegetables should be stored in a cool, dry, dark place.

Whole Grains and Flours

Most of us don't realize how many delicious grains are available. The standard choices for most families are still white rice and white all-purpose wheat flour. But nutritional experts confirm that a variety of *whole* grains are essential to an optimal diet.

Grains are seeds of plants, the nutrient storehouses that produce the next plant generation. They are low in fat (unlike nuts and seeds) and high in complex carbohydrates (70–85 percent in most grains), proteins (an average of 5–10 percent), fiber, vitamins, and minerals. Grains provide an almost limitless source of low-cost, high-nutrition eating enjoyment. Along with legumes, grains are a traditional staple food of healthy, long-lived people throughout the world.

Grains are best when organically grown and can be cooked, soaked, sprouted, or stone-ground into meal or flour and baked. Modern civilizations have managed an amazing destruction and denaturing of grain for bread. Commercial mills produce white flour by grinding off the outer fiber-rich bran, removing the high-nutrition germ, and then chemically bleaching and treating what is left — in the process eliminating most nutritional value. Traditional whole-grain recipes offer a wide range of delicious tastes and textures, and we can each benefit by expanding the variety of dietary whole grains that we consume.

Whole wheat is now cultivated on more acres than any other grain in the world, and America has made it the most popular grain. But wheat's nutritional profile is insufficient to warrant choosing it as the solitary grain in anyone's diet. The key once again is *variety*. In addition to wheat, how many of the following whole grains are a regular part of your diet each week?

Rye and *buckwheat* are the primary grains for more than one-third of the countries in northern Europe, including Scandinavia and the Soviet Union. *Amaranth* was a staple grain of the Aztec civilization and is used by the country people of Mexico, South America, China, India, and Africa. *Millet,* a staple grain of the ancient Egyptians, has been eaten for more than a thousand years in northern China, the Himalayan region, and parts of Russia, India, and Africa.

Barley, a favorite in ancient Egypt, Rome, and Greece, was cultivated in China as early as 2000 B.C. It is favored today in western China, Tibet and other Himalayan countries, and the mountainous regions of the southern and southeastern Soviet Union. *Brown rice* has been cultivated for centuries in China and surrounding countries, and *corn* originated in Central and South America.

Oats are a relative newcomer to the grain family, thriving in cooler countries such as Scotland, Ireland, Great Britain, the northern United States, and Canada. *Quinoa* (pronounced keen-*wa*) is botanically a fruit, yet, like buckwheat and wild rice, it has been consumed for centuries as a cereal grain. It's an ancient staple food from the South American Andes and the mountainous regions of Ecuador, Peru, Bolivia, southern Colombia, northern Argentina, and Chile.

Triticale is a hybrid of wheat and rye. *Wild rice* is botanically related to brown rice. It grows in cool freshwater lakes and rivers of the northern Midwest United States, New Brunswick (Canada), and some areas of the Rocky Mountains.

Each of these popular whole grains offers a special taste, texture, and nutrient profile. All are available in natural food stores and grocery stores in Europe and America.

One of the most popular whole-grain foods of all is pasta — a delightful staple made from flour dough using various grains. "Pasta is a food that comes closer to being universally adored than any other single food," writes health columnist Jane Brody. "American consumption of pasta lags behind that of nations that, incidentally, lack our problems with rampant heart disease and obesity."[193]

Contrary to the popular belief that pasta is fattening "filler" food, when properly prepared it is a very nonfattening, nutrient-rich food. What usually makes pasta meals fattening are the rich, abundant sauces many of us love. The nutritional value of pasta is determined by what it's made of. Look for good-quality, whole-grain ingredients whenever possible. Pasta is a wonderful food as part of a varied, optimal diet. Find new ways to enjoy it!

Legumes

Legumes, by definition, are the edible mature seeds that grow inside the pods of leguminous plants. This important food group includes dried beans, peas, and lentils. Known for centuries as a "poor man's food," legumes are a staple of many of the world's healthiest, longest-lived peoples.

Easily grown, dried, and stored, legumes provide wonderful opportunities to break meal plan boredom. They are an inexpensive, nutrient-rich food source, high in complex carbohydrates, fiber, good-quality proteins (deficient in one or more essential amino acids but ideal as complementary proteins when eaten with grains), minerals (especially iron, potassium, zinc, magnesium, and copper), and several B vitamins. They are free of cholesterol, low in simple sugars and sodium, and, with the exception of soybeans, very low in fat (an average of only 3 percent).

Recent medical research indicates that legumes are beneficial for diabetics because they have a remarkable balancing effect on insulin that lasts for hours, helping the body stabilize blood-sugar levels, metabolize excess fat, and keep LDL serum cholesterol levels lowered.[194] Legumes may also be helpful in protecting against certain cancers, according to researchers at the Harvard University School of Public Health and other institutions.[195]

One of the reasons some people don't eat beans is that they produce "gas." Most legumes, particularly baby lima beans, aduki beans, split peas, and lentils generally don't cause flatulence. Others (especially kidney, fava, and soy beans) contain small amounts of carbohydrates called alphagalactosides or trisaccharides, which are not easily broken down by the routine enzymatic processes in the intestinal tract. These sugars combine with intestinal bacteria, ferment, and produce by-products such as carbon dioxide, hydrogen, and a few other gases. There *is* a solution for those sensitive to this effect.

Biochemists with the USDA research centers have found that up to 90 percent of the gas-forming sugars in selected legumes can be eliminated with several simple steps.[196] First, rinse the beans, picking out all foreign matter (small pebbles may occasionally be present). Second, soak the beans for at least 4 hours — overnight in the refrigerator is one convenient way. Discard the soaking water. Third, add fresh water and cook the beans.

Easily digested legumes such as lentils, split peas, and lima beans generally don't require these preparatory steps, although *all* beans must be thoroughly cooked to make them digestible.

There are hundreds of varieties of legumes grown throughout the world. Some, such as green peas and lima beans, may be eaten fresh as vegetables. Dried legumes should be stored in a cool, dry place in tightly covered containers. Even though cooking time for some of the legumes is fairly long, they require little attention during cooking. And once cooked, they can be stored for a few days in the refrigerator or frozen for later use. When buying dried legumes, choose those that have been organically grown, and look for uniform size (which helps prevent the problem of small legumes being overcooked and exceptionally large ones being undercooked) and avoid legumes that are cracked or shriveled or have pinholes (which can indicate insect damage).

How many of these popular legumes do you eat? Aduki beans, blackeyed peas (cowpeas, China beans), chickpeas (garbanzo beans), fava beans (broad beans, Windsor beans, scoten beans, English beans), lentils, lima beans (butter beans), mung beans, navy beans (pea beans), pinto beans, small pink beans, small red beans, soybeans (tofu, tempeh, grits, flour), split and whole dried peas.

Nuts and Seeds

Nuts and seeds, in very limited quantities, can be a delicious part of a good diet. Because of their high fat content, however, nuts and seeds should be eaten fresh and raw and usually not more than once or twice a day with meals or snacks.

Each seed and nut contains within it all of the nutrients needed to nourish and sustain a new plant. Fresh, raw nuts and seeds can be good sources of protein (incomplete), essential fatty acids, carbohydrates, fiber, vitamins, and minerals. They may be chopped or ground and sprinkled on salads, yogurt, and other whole-food recipes. Once shelled, nuts and seeds should be stored in the refrigerator away from light. Buy in small quantities and eat promptly.

In terms of fat, one tablespoon of peanuts or filberts (hazelnuts) contains more than 7 grams of fat, almonds 5 grams, and chopped walnuts 4.8 grams! Peanut butter (or other nut butter) sandwiches should be spread-it-thin-and-have-it-only-once-in-a-while treats in a low-fat diet.

One delightful exception for all of us who love the crunch of nuts is chestnuts. Unlike other nuts, they are high in carbohydrates, low in fat, and low in calories. In fact, two large chestnuts contain only 0.2 gram of fat. Fresh chestnuts are available in some parts of the country during the fall and winter. They are usually sold in the shell and may be prepared at home by heating in the oven at 350°F for one hour, then cracking the shell, and eating them.

Sesame seeds are popular in many parts of the Orient and the Middle East. Although high in protein (approximately 20 percent), vitamins, and minerals, sesame seeds contain nearly 50 percent fat and should therefore be eaten raw and in very small quantities. For ease in digestion, buy sesame seeds with the hulls removed — and choose those dehulled mechanically rather than chemically.

Other seeds can be eaten on occasion, too. Sunflower seeds, which contain about 45 percent of their calories as fat, should also be selected with care. Pumpkin seeds (pepitas), pinenuts (really seeds), and flax seeds are popular choices. Alfalfa seeds and chia seeds are among those recommended for sprouting.

Dairy Products

It is widely recognized that dairy products are rich in nutrients. Three-fifths of the world's population consumes and enjoys milk, yogurt, kefir, whey, cheeses, or butter. Americans are experiencing a long-overdue trend away from high-fat, disease-promoting dairy products and toward low-fat and nonfat varieties.

The amino acid profile in milk protein is excellent, and dairy products complement vegetables, grains, and legumes in the diet. Research suggests that certain dairy products may even offer minor protection against cancer.[197]

Studies also suggest that regular consumption of milk during childhood helps protect against osteoporosis later in life.[198] Saturated, long-chain fats like those found in beef and pork are likely to react with calcium to form insoluble "soaps" that are excreted in the feces, preventing the calcium from being absorbed and used by the body. Medium- and short-chain fatty acids, like those found in dairy products, are less likely to interfere with calcium absorption.[199]

Reports suggest that milk drinkers may generally have healthier colons, with less risk of colorectal cancer, than non–milk drinkers have.[200] Nonfat milk may help reduce serum cholesterol levels,[201] and dairy products have a beneficial effect on bone mineralization, which is reportedly superior to the effect of calcium supplements.[202]

Yogurt and other cultured dairy foods (such as kefir, koumiss, acidophilus milk, and nonfat buttermilk) are receiving scientific praise. Two beneficial bacteria in fresh yogurt are *Lactobacillus bulgaricus* and *Streptococcus thermophilus*. Khem Shahani, professor of food science at the University of Nebraska, has researched the nutritional aspects of cultured dairy foods for more than twenty-five years. According to Shahani, these bacteria help the body by producing several B vitamins (B_{12} and biotin) and enzymes that aid in the digestion of fats, carbohydrates, and proteins, produce natural antibiotics, and retard the growth of certain cancer cells.[203] Kefir, koumiss, and buttermilk have active cultures much the same as yogurt and presumably provide similar benefits.

Lactobacillus acidophilus, another beneficial strain of bacteria that curdles milk, has recently been shown to survive the intestinal tract better than *L. bulgaricus*. Because of this, it may be more effective in aiding digestion and helping prevent colon cancer (as part of a low-fat, high-fiber diet). When they are present together, *L. bulgaricus* inhibits the growth of *L. acidophilus,* and therefore yogurt rarely contains viable acidophilus culture. Acidophilus is reportedly available in some brands of kefir and koumiss although the best source may be sweet acidophilus skim milk, available in a growing number of grocery stores and natural food markets.

In spite of all this good news, there are some well-recognized disadvantages to many dairy products. First, many people begin to lose their ability to digest the carbohydrate in milk (lactose) beginning between the ages of two and four. This happens because the production of the enzyme lactase, which digests the lactose, diminishes. Although most adults would experience some stomach upset and gas if they drank a full quart or more of milk at a single sitting, only one in twenty has problems with an 8-ounce serving.[204]

So long as dairy products make up no more than 5 to 10 percent of the overall diet, most adults tolerate them well. For those who don't, yogurt and other cultured products can often help circumvent lactose-intolerance problems.[205]

Another concern about dairy products is fat and cholesterol. Whole milk contains 9 grams of fat per 8-ounce serving. Two percent low-fat milk has 5 grams, 1 percent low-fat milk between 2 and 3 grams, and nonfat skim milk only a trace. The best advice for most of us: gradually phase into consuming low-fat and then nonfat milk, yogurt, and other dairy foods.

Be certain to read the labels on cheeses. One ounce of American cheese contains nearly 9 grams of fat! In contrast, some part–skim milk cheeses have 2 grams or less. Whole milk cottage cheese contains almost 10 grams of fat per cup. Two percent low-fat cottage cheese has only 4½ grams of fat, and 1 percent cuts it down to about 1½ grams.

In limited quantities, low-fat and nonfat cottage cheeses can be part of a good diet, but avoid "processed" and "imitation" cheeses made from space age ingredients. If you enjoy traditional hard or soft cheeses, choose them with care, keep servings very small, and reduce fat and sodium elsewhere in your diet.

Ice cream remains America's favorite dessert, but it's often loaded with fat, sugar, and a smorgasbord of chemicals. And some of the popular "frozen tofu" desserts contain more fat and sugar as ingredients than they contain tofu! Far better choices are fat-free fruit sorbets and nonfat frozen yogurts.

Safe, Clean Milk

Today's dairy farms use modern equipment to produce good-quality dairy foods. But the truth is that some commercial milk may be laden with toxic chemicals including pesticides, antibiotics, and detergent residues from washing milking machines and utensils. In some cases, cows are fed chemical-laden feeds to boost milk production and are kept alive with drugs.

Pasteurization, the process of heating milk to 145°F for 15 seconds, was implemented in 1895 to protect consumers from disease-causing bacteria that may be transmitted in milk. While it is a commendable public health concept, ensuring *highest-quality* dairy products requires more than pasteurization alone. The milk must come from healthy, drug-free animals and be handled in accordance with stringent safeguards for milking procedures, milking equipment, milk cooling requirements, handling, and processing. Groups such as Americans for Safe Food (1501 16th St., N.W., Washington, DC 20036; 202-332-9110) are lobbying for strict enforcement of the highest-quality dairy standards. They deserve our support.

Eggs

Each year in America, more than 260 million chickens lay 62 billion eggs. Eggs, high in protein, saturated fat, and cholesterol, have been heavily criticized as contributing to elevated blood cholesterol levels.

There is no doubt that eggs are high in food cholesterol — a single yolk from a large egg contains between 250 and 275 milligrams of cholesterol, and major health organizations now recommend a *maximum* of 300 total milligrams of dietary cholesterol per day.

Studies show that as eggs are added to the diet, LDL serum cholesterol levels (the kind you don't want to be elevated) tend to rise. A recent study by the National Heart, Lung and Blood Institute in Bethesda, Maryland, indicated that even in cases where the total serum level of cholesterol did not increase in response to eating eggs, the balance among the cholesterol-transporting lipoproteins (HDL, VLDL, and LDL) may be adversely affected. On the other hand, studies at the University of Illinois and UCLA suggest that eating eggs may have little effect on serum cholesterol if overall dietary fat levels are low.[206]

Other egg-related problems are the result of questionable practices in the commercial egg production industry in America. Groups such as Americans for Safe Food and FACT (Food Animal Concerns Trust, P.O. Box 14599, Chicago, IL 60614) are working to upgrade egg quality standards and their enforcement.

If you choose to eat eggs, buy them fresh from local sources and cut back on the number you consume. With all the research supporting the need to limit intake of fat and protein, reducing egg quantities makes good sense. A weekly average of not more than two or three is prudent. If you have elevated serum cholesterol levels, you may be asked by your physician to eliminate eggs from your diet entirely. If you do eat them, be certain to cook them well to avoid problems with salmonella bacteria and avidin, a protein in egg whites that can bind with the vitamin biotin and prevent its absorption.

For greatest safety, avoid eating raw or partly cooked eggs. A recent Centers for Disease Control report recommended that when cooking eggs, you should boil them for seven minutes, poach for five minutes, or fry on each side for three minutes.[207] Don't fry eggs in polyunsaturated oils or lard. If necessary, use a *very* small amount of olive oil; better yet, hard-boil the eggs in water, or scramble tofu and save the eggs for baking.

If you cannot find top-quality eggs or choose not to eat them at all, try a natural "egg substitute" in recipes calling for eggs. Some of these products are available at grocery and natural food stores. Their basic ingredients are soya, potato, and tapioca flours and arrowroot. The best egg substitutes are inexpensive and contain no preservatives, artificial flavorings, or sweeteners.

Seafood, Poultry, and Meat

As noted in Chapter 21, vegetarian diets can provide us with all vital nutrients, many of them limited or unavailable in flesh foods. Semi-vegetarian diets — in which seafood, poultry, or meats are eaten only on occasion — also provide significant health benefits over the traditional American diet heavy with meat.

Seafood

Americans are eating more fish and shellfish than ever before, in part because seafood is receiving increased publicity as a health-promoting food. A recent editorial in the *New England Journal of Medicine* stated that research findings "support the possibility that the consumption of fish may be of special benefit to human health."[208]

Current studies indicate that one to three weekly meals with a small portion of fish — an average daily serving of 30 mg (just over 1 ounce) — may supply a safe, beneficial amount of omega-3 fatty acids (discussed in Chapter 22).

But don't go overboard. "Before you go out and fill your freezer with oily fish, you should know that many environmental contaminants, such as DDT, dioxin, and PCBs, collect in the oil," warns Michael Jacobson of the Center for Science in the Public Interest. "These chemicals, chlorinated hydrocarbons, are suspected of causing cancer and birth defects. Most likely to be contaminated are the fattier freshwater fish, such as carp, lake trout, catfish, and yellow perch, as well as the fatty migratory species, like bluefish. Least likely to be contaminated are saltwater fish such as salmon, shellfish, and freshwater fish grown on farms or caught in unpolluted mountain streams. . . . If you want to eat fish and not worry about the fat or contaminants, choose cod, haddock, flounder, sole, turbot, ocean perch, halibut, tuna, pollock, clams, scallops, or other lean species."[209]

Recent research at MIT indicates that canned salmon, sardines, mackerel, and albacore (white) tuna packed in water retain plenty of beneficial omega-3s.[210]

You may have heard that shellfish are high in cholesterol and should be avoided. The original researchers made a mistake, however, and this warning is overstated. New, sophisticated scientific techniques reveal that most shellfish is fairly low in cholesterol. In a 3½-ounce serving, clams have only 34 mg of cholesterol, mussels 28 mg, oysters 55 mg, scallops 33 mg, Alaskan king crab 42 mg, Dungeness crab 59 mg, northern lobster 95 mg, and shrimp 152 mg.[211]

In addition, evidence shows that much of what scientists formerly thought to be cholesterol in mollusks (clams, mussels, oysters, and scallops) turns out to be a composite of several different types of noncholesterol sterols. Rather than raising serum cholesterol, this type of shellfish actually seemed to lower cholesterol absorption by about 25 percent in one human study.[212] Shellfish have the added benefit of being low in fat (in a 3½-ounce serving, scallops have only 0.2 gram of fat, shrimp 0.8 gram, and lobster 1.9 grams). Much of what little fat there is in shellfish is omega-3 fatty acids, reports Jacob Exler, an expert on shellfish for the U.S. Department of Agriculture.[213]

Variety and freshness are the watchwords with seafood. While United States regulatory agencies are confident about the safety and wholesomeness of fish and shellfish sold in America, other organizations are calling for more stringent inspections. Stay informed of water pollution problems in your area if you eat local fish. When possible, buy smaller fish and trim away the dark meat, usually the fattiest tissue where contaminants accumulate.

What about eating raw fish or sushi? Dangers include viruses, bacteria, and toxic pollutants. Outbreaks of disease caused by eating raw shellfish have occurred across the United States. Dangers result from a lack of adequate methods for detecting human pathogens in shellfish and from unscrupulous suppliers taking clams and oysters from illegal waters loaded with human sewage.[214]

"Eating poorly cooked shellfish is a high-risk adventure at best," reports the *New England Journal of Medicine*.[215] Other authorities advise against eating raw animal flesh foods of any kind and extend the risks to include all types of raw fish.[216]

Poultry

Poultry sales in the United States have boomed in recent years as millions have heeded medical warnings and reduced their intake of red meat. Until the 1960s, poultry — chicken, turkey, game hen, duckling, pheasant, and goose — was traditionally reserved for holiday feasts or special weekend dinners in America. Skinless breast of chicken or turkey is often recommended these days as a dietary substitute for beef, pork, and other high-fat meats. As noted earlier in our review of the scientific and medical evidence supporting semi-vegetarian and vegetarian diets, if you choose to eat poultry, keep the portions small and eat it infrequently.

And remember to follow strict kitchen hygiene guidelines, cooking poultry thoroughly to kill harmful bacteria and cleaning your work space and your hands before handling other foods. More than one-third of the chickens tested by government inspectors in or on their way to stores during 1982–1984 were contaminated with salmonella bacteria.[217]

Beef, Veal, Pork, Lamb, and Other Meats

Beef, veal, and pork have come under increasing criticism by nutritional scientists and medical researchers. Many of the problems discussed in Chapter 23 — chemical residues, antibiotics, hormones, and pathogenic microbes that may be concentrated in beef, pork, and veal — can be overcome by insisting on contaminant-free, "organic" meat from healthy animals. But that doesn't change the fact that these meats are high in saturated fat, cholesterol, and protein, all of which are overconsumed in America. Diets with a large meat content also tend to be deficient in complex carbohydrates and fiber.

Studies suggest a direct correlation between beef consumption and cancer of the colon.[218] Researchers have also linked eating pork[219] and beef[220] to hypertension (high blood pressure). In addition, the tissue residues that result from a diet high in beef or pork are acidic. Some researchers believe that the change in body chemistry resulting from consuming those meats contributes to calcium loss[221] and the development of osteoporosis.[222]

If you choose to eat beef or pork on occasion, be certain to select the leanest cuts, such as top round of beef, flank steak, chuck arm pot roast, short loin of beef, center loin of pork, and shoulder roast of veal. Always trim off all excess fat and eat very small portions.

Eliminating beef, pork, and other meats from the diet — or at least cutting back on them and insisting on lean, contaminant-free sources — makes good health sense.

25 Meals and Snacks

Great Nutrition Where It Counts

All the nutrition guidelines in the world won't result in better health and performance if you can't bring those dietary principles to life in your kitchen — with fast, enjoyable meals and snacks.

Priority number one is to plan your meals and snacks as far in advance as possible, never less than a full day ahead. This is the best way to take charge of your daily nutrition, to be certain you are eating a widely varied diet that meets the goals you have set. On your planning sheets, list six spaces each day: a small to moderate breakfast, a light midmorning snack, a moderate lunch, a light midafternoon snack, a moderate supper, and a very small evening snack.

With the right recipes, you can quickly and inexpensively implement the *Health & Fitness Excellence* nutritional guidelines, such as cutting back on fat, cholesterol, and salt, increasing complex carbohydrates and fiber, and so forth. At the same time, you can preserve the delicious flavors you love and can introduce new ones.

This all begins with your selection of a cookbook, choosing from among the thousands in print. There are several solid options. First, use whatever favorite cookbooks are already on your kitchen shelf — preferably one of the new lower-fat, higher-carbohydrate classics such as *Jane Brody's Good Food Book* (Norton, 1985) — and begin reviewing and modifying recipes using *Health & Fitness Excellence* nutrition principles.

To calculate total daily nutrients — protein, fat (monounsaturated, polyunsaturated, and saturated), carbohydrate, fiber (soluble and insoluble), cholesterol, salt, and other nutritional factors — you'll want to use a scientific manual. The standard in the field is *Nutritive Value of Foods* by the U.S. Department of Agriculture, H & G Bulletin No. 72 (U.S. Government Printing Office, Washington, DC 20402; 202-783-3238). For advanced analysis, the government's revised Agriculture Handbook No. 8 series is excellent.

To handle this whole process at top speed, I recommend the computer software program called *Nutrition Wizard,* designed by Dr. Michael F. Jacobson (Center for Science in the Public Interest, 1501 Sixteenth St., N.W., Washington, DC 20036; 202-332-9110). *Nutrition Wizard* includes data on more than two dozen key nutrients and nutritional profiles for nearly two thousand foods, with provisions for you to enter any additional foods you may choose.

But the fastest way to bring *Health & Fitness Excellence* to life in your kitchen is by using *The Health & Fitness Excellence Cookbook* by Leslie L. Cooper (Advanced Excellence Systems, P.O. Box 1085, Bemidji, MN 56601; 218-854-7300; 1989). My wholehearted endorsement of this book is confirmed by the many people who have attended courses taught by my wife, Leslie, or who have tested the menus and recipes in her book or sampled them at our center. The cookbook includes a full 28-day menu with 14-day cool-weather and 14-day warm-weather meal/snack plans and more than two hundred recipes.

The Health & Fitness Excellence Cookbook also includes up-to-date information on a variety of foods, spices, and seasonings, guidelines for cooking with whole grains and legumes, fruits, vegetables, and low-fat/nonfat dairy products. Most recipes are vegetarian but delicious options are included for meals with seafood or poultry. There are chapters on shortcuts for baking your own whole-grain breads and other recipes, suggestions on packing lunches for children and adults, and the best nutritional bets for where and what to eat when dining out. Each individual recipe, meal, snack, and complete day's menu has a full nutritional analysis. The book also lists preparation times for each recipe and features an index noting recipes that can be prepared in 5 to 30 minutes.

26 Dining Out

OUR HEALTH IS not only in our own hands but in the pots, pans, and buffets controlled by chefs in America's 620,000 restaurants. Less than twenty years ago, eating out was still considered a luxury by most families. It was a way to splurge once or twice a month and to celebrate special occasions. But in response to changing lifestyles and a two-decade food industry advertising campaign, Americans now eat away from home an average of four times a week and spend almost 40 percent of their monthly food budget at restaurants.

Chances are, your busy lifestyle often makes it necessary to eat meals and snacks away from home. Some health writers flatly condemn dining out. But there is no reason why eating away from home has to be a dietary disaster. While there's no doubt that many restaurant menu items are loaded with fat and cholesterol, making healthy choices is becoming easier.

Restaurants are adding more fresh salads, seafood, baked potatoes, grain-legume casseroles and side dishes, whole-grain breads, and lower-fat pasta recipes to their menus. Nonetheless, we still need to watch out for hidden fats, especially in prepared cookies, muffins, pie crusts, cream sauces and soups, and cheeses.

High-quality, low-fat dining begins with your selection of restaurant. Skip all-you-can-eat buffets and smorgasbords. Order à la carte since full-course bargain dinners encourage overeating and tend to be too high in fat and protein. If possible, look over the menu in advance or call ahead to ask about featured recipes and daily specials.

Don't be shy about making requests over the phone or in person to the waiter, waitress, or chef — many restaurants will eliminate salt, cook with half the amount of fat (or no added fat at all), and cut back on cheese, eggs, and whole-milk dairy products. Many regional offices of the American Heart Association (7300 Greenville Ave., Dallas, TX 75231) print lists of local restaurants serving low-fat meals. Write for details.

Choose entrees that are steamed, poached, broiled, roasted, baked, or cooked in their own juices. Pass up anything fried or sautéed. Good restaurants will broil seafood or poultry dry (without fat) and unsalted and have or will create a special low-fat sauce to your liking. Salads and salad bars can be good choices if the vegetables are *fresh,* but steer clear of prepared salads with a cream or heavy oil base since they are usually high in fat. Instead, choose a variety of fresh raw vegetables or fruits, legumes, and whole-grain bread. As a salad dressing, use a very small amount of olive oil with vinegar or lemon added.

The best restaurant soups are vegetable-based since cream- and meat-based soups are usually high in fat. Pasta can be a good choice if served with tomato, wine, or other low-fat sauces. Whole-grain breads, rolls, bagels, and low-fat muffins are delicious sources of fiber and complex carbohydrates, but skip the nut spreads, mayonnaise, butter, or margarine. Hot cereals such as oatmeal, oat bran, and multigrain varieties and whole-grain dry cereals can be a good breakfast choice when served with skim milk and fruit. Original Swiss Bircher-Benner muesli (made with fresh fruits, soaked oats or other whole grains, and low-fat or nonfat yogurt) is also excellent.

Remember that desserts are a treat, not a necessity. When you choose them, make the portion small. A slice of home-baked pie or cake is all right as a once-a-month option, but on a more frequent basis fresh fruit, fruit-based frozen sorbet, nonfat yogurt, and low-fat or nonfat puddings top the list.

If you eat out often, you run the risk of excessive fat and protein. Watch quantities — many eateries serve extra-large portions of food. If you are dining with other people, consider having a fresh salad, vegetable/grain/legume side dish, and a piece of whole-grain bread and then splitting a main dish with at least one other person. Don't hesitate to ask for a "people bag" to take leftovers home for a meal or snack the next day. And remember to select a wide variety of meals from week to week.

Many ethnic restaurants offer exquisite-tasting cuisine featuring whole grains, legumes, vegetables, and fruit and recipes supplemented with fish or poultry. Here are several quick insights:

Italian. Delicious, low-fat foods with a fabulous array of tastes can make Italian restaurants a good choice for dining away from home. Pasta with meatless marinara (tomato-based), vegetable, red clam, or wine sauces is first-rate. Shrimp al vino bianco (sautéed in white wine) gets high marks, too, for its low fat content. Polla cacciatore (boneless chicken breast served in a tomato and mushroom sauce) is another option. The list also includes nonmeat (vegetable) lasagne, and cioppino — fisherman's stew with a variety of seafood and vegetables in a tomato-base stock (make certain it's low in fat). If you enjoy pizza, order it vegetarian style (go very light on the olives) with extra vegetables and half or one-third the cheese (ask for part-skim mozzarella). Onions, green peppers, and mushrooms are standard, but try fresh spinach, garlic, tomatoes, artichoke hearts, beans, seafood, and other ingredients for a delightful change of pace.

Mexican. When chosen with care, Mexican food is inexpensive, delicious, high in complex carbohydrates, and low in fat. Beans, rice, unfried corn tortillas, fish, and salads are common staples. Vegetable-bean burritos, fresh fish marinated in lime sauce, and beans with rice are low-fat specialties. A good practice when selecting a new Mexican-style restaurant is to call ahead and ask if they use lard, coconut oil, or other oils in the refried beans. Many establishments have switched to small amounts of soybean oil or, ideally, no added fat at all. Skip the sour cream, guacamole, meat/egg dishes, and fried foods, and request no more than half the amount of cheese.

French. Traditional French restaurants offer rich, delicious foods that are high in fat, calories, and cholesterol. Fortunately, more and more French chefs are preparing nouvelle cuisine, including a special variety called cuisine minceur ("cuisine of slimness"). Cuisine minceur uses culinary techniques such as steaming or poaching seafood or poultry in vegetable juices and wine and serving side dishes of fresh vegetables, potatoes, and grains. For dessert, skip the usual fare and request fresh fruit or fruit (usually peaches or pears) poached in a light wine sauce — which gives a delightful taste with few calories.

Indian. The recipes used in Indian restaurants often include vegetables, legumes, yogurt, and lots of spices. Avoid the dishes soaked in coconut oil or ghee (clarified butter). Before ordering, ask the waiter or waitress how the various dishes are prepared. One popular recipe is murg jalfraize — chicken or legumes flavored with fresh spices and sautéed (request no butter or oil) with onions, tomatoes, and bell peppers.

Chinese. Some menu items at Chinese restaurants are good choices because of the emphasis on rice and vegetables with only small amounts of seafood or poultry. Bypass the fried appetizer dishes like egg rolls and spring rolls. And don't choose duck — a 3½-ounce serving of Peking duck has 30 grams of fat. Stir-fried dishes like moo goo gai pan — a combination of mushrooms, bamboo shoots, water chestnuts, and chicken, seafood, or tofu served over rice — generally get good ratings. At Chinese restaurants, stir-fried dishes tend to be cooked quickly in a lightly oiled, very hot wok, and vegetables retain more vitamins than those cooked the traditional American way. The oil is usually peanut, which is high in monounsaturates. Choose restaurants that will honor your request for less oil, little or no salt, and no monosodium glutamate (MSG), the flavor enhancer that gives some people headaches.

Japanese. Generally low in fat, Japanese cuisine is based on protein-rich soybean products (such as tofu and tempeh), seafood, vegetables, noodles, and rice. The seaweed used in Japanese soups and stews is high in minerals. One top entree choice is yosenabe, a vegetable dish with seafood.

American. Traditional American restaurants have contributed some healthful dishes to the array of dining options, including New England and West Coast seafoods, fresh salad bars, Cajun gumbos, and a variety of new "California cuisine" specialities.

Vegetarian. Although vegetarian restaurants serve nonmeat and even nondairy meals, many dishes tend to be high in fat. Limit cheeses and avoid items heavy with oil, butter, or cream. Choose fresh whole-grain breads, cooked grain/legume casseroles and side dishes, and rice or pasta with low-fat sauces and a variety of vegetables.

On the Road

When you have to be out of town for a few days, consider bringing along some basics, such as dry cereals, fruit, and nonfat yogurt for breakfasts and whatever you favor for light snacks. Brown-bagging can save you time, money, and needless calories. A small cooler in your car or a hotel room refrigerator can help keep perishables fresh.

If you travel by plane, call ahead to order a special meal. You can often choose from seafood, vegetarian, kosher, and other options. Some major carriers now offer a seafood platter with vegetables, whole-grain bread, and tomato cocktail sauce; or a vegetarian platter with vegetables over rice or legumes, a salad, whole-grain bread, and a piece of cheese or fruit; and even a fresh fruit plate. Remember to drink plenty of water between meals in the air since aircraft cabin air rapidly dehydrates your body. In general, skip alcoholic beverages, coffee, and tea, since they make the water loss even worse. A number of air carriers now offer a variety of spring waters.

27 Gaining Greater Control of Your Mind and Emotions Through Food

SCIENCE HAS BEGUN to unravel the complex connections among food, mind, and emotions. No matter how good your food choices are, compelling new research suggests that the foods you choose for meals and snacks may influence production of brain messenger chemicals called neurotransmitters, which in turn affect your mental energy, concentration, attitude, mood, behavior, and performance.

New studies at Harvard, MIT, the National Institutes of Health, and other research centers have been published in specialized scientific and medical journals.[223] Discoveries in those studies were recently brought to the public's attention by Judith J. Wurtman, nutritional research scientist at MIT, in her book *Managing Your Mind and Mood Through Food*. Continued research has shed further light on this exciting subject.[224]

The emerging picture on the mind-mood-food connection suggests the following:

▶ The *wrong* personal choices and timing of foods for meals and snacks may create or contribute to loss of enthusiasm, mental and physical fatigue, increased body fat, and poor performance *or* tension, anxiety, and irritability.
▶ The *right* personal choices and timing of foods for light meals and snacks may create or contribute to a more alert, faster-reacting, more focused, more productive mind *or* the calm composure for clearest thinking, problem solving, and stress management.

According to Wurtman and other researchers, mental behavior can be modified, often within 30 to 45 minutes, when the right kind of light snack or small meal is eaten. Neurotransmitters are manufactured by the brain from or in response to constituents of the food we eat.

Before we go any further, one point needs to be made absolutely clear: It would be an egregious oversimplification of human behavior to suggest that mental and emotional states can be controlled by the manipulation of a single aspect of life — *any* aspect. Food is an important consideration, but only one of many. Chapters throughout *Health & Fitness Excellence* provide you with scientifically based ways to manage stress and improve your brain/mind power, emotional/attitudinal control, and performance. So by all means test the principles in this chapter, but be certain not to overlook the many other aspects of *Health & Fitness Excellence*.

Alertness Neurotransmitters

According to researchers, dopamine and norepinephrine are two brain neurotransmitters that promote alertness — faster thinking, greater reaction speed, attentiveness, energy, and motivation. The amino acid tyrosine is a principal constituent of dopamine and norepinephrine. When tyrosine from a food enters the brain, production of dopamine and norepinephrine increases, enhancing alertness.

Foods rich in protein and low in fat reportedly work best to provide the brain with tyrosine. Examples include fish, shellfish, skinless white meat chicken or turkey breast, tofu, skim milk, low-fat or nonfat cottage cheese or plain yogurt (fruit may be added), lentils, and dried peas and beans. High-fat foods cause fatigue, says Wurtman, and therefore are not recommended. "Fat seems to slow other processes, like thought or movement. It makes people very lethargic. During the long digestive process that follows a high-fat meal, more blood is diverted to the stomach and intestines and away from the brain."[225]

The quantities of protein-rich foods necessary to help many people increase mental alertness are very small — 2 to 4 ounces are usually enough, and that is generally consistent with the nutritional wellness principles in *Health & Fitness Excellence*.

Adding carbohydrate-rich foods — such as grains, fruits, and vegetables — to the small snack or meal doesn't appear to interfere with the tyrosine available to the brain.

Calmness Neurotransmitter

Serotonin is a neurotransmitter that promotes calmness — an easing of the feelings associated with negative stress and tension, less distraction from environmental stimuli, and a relaxed ability to focus more clearly on a job at hand. In some people, depending on the time of day, serotonin slows reaction time and contributes to drowsiness.

Tryptophan is the principal amino acid from which serotonin is made, and carbohydrate-rich foods — eaten alone, without a high-protein food — increase the brain's access to tryptophan. When tryptophan is forced to compete with tyrosine for access to the brain, it loses; that's why eating protein- and carbohydrate-rich foods together tends to make tyrosine — not tryptophan — available to the brain for increased alertness and energy.

Therefore, for a calming, focusing effect, try eating low-fat, carbohydrate-rich foods alone as a light snack or small meal. Examples include cooked whole grains (rice, wheat, oatmeal, corn, buckwheat, barley, and so on) eaten with fruit or a sweetener but without milk; breads, pastas, cereals, dry popcorn, crackers, low-protein cookies and muffins, baked potatoes, corn, and so on. Very small amounts of sweets and starches — 1 to 1½ ounces for most people — usually permit enough tryptophan to enter the brain for a calming, focusing effect. Exceptions include people 20 percent or more overweight and women in the days just preceding menstruation, when 2 to 2½ ounces of carbohydrate-rich food may be required.

Note: A few people have a biological craving for carbohydrates and, rather than being calmed by them, find them energizing. For this small group of individuals, the "sugar buzz" is real. But contrary to popular belief, carbohydrates do not cause hyperactivity or increased energy or aggressiveness in most normal healthy people, including children.

Psychologist Bonnie Spring, from Texas Tech University, has conducted much of the research debunking common carbohydrate myths. It turns out that sugar consumption and hyperactive behavior in children may be coincidental. Spring reports that sugar does not increase physical activity or aggression in normal *or* hyperactive children.[226]

Some highly active children may consume lots of carbohydrates because these foods are calming or because they quickly replenish calories for physical energy. This is not to say, of course, that it's fine for children or adults to eat large amounts of refined sugar. It isn't. But the decision not to do so should be based on sound dietary rationale — as noted in Chapter 22 — rather than on the assumption that it will alleviate a behavior problem.

Fruits (including the sweetener fructose) and vegetables (except potatoes and corn) appear to be mind-mood neutral, say researchers. That is, these foods don't directly affect either alertness or calmness neurotransmitter production and therefore can generally be eaten with either protein-rich or carbohydrate-rich foods.[227] Another important discovery: Amino acid supplements, such as pills or capsules of concentrated tyrosine or tryptophan, are not a short cut to better mind-mood control. In fact, they are potentially harmful, and you should get qualified professional advice before taking them. Your *food* choices are the key.

Test It Yourself

Your success in choosing the right foods and combinations of foods that help you manage your emotions and mind depends on careful observation of your body's responses and habits over the next weeks. Take notes on your state of mind and mood 10 to 15 minutes before meals and snacks. Do you feel alert and motivated; or calm and focused; or tense and irritable? One hour after eating, reassess your state of mind and emotions, and then quickly and honestly write down your observations.

Review your appraisals to create a list of the food choices that seem best for you and use it as a helpful tool in your day-to-day eating patterns and as one of many self-care aids.

The questions surrounding the mind-mood-food connection are complex. The preliminary answers are intriguing and further investigation is ongoing. To learn more about this exciting theory and its supportive research, see *Managing Your Mind and Mood Through Food* by Judith J. Wurtman, Ph.D. (Harper and Row, 1987).

28 Nutritional Supplements

A poor diet plus vitamins is still a poor diet.

—*ART ULENE, M.D.*

Nutritional supplements are a multi-billion-dollar annual industry in the United States and part of a dizzying controversy. A bombardment of advertising claims, contradictory opinions, and conflicting research reports leaves many consumers bewildered and confused.

The truth is this: You cannot purchase high-level wellness in a bottle of tablets. Contrary to widespread myths, there is no lazy person's short-cut, no miracle pill just around the corner, no space age elixir that gives you well-being, immunity, or peak performance. It is a step-by-step, multifactor process. Let's keep everything in perspective: An optimal diet is only one of the seven steps to *Health & Fitness Excellence*. And nutritional supplements are only one of many considerations *within* that one step.

Keeping those facts in mind, the overall evidence indicates that even if you eat a well-balanced diet, manage stress, and lead an active lifestyle, you may still want to take a vitamin and mineral supplement, if only as a form of nutritional insurance.

Are Nutritional Supplements Necessary?

Recent surveys indicate that up to one-half of the American population regularly takes some form of daily vitamin or mineral supplement, and, contrary to fears expressed by some professionals, most people seem to realize that a basic vitamin-mineral pill is no substitute for a good diet. Apparently, Americans are using supplements as part of an overall approach to a healthy lifestyle. In this respect, supplements may be appropriate.

When I first began studying about health and fitness twenty-five years ago, vitamin-mineral supplements were considered strictly faddism. But over the years, scientific research has pinpointed some specific benefits to moderate, balanced supplementation.

"Dietary/nutritional imbalances and deficiencies contribute significantly to the premature deaths of millions of Americans annually," says Dr. Sheldon Saul Hendler, biochemist, internal medicine specialist, and professor at the University of California at San Diego School of Medicine and author of *The Complete Guide to Anti-Aging Nutrients*. "Moreover, our changing world has placed new demands on our bodies, exposing them to environmental stresses and insults that were not previously so prevalent, stresses and insults that deplete our tissues of protective micronutrients as never before."[228]

One reason for public confusion about vitamin-mineral supplements is the pure emotion of the issue. It has become a battle. "On the one side [of the dietary supplementation question], legions of lay and semilay faddists and commercial interests line up to promote their advice or their products with little understanding of or regard for real evidence," observes Dr. Roy L. Walford, professor of pathology at UCLA School of Medicine, life extension specialist, and author of *The 120-Year Diet*. "On the other side stand cadres of otherwise quite good scientists and physicians who, because establishment medicine is dead set against *any* [dietary] additives in excess of the holy RDAs, accept mediocre evidence uncritically if it seems to support their views."[229]

Government Recommendations

What is the ideal quantity of individual vitamins and minerals for each of us on a daily basis? There are a number of variables. The Food and Nutrition Board of the National Academy of Science (NAS) appoints a committee every five years or so to update the Recommended Daily Dietary Allowances (RDAs), which include many vitamins and minerals. The U.S. Department of Health and Human Services (5600 Fishers Lane, Rockville, MD 20857) publishes the U.S. Recommended Daily Allowances (U.S. RDAs) used for food labeling. These values are set by the federal Food and Drug Administration and feature single numbers representing the highest level of a nutrient recommended, regardless of age or sex. Both versions are sometimes referred to simply as "the RDAs."

RDA decisions are a political fulcrum affecting hundreds of corporate, federal, and state programs. Government welfare funding hinges on the RDA levels. At the same time, the lower the RDA figures, the more easily vitamin and food package labels can claim higher RDA percentages at no additional cost. A heated debate continues about choosing RDAs that prevent dire clinical deficiencies versus establishing those that may also safely promote best health.

"*Optimal* dietary allowances for *optimal* health and *maximum* longevity . . . have not been determined by any federal agency," writes Dr. Hendler. "There is growing evidence that micronutrient intake . . . in amounts *higher* than the RDAs may be protective against various diseases or aging, such as cardiovascular disease, cancer and bone disease. . . . The current Recommended Dietary Allowances simply do not deal with the maximization of life span."[230]

The conservative American Dietetic Association has maintained the official position for many years that nutritional supplements are unnecessary for people who eat a normal, "balanced" diet. However, a recent survey of 900 registered dietitians revealed that 60 percent of this professional group took some kind of nutritional supplement.[231]

The "researchers didn't ask *why* the dietitians were taking pills, but other studies have," reports *Nutrition Action Healthletter*. "The most common reason: insurance. People want to play it safe. When the cost is minimal and the possible benefit is better health, that approach makes sense."[232]

The RDAs can serve as a helpful starting point for nutritional supplementation and underscore the fact that safe limits for vitamins and minerals vary. There is evidence that supplements with nutrient levels at — or moderately above — the current RDAs may be advisable for many people. But remember that taking nutritional supplements in excess of your needs is a waste of money and can create a false sense that other aspects of a health and fitness program are less important than they really are. Second, in megadoses some vitamins and a number of minerals *can* be dangerous to health.[233]

Priorities in Selecting a Nutritional Supplement

Comprehensive, Synergistic Formula

As nutritional biochemist Roger Williams points out: "Nutrients always act as a team. Comprehensive nutritional science must rise above the traditional piecemeal approach."

For greatest benefits and safety, vitamins and minerals should be taken together in a balanced formula. Taking large doses of isolated nutrients puts you at risk of developing an imbalance in nutrients not being supplemented. Although each vitamin and mineral has its own biochemical functions in the body, they work *synergistically* — they help each other. Until the recent advent of powerful laboratory computers, it wasn't possible to do the complex analyses that make this truth obvious. Unfortunately, ultraconservative advice on vitamins and minerals is often still based largely on obsolete, single-nutrient experiments, usually done *in vitro* (in the test tube), outside the body.

Certain broad-spectrum vitamin-mineral formulations have been designed to maximize the efficient functioning of individual nutrients through their balance with "helper" nutrients present in the formula. For example, vitamin E has at least double the effectiveness in the body when it is present with other antioxidants such as vitamins A and C and the trace minerals zinc and selenium.[234] A well-balanced supplement is a highly efficient supplement, one in which dosages of all nutrients can be kept optimal but as low as possible and costs can be minimized.

Continuous Biochemical Availability

To help the body best utilize nutrients from supplements, it is important to take them at regular intervals throughout the day along with meals or snacks. This may also help protect the gastrointestinal tract, since extra antioxidants will be present during digestion.[235]

Appropriate Nutrient Levels

Begin with nutrient levels that are equal to or moderately above the RDAs. "My own opinion," says Hans Fisher, chairman of the nutrition department at Rutgers University and contributing editor to *Nutrition Reviews* and associate editor of *Nutrition Reports International,* "is that while the experts are busy wrangling over the issues, we should take the pragmatic approach. A good, multivitamin supplement that provides all the important vitamins and minerals in amounts equal to the U.S. R.D.A. for each nutrient is worthwhile under most conditions for most people."[236]

Most health authorities seem to agree that there is no harm in taking a broad-spectrum multivitamin-mineral supplement that provides up to 150 percent of the RDAs for nutrients.[237] For advice on specific nutritional supplement formulations that take into account new research on *optimal* health and longevity, see *The Complete Guide to Anti-Aging Nutrients* by Sheldon Saul Hendler, M.D., Ph.D. (Simon and Schuster, 1989). This is one of the best books written to date about the fads and facts of nutritional supplements.

There are hundreds of different formulas available and they differ in quality, ingredient sources, quantities, balance, extra additives, recommended dosages, and cost. It is up to you to comparison shop, reviewing nutrient balances compared with the RDAs. Contact companies suggested to you by qualified professionals. Request supportive research, full ingredient disclosure information, freshness standards, recommended dosage, costs, availability (where to purchase in your area or by mail), and endorsements by reputable nutrition scientists.

And do your best to stay abreast of scientific information on supplements by subscribing to the nutrition periodicals listed at the end of this book or reading them regularly at your local library.

Freshness Matters   Choose a supplement with an expiration date on it. Certain nutrients interact with others (for example, thiamine may hasten the decomposition of folic acid and vitamin B_{12}). Because of this, vitamin formulas can lose potency over time. Store supplements in a cool, dark, dry place but not in the refrigerator.

Vitamin C

It is easy to get carried away by advertising claims and end up spending too much money on too many different nutritional supplements. The best advice is to keep it simple. In addition to, or as part of, a broad-spectrum multivitamin-mineral formula, consider an amount of vitamin C moderately above the RDA.

Ascorbic acid, as vitamin C is known to chemists, is an essential nutrient and antioxidant, aiding the immune system and virtually every cell in the body in neutralizing dangerous free radicals. Along with other nutrients, vitamin C also helps protect the body from certain carcinogens and toxic environmental chemicals.

"There is good evidence that supplements of ascorbic acid greater than the amount needed for its vitamin function may be useful in combating some of the effects of both physical and emotional stress," says Hans Fisher of Rutgers University. "There is evidence that emotional stress can reduce blood ascorbic-acid levels, suggesting the body has a greater need for vitamin C at that time. A potentially important finding has been the report by researchers at the prestigious Massachusetts Institute of Technology that ascorbic acid at levels of two grams [2,000 mg] a day blocked the formation in the intestine of potent cancer-forming compounds called nitrosamines."[238]

The National Research Council itself now recommends a diet with "plenty of vitamin C–containing materials," which seems to be a recommendation of more than its own official RDA of a mere 60 mg per day.[239]

According to Dr. Oliver Alabaster, director of Cancer Research at George Washington University Medical Center: "Since it is very difficult to achieve levels of vitamin C much above 250–500 milligrams with modern dietary habits, we probably should be taking supplements to achieve the cancer-protecting levels of vitamin C that we need. . . . After considering all the evidence carefully, I have come to the conclusion that a reasonable vitamin C intake, which might lower your cancer risk and is completely safe, is 1 gram [1,000 mg] a day, preferably in divided doses

(250 milligrams four times a day). This should be achieved by combining a 1-gram daily supplement with a diet that is rich in vitamin C."[240]

"The best available data," says Dr. Sheldon Saul Hendler from the University of California at San Diego School of Medicine, "suggest that adults and children over ten years of age may benefit from a daily intake of 250 milligrams to 1,000 milligrams of vitamin C. . . . Vitamin C will be best utilized by the body if taken in divided doses, preferably with each meal."[241]

Optimum Diets and Supplements for Children

In general, the principles of nutritional wellness discussed in *Health & Fitness Excellence* apply to children as well as adults. Consult with, and follow the advice of, your trusted pediatrician and family physician. Lifelong habits begin at an early age. Overall, *the single most important influence on children's eating habits is the example set by their parents.*

Parents have a great responsibility for educating their children about nutritional wellness — by example, discussions, patience, and support. First, see that mealtimes are a very happy experience and a time when all family members are present. Arguments and scolding shouldn't be permitted during meals. The best diets feature a wide variety of foods and recipes — diverse tastes, textures, and colors make eating fun.

Children can best learn about healthy foods by being actively involved in choosing and preparing them at home. Force-feeding children (of any age) should be avoided — it undermines their confidence. Foods shouldn't be offered as rewards, bribes, or solace. Nonfood rewards (a hug, spending some extra time with your child, a trip to the movie, and so on) are superior. Moreover, food should never be withheld as punishment. Parents should also do their best not to express their own food dislikes in front of their children. If your children are currently picky eaters, don't despair.

In addition to the publications recommended in the preceding chapters and the periodicals listed at the end of this book, the following resources may prove very helpful in working with your physician in planning optimum nutritional programs for infants, children, and adolescents.

▶ *Child of Mine: Feeding with Love and Good Sense* by Ellyn Satter, M.S., R.D. (Bull Publishing, P.O. Box 208, Palo Alto, CA 94302; 1983). A conservative book for expectant and new parents that encourages seeking a middle ground for teaching healthy eating habits without dominating the child's own perceptions about food choice and quantity.

▶ *Creative Food Experiences for Children* (Center for Science in the Public Interest, 1501 16th St., N.W., Washington, DC 20036). A wonderful book for teaching three-to-ten-year-olds basic awareness of good nutrition.

▶ *Eat, Think, and Be Healthy!* (Center for Science in the Public Interest, 1501 16th St., N.W., Washington, DC 20036). A guidebook filled with fun activities designed to teach good nutrition to children ages eight to twelve.

▶ *The Health & Fitness Excellence Cookbook* by Leslie L. Cooper (Advanced Excellence Systems, P.O. Box 1085, Bemidji, MN 56601; 1989).

▶ *Jane Brody's Good Food Book* by Jane E. Brody (Norton, 1985).

▶ *Jane Brody's Nutrition Book* by Jane E. Brody, revised edition (Bantam, 1987).

▶ *Nutrition Action Health Letter* (available from CSPI, 1501 16th St., N.W., Washington, DC 20036; 202-332-9110). Prospective and expectant parents should subscribe to this excellent periodical and be certain to read the April 1987 issue. It features well-documented articles such as "Eating for Two" and "Playing It Safe While You're Pregnant." Topics covered include healthful eating, selecting the best nutritional supplements, and avoiding a host of environmental hazards.

▶ *The Stoplight Diet for Children* by Leonard H. Epstein, Ph.D., and Sally Squires, M.S. (Little, Brown, 1988). An innovative weight control program that pairs parents and children (ages six to twelve) as partners for psychological support. Solid advice, color-coded food choices, helpful quizzes. An 8-week plan that can give lifelong benefits.

Step 4

BODY FAT CONTROL

29 Introduction

MYTH: To lose weight, you need to skip some meals and ignore your hunger.

FACT: Hunger is a body signal — like pain or tension — that shouldn't be ignored. Skipping meals and struggling to resist feelings of hunger push you toward overeating binges. And fad "crash diets" fail; any pounds lost are usually water or vital muscle tissue, *not* excess body fat, and actually make it easier for you to gain more body fat with every new diet you try. Now you can cut through the dieting myths with a five-part scientific formula to help eliminate excess body fat once and for all.

MYTH: Obesity is inherited — some people are just born to be fat.

FACT: While certain people may genetically inherit the *tendency* to form extra fat cells, obesity itself isn't inherited. It is caused by eating too much fat-laden food, skipping meals, and forgetting about exercise and stress management. Result? Fat cells load up with fat, and when they're full your body makes more fat cells to handle the overflow. A solution — no matter what genes you have — is explained in detail in this section of *Health & Fitness Excellence*.

MYTH: Food allergies cause obesity.

FACT: There is no scientific evidence that food allergies cause obesity. In fact, government investigations show that many food allergy testing methods are a fraud.

MYTH: Emotional problems force people to become fat.

FACT: It's a negative spiral: emotional distress pushes people toward making poor choices — selecting low-quality foods, overeating, and skipping regular exercise. In turn, struggling with and failing in weight loss efforts cause emotional and mental stress. Learn ways to break out of this trap. (*See Chapter 32.*)

MYTH: If you want to trim down one place — such as the waist, hips, buttocks, or thighs — all you need to do is "spot reduce."

FACT: Contrary to popular opinion, you can't spot reduce. Special exercises or gadgets won't burn fat in isolated areas of the body. To help you become fit, lean, and toned — and stay that way — the best exercises are aerobics (which burn excess fat throughout the body), abdominal exercises (including the little-known transpyramid exercise), posture exercises (which help you look slim and move with ease), and muscular strength and endurance exercises (which firm and tone the body). (*See Chapter 30.*)

MYTH: Watch out for extra fluids. If you drink too much water you'll retain it and get even heavier.

FACT: Don't get trapped by the myth that drinking water will cause bloating or puffiness and then you'll look fatter. The fact is that by not drinking enough water you can slow down fat loss. (*See Chapter 31.*)

MYTH: To lose weight, you just pick an aerobic exercise — running, swimming, dance, or cycling — and do it every day.

FACT: Aerobic exercise is essential to body fat control, but it can be ineffective unless you follow seven key guidelines. And there's no need to do aerobics every day. Moreover, certain aerobic sports like swimming may burn less fat than others. (*See Chapter 30.*)

Diets — you've probably heard about hundreds of them and may have tried dozens yourself. Fiber diets, grapefruit diets, all-fruit diets, and no-fruit diets; food-combining diets, food allergy diets, and miracle pill diets; liquid protein diets, starch-blocker diets, celebrity diets, and sucrose polyester diets. There are more than thirty thousand diets on public record in America.[1] And because so very few of them are safe or successful, the list keeps growing — and so does the number of frustrated people who fail again and again in their efforts to lose excess fat.

If you're among the 98 percent of the 80–115 million Americans who are currently dieting,[2] statistics show that you'll fail, not only gaining back any weight you lose and then some[3] but making it easier to gain more body fat with every new diet you try. At the same time, you are increasing your risk of disease and a shortened life. Is there a way out of this dilemma? Yes. The next three chapters present a step-by-step scientific way to help control excess body fat, once and for all.

Despite the innumerable gimmicks and fad diets in America, more Americans are overweight than a generation ago. Studies show that about 50 million men and 60 million women between the ages of eighteen and seventy-nine are "too fat" and need to reduce excess weight.[4] As amazing as it may sound, the old principles of "dieting" — weighing yourself, eating low-carbohydrate/high-protein meals, and going to extremes counting calories — turn out to be among the surest ways to gain more fat rather than lose it.

Diet and diet-related materials are a $10 billion annual industry in the United States. It's a classic paradox: ever-greater investments of time and money, fueled by a wave of consumer frustration with "old diets" and clamor for "new diets." Nowhere is the golden circle of *Health & Fitness Excellence* more needed than right here. Actually, this whole book is a resource guide for sensible, permanent body fat control. The next few chapters highlight new discoveries and draw your attention to priorities in launching a successful program.

Health Risks from Excess Fat

"The evidence is now overwhelming that obesity, defined as excessive storage of energy in the form of fat, has adverse effects on health and longevity," reports a panel convened recently by the National Institutes of Health (NIH).[5] Obesity is linked to heart disease, congestive heart failure, diabetes, cancer, bone and joint diseases, respiratory diseases and distress, menstrual irregularities, pregnancy difficulties, a wide range of psychological problems, and premature death.[6]

"Yo-yo" dieting — going on a diet, losing some weight, then going back to normal eating, and regaining weight — alters your metabolism, causing fewer calories to be burned as fuel and more to be converted into fat. This results in slower and slower weight loss followed by more rapid body fat gains after each new diet is discontinued.[7] Yo-yo dieters lose "weight" (pounds on the scale) primarily from water and muscle mass, while the weight gained back is more fat. Repeat dieters may be condemning themselves to a lifelong struggle with obesity.

The regaining cycle of on-again-off-again dieting not only increases the size of existing fat cells in the body, but it *adds new fat cells* that are never lost, as well as strengthening the fat-preserving mechanisms in your body.[8]

And yo-yo dieting stimulates excessive production of stress hormones such as epinephrine that cause blood pressure to rise. In addition, researchers have suggested that body fat can serve as a storehouse for carcinogenic chemicals.[9] And, according to a recent NIH report, many overweight people suffer most from the psychological effects of obesity — such as poor self-image, social stress, and self-doubt.[10]

Crash Diets Can Be Deadly

"Crash diets" severely restrict caloric intake in hopes of producing rapid weight loss. But ironically these popular diets actually decrease the body's metabolic rate and increase the body's tendency to convert foods into, and store them as, fat. A recent European study suggests that strict weight loss programs — like many popular crash diets — may also cause neurological problems.[11]

An Australian-Canadian study reported that crash dieting disrupts muscle function.[12] After two weeks, the subjects had muscle cells too weak to pump essential minerals out of the cells as fast as they came in. Then, according to the researchers, "the muscles can't relax properly after they've contracted." This contributes to chronic fatigue.

Don't Be Gullible!

Although they have been America's favorite weight loss method for many years, high-protein/low-carbohydrate diets are ineffective and dangerous. In Chapter 22, we discussed the need to ensure enough high-quality protein in the diet and the dangers of too much. But a great number of Americans eat at least twice as much protein as they need for good nutrition. The point is that you can actually get fatter by eating too much protein, since the body cannot store the excess and must convert it to fat or eliminate it as toxic wastes. Even worse, high-protein diets strain the kidneys and liver, contributing to dehydration, electrolyte imbalance, and muscle-tissue loss.[13]

Food combination diets and modified fasting diets, which emphasize high fruit intake and the absence of all dairy foods or rigid food combination rules for everyone, are scientifically unsubstantiated and potentially dangerous.[14]

What about fasting and low-calorie "formula diets"? Studies show that after less than 24 hours on a fast, the body begins to break down muscle tissue as a source of energy.[15] "Prepackaged formula diets, such as Metracal, Sego, Cambridge, Shaklee and liquid protein diets, have been around for many years," says Dr. Peter Lindner, past president of the American Society of Bariatric Physicians.[16] "Since most contain less than 800 calories, they may produce a rapid weight loss, but a good percentage of that loss is muscle, vital organ tissues, and water — not fat. Huge losses of both water and muscle tissue are potentially dangerous. And, of course, claims of long-term weight reduction maintenance simply aren't true."

How Much Should You Weigh?

"Being mildly or moderately overweight may be more harmful than generally believed," concluded a recent Harvard University Medical School study.[17] In fact, people who weigh at least 10 percent *below* the average for adults in the United States have the lowest death rates. A recent conference sponsored by a National Institutes of Health committee and the

Centers for Disease Control reached the same conclusion: *The weights associated with the greatest longevity are below average weights of the population,* as long as such weights are not associated with illness.[18]

For many years health professionals have relied on the 1959 "ideal" weight figures calculated by Metropolitan Life Insurance to match the weights and heights for male and female policyholders with the lowest mortality rates. Over the years, the Metropolitan weight tables were criticized for failing to account for body type, age, ethnicity, and body fat percentage. The tables were revised in 1983 by simply increasing the "desirable" weight listed for each height.

The NIH cautions against using *either* Metropolitan Life table as the sole indicator of your ideal weight.[19] After reviewing twenty-five major studies on weight and longevity, a Harvard research team reported that most of the studies used to establish these weight tables in the first place underestimated the risk of being overweight and contain biases that allow "desirable" weights to creep up.[20]

Fat percentage, not weight in pounds or kilograms, is the key to finding your desirable body fat level. Unfortunately, to most accurately measure fat percentage it's necessary to go to a high-tech physiology laboratory for underwater weighing. An easier, quite reliable way to estimate body composition is skinfold caliper measurements — but only when the measurements are taken by a skilled professional. If you don't have ready access to either of these assessment procedures, the next best choice is to estimate *body mass index* (BMI). This method is only moderately reliable. The NIH suggests setting initial body fat goals by using the BMI, which compares weight with body fat, generally accounting reasonably well for variations in height.[21]

Here's how to calculate your BMI: (1) Convert your weight into kilograms by dividing your weight in pounds (without clothes) by 2.2. (2) Convert your height to meters by dividing your height in inches (without shoes) by 39.4 *or* multiplying your height by 2.54 and then dividing that number by 100. Next, square that figure (multiply it times itself). (3) Divide your weight in kilograms by your height in meters. This final figure is an approximation of your body mass. Let's use an example of a 5'10" male who weighs 160 pounds: (1) 160 divided by 2.2 = 72.72 kg. (2) 70 divided by 39.4 = 1.78; 1.78 squared = 3.168. (3) 72.72 divided by 3.168 = 22.95 BMI.

The NIH suggests that for women, a BMI above 23 often indicates excess fat. For men, excess body fat is suggested by readings above 24. Strictly defined obesity (20 percent above the top of the normal range) begins at 27.2 for men and 26.9 for women.

Don't get trapped in the math, though. It's far from the whole story. A healthy, active body has well-toned muscles, sparkling eyes, and a strong heart. When you look in the mirror, leave the numbers behind and look beyond slimness — to *fitness*.

Basic Calorie Facts

The traditional approach to weight reduction centers on the idea that you can count calories and then determine, by weight and age, how many calories to cut to produce a given weight loss.[22] According to this theory, you simply use printed "caloric value tables" to calculate calories of food intake and subtract activity output, arriving at a net daily figure.

However, as weight control authorities now realize, 3,500 calories may equal a pound of fat in the chemistry laboratory but in the real day-to-day world of "adaptive metabolism," the equation doesn't hold up.[23] Sedentary, overweight people struggle with a metabolism that works against them, often failing to achieve desired results even when they closely follow traditional weight management rules. Before long, in confusion or frustration, they turn to fad diets, hoping for an answer.

"If weight loss were merely a reflection of total caloric intake, it would be a simple matter to lose weight by simply missing breakfast and eating normally the rest of the day," say Dr. Dennis Remington, Garth Fisher, and Edward Parent in *How to Lower Your Fat Thermostat*. "Theoretically, this should result in a 30 to 50 pound loss each year. With more drastic changes in eating patterns, we would expect to see even more dramatic weight changes."[24] But that's not what happens.

Two variables determine what you weigh: *energy balance,* the number of calories you consume each day (energy input) in contrast to the number of calories you burn off (energy output), and *body composition,* your percentage of body fat compared with lean tissue.

Energy output depends on body composition and basal metabolic rate (BMR). Lean tissue is *active* tissue, producing and using energy by metabolizing — "burning" — calories. In general, the greater your body percentage of lean tissue, the more energy you automatically expend and the more calories you can usually eat in small meals throughout the day without becoming fatter. Body fat, in contrast to lean tissue, *uses very little energy*. The greater your body's percentage of fat, the less energy you expend and the less food you can eat without gaining fat.

What about following a 1,200–1,800 calorie daily target, as recommended by a number of doctors and qualified nutritionists? For many people it still makes good sense. (Diets with total daily intake less than 1,200 calories *always* require medical supervision.) But even if you count calories, be certain to follow the *Health & Fitness Excellence* nutritional principles — frequent small meals and light snacks from a wide variety of fresh, wholesome, low-fat, high-carbohydrate, high-fiber foods: vegetables, fruits, whole grains, legumes, fish, lean poultry, and low-fat/nonfat dairy products.

Body Fat Theories

Ten basic scientific theories address the body fat issue.

Genetics Theory

To some extent, the *tendency* to gain excess fat may be inherited.[25] Compared with children of normal-weight parents, children of obese parents are more likely to become obese themselves. A child with one or both parents overweight has an increased chance — by about 40 and 80 percent, respectively — to become obese.

Fat Cell Theory

Some researchers have found that the number of fat cells in the body increases from overeating patterns early in life.[26]

Environment Theory

The most popular theory is that obesity results from environmental factors such as behavior patterns learned from parents, stress-induced eating, overreaction to advertising cues such as television commercials, inadequate discipline, lack of exercise, and peer pressure to overeat.[27]

Setpoint Theory

Scientific support is growing for the theory that proposes that the body has an internal "weight-regulating mechanism" or "setpoint."[28] The setpoint — believed to be controlled in the brain's hypothalamus area — "chooses" the amount of body fat it considers ideal for your needs and then defends that level. "The weight-regulating mechanism controls body weight in two ways," say Remington, Fisher, and Parent. "First, it has a profound influence on the amount of food that you eat, dramatically increasing or decreasing your appetite as needed to maintain the setpoint weight. Second, it can actually trigger systems in the body to 'waste' excess energy if you overeat, or to 'conserve' energy if you eat too little."[29] Frequent small, balanced meals, regular aerobic exercise, and behavior changes lower the setpoint and improve your body's ability to burn excess fat.

Amount of Food Consumed

Ironically, starving yourself by severely restricting calories or skipping meals drives up the setpoint and makes it harder to lose fat — and easier to gain it — from eating less and less food.

Brown Fat Activity Theory

Scientists have discovered that the body contains more than one kind of fat tissue. Yellow (sometimes called white) fat — yellow adipose tissue — is the type stored in about 99 percent of your body's fat cells.

Brown fat — brown adipose tissue (BAT) — accounts for approximately 1 percent of your total body fat but plays a key role in metabolism.

The primary mechanism that allows metabolism to eliminate calories is thermogenesis, the production of heat.[30] The principal site of thermogenesis is brown adipose tissue. Brown fat is located between the shoulder blades, in the armpit area, surrounding the kidneys, and around the large arteries and veins that are near the heart. BAT cells act like minifurnaces, generating tremendous amounts of heat to warm your internal organs, especially the heart. The heat-generating fuel used by brown fat is yellow fat.

Brown fat activity can be increased by regular aerobic exercise. "When it comes to exercise, brown fat seems to follow the evolutionary logic that equates inactivity with fat storage," says Dr. Gabe Mirkin, *New York Times* columnist, sports medicine researcher, and author of *Getting Thin*. "If you're inactive, brown fat burns calories sluggishly. But when you're very active, brown fat assumes you have no need for a great amount of stored fat, and it sets about burning off some of the excess."[31]

Frequent small, low-fat meals and light snacks also help keep the calorie-burning activities of brown fat high. This is called "diet-induced thermogenesis."[32] Compared with sedentary people with excess fat, active people of ideal weight produce more heat — burn more calories — as a result of eating the same number of calories.

When active, ideal-weight people do overeat on special occasions, the heat produced during digestion, absorption, and metabolism is increased to compensate for the food overload.[33]

Sodium-Potassium Pump Theory

Quadrillions of sodium-potassium pumps are spread throughout the cells of your body, actively pumping sodium out of each cell and potassium in. This exchange serves many purposes, including nerve impulse conduction.

Sedentary people with excess body fat have sodium-potassium pumps that are at least 20 percent less active than those of thinner people who exercise adequately and often, reports Dr. George L. Blackburn, professor at Harvard University Medical School and a top obesity expert.[34] He has demonstrated that proper exercise can help bring sluggish sodium-potassium pumps back up to more ideal function and aids in metabolism of excess fat.

Enzyme Theory

This theory suggests that some people have more enzymes that stimulate depositing — rather than burning — excess dietary fat, "locking" it into the yellow adipose tissue areas.[35] Regular aerobic exercise may alter the enzyme levels in obese people to approximate those of lean, active people.

Carbohydrate Balance Theory

For many years, carbohydrates were condemned as fat-promoting foods. However, recent research shows that regular dietary intake of complex carbohydrates *reduces* the incidence of obesity and other diseases.[36]

"Gland/Hormone Problems" Theory

Hormones play a pivotal role in directing the body's energy storage and expenditure processes. But true glandular obesity is very rare — less than 3 percent of all obesity can be attributed to glandular imbalances such as "underactive thyroid syndrome."[37] Malfunctioning hormones are usually the result, not the cause, of being fat, and glandular functions are almost always correctable through a balanced health program.

Insulin is generally considered the most powerful of the hormones promoting fat storage in the body (others include cortisol, estrogen, progesterone, and testosterone). Insulin's main task is to reduce levels of blood sugar and fat by forcing them out of the bloodstream into your cells while, at the same time, stimulating the liver to convert sugar to fat at an accelerated rate. Whereas some body cells try to pick up fat from the bloodstream to burn for energy, insulin works to force the free fat *into* fat cells, acting directly on fat cell membranes to "lock" the fat inside, preventing its escape back into the general circulation.

Your body's response to insulin is based on how many "insulin receptors" your cells have. They are located on the outer cell membranes and serve as attachment surfaces for insulin and help transport it into the cells. The more insulin receptors your body has, the more sensitive you are to insulin, and the less insulin your body needs to produce. With decreased insulin, there follows a reduction in the amount of fat being forced into your fat cells, as well as a reduction in the amount of excess fat produced by your liver.

The number of insulin receptors can be increased by reducing body fat levels, exercising, and eating more high-fiber/high-complex-carbohydrate food and less fatty food. Frequent small meals and light snacks help keep glucose and insulin levels balanced.

Children and Obesity

American children are fatter now than ever before.[38] In fact, the prevalence of obesity has increased by 54 percent among six-to-eleven-year-olds and by 39 percent among twelve-to-seventeen-year-olds over the past fifteen to twenty years.[39]

When obesity begins in childhood, the chances for adult obesity are more than three times greater than for adults who were of normal body weight as children.[40] Assuming that a youngster will simply "outgrow" excess body fat may sentence him or her to a life of obesity, according to researchers at the National Institutes of Health.[41]

Obesity, elevated blood pressure, high cholesterol level, or inactivity — all heart disease risk factors — are now evident in nearly 40 percent of American children between the ages of five and eight.[42] Overweight children need to do more than eat the right foods and get regular aerobic exercise. They need to trim television viewing hours.[43]

Children ages six to eleven watch an average of 24 hours of television every week, seeing an average of 10,000 food commercials a year.[44] And the more they watch TV in their younger years the more likely they are to become obese teenagers and adults. Citing a "highly significant association" between television viewing and obesity in both children and teenagers, Harvard researchers warn that the prevalence of obesity increases by 2 percent for each weekly hour of TV viewed by twelve-to-seventeen-year-olds.

A Stanford University study recommends changes in family lifestyle, including reduced television viewing time for children and teenagers, increased daily time spent exercising, and — with safety-conscious friends — more frequent walking or cycling to school or on errands instead of riding in a car or bus.[45]

Societal and peer pressures have caused younger and younger children to try fad diets. A recent study at the University of California at San Francisco reports a high percentage of girls from grades four through twelve are dieting to lose weight — almost half of the nine-year-olds and close to 80 percent of the eleven-year-olds in one study.[46] It's time for all of us, as concerned parents and health-conscious adults, to take action to end this tragic trend.

True Indicators of Success

Most dieters evaluate progress by weighing in each morning on the bathroom scale. This measurement often determines the day's emotional tone. Don't let false discouragement tempt you to abandon your program. *Get rid of your bathroom scale.* "Body weight" reflects an intricate combination of water, muscle, fat, bone, and related tissues in your body. It varies from minute to minute, hour to hour, day to day. It can be manipulated with remarkable ease, even with no fat loss occurring. Bathroom scales cannot distinguish between water weight and fat weight. A sudden added pound or two may be just water and may vanish in a day or so.

A good basic goal here is (1) to improve your overall health and fitness, while (2) losing excess body fat and then keeping it off. As you become more physically fit, you will increase lean tissue mass, gaining muscle. Muscle weighs more than fat and, to no surprise, you may actually gain weight on the scale while losing fat, changing body proportions, improving health, and increasing your energy.

If you're a stickler for mathematical progress checks, you may want to schedule regular body composition assessments at a sports medicine facility. Other indicators include measurements of your waist, hips, thighs, arms, and other body areas — which will begin to change as you lose excess fat. Checking these measurements every month or two can provide a simple indication of progress. The fit of your clothing is, in many cases, a valid sign of improvement. Use a specific article of clothing as a reference. You may want to try on a tight pair of jeans now, and put them away, without washing or wearing them again, for future comparison.

Should You Begin a Body Fat Loss Program Now?

If you are pregnant, a nursing mother, or diabetic, have any medical condition that might be adversely affected by weight loss efforts, or are "binging and purging" by self-induced vomiting, it's essential to consult your physician before beginning this, or any other, program. Children should have a health-and-fitness-oriented lifestyle but should not undertake body fat loss programs without medical supervision. This is especially crucial for infants and young children, since fat-loss-conscious parents can inadvertently harm the health of younger family members by putting them on a rigid, overrestricted diet.[47]

If you have medical questions about weight loss, contact the American Society of Bariatric Physicians (7430 E. Caley Ave., Suite 210, Englewood, CO 80111), an organization specializing in education for physicians on the medically supervised management of obesity.

RESOURCES

To remain up to date on scientific advances in body fat control, refer to the periodicals recommended in the Resource list at the end of this book. The following publications are excellent.

▶ *Controlling Fat for Life* by Robert E. T. Stark, M.D. (Arizona Bariatric Physicians, 444 W. Osborn Rd., Phoenix, AZ 85013; 1985). This basic book focuses on the nutritional aspect of controlling body fat. Written by the president of the American Society of Bariatric Physicians.

▶ *The Dieter's Dilemma: Why Diets Are Obsolete — The New Setpoint Theory of Weight Control* by William Bennett, M.D., and Joel Gurin (Basic Books/Harper Colophon Books, 1982). A look at the setpoint theory.

▶ *Getting Thin: All About Fat, How You Get It, How You Lose It, How to Keep It Off for Good* by Gabe Mirkin, M.D. (Little, Brown, 1983). One of the best general books on body fat control.

▶ *The LEARN Program for Weight Control* by Kelly D. Brownell, Ph.D. (Department of Psychiatry, University of Pennsylvania, 133 S. 36th St., Philadelphia, PA 19104). LEARN stands for Lifestyle, Exercise, Attitudes, Relationships, and Nutrition. This balanced manual provides lessons in each area.

▶ *Maximize Your Body Potential* by Joyce D. Nash, Ph.D. (Bull Publishing, 1986). A first-rate, comprehensive program for body fat control.

▶ *Nutrition, Weight Control, and Exercise* by Frank I. Katch, Ed.D., and William D. McArdle, Ph.D. (Lea & Febiger, 1988). This highly competent textbook, now in its third edition, provides clear, technical guidelines based on research facts in biochemistry and applied physiology.

30 Exercise Priorities

EXERCISE, ESPECIALLY AEROBIC EXERCISE, is of critical importance in body fat control. It helps your body metabolize ("burn") excess fat by lowering the setpoint to a more optimal level,[48] increasing brown fat activity, reducing insulin-related fat storage abnormalities, encouraging hormonal balance, protecting and increasing lean body weight, raising basal metabolism for more effective utilization of calories from your diet, and increasing the number and activity of fat-burning enzymes — dramatically increasing the muscle cells' capacity to burn fat as a fuel to make energy.[49]

Stress-related hormones such as adrenaline and cortisol can actually be metabolized by exercise, and this may also affect fat storage.[50]

Calories Continue to Be Burned After Exercise

Aerobic exercise raises basal metabolic rate for between three and twenty-four hours, so you continue to burn extra calories long after you finish each exercise session.[51]

"Muscle is all active metabolic mass," says David Levitsky, nutritional scientist at Cornell University. "The exerciser whose body fat has been replaced by muscle will experience an increase in basal metabolic rate (BMR), the energy the body uses at rest."[52] This increase reduces the body's tendency to store calories as fat.

Exercise Helps Control Appetite

Aerobic exercise also contributes to the normal functioning of the brain's feeding control mechanisms and helps keep the body's appetite stabilized.[53] Sedentary people often complain of appetite pressures that drive them toward overeating and "creeping obesity."

Although exercise doesn't necessarily reduce hunger, it boosts metabolism, often dramatically. "It astonishes people," says Peter Wood, associate director of the Stanford University Center for Research in Disease Prevention. "They can't believe it's possible to eat more and lose excess body fat at the same time. But that's what happens as you get more active."[54]

Sit-ups Don't Melt Fat

Contrary to popular myths, you can't "spot reduce." It doesn't work to use special exercises or gadgets to cut down fat in an isolated area of the body. Fitness is developed from balanced exercises for the entire body — aerobics, breathing, abdominal exercises, posture and flexibility, and muscular strength.

But what about traditional sit-ups and leg-lifts? many people wonder. Surely, *those* tried and true exercises cut fat from the stomach area, don't they? A University of Massachusetts research team recently studied people performing traditional sit-ups, with some individuals doing as many as 5,005 sit-ups over a 27-day period.[55] Result? No extra loss of body fat in the abdomen.

A slim, strong waist comes from exercising five equally important abdominal muscles, including the little-known transversalis and pyramidalis. Traditional sit-ups and leg-lifts simply don't work; in fact, they often create — or worsen — lower-back pain. To learn key exercises — transpyramid, roll-ups, and reverse trunk rotations — see Chapter 14.

Aerobics Success Formula

Millions of Americans have started exercise regimens. Many of these people are doing regular "aerobic exercise" — vigorous activities such as cycling, swimming, walking, running, rowing, cross-country skiing, skating, dancing, and the like. Without knowing it, the majority of these exercisers are missing many — some authorities say most — benefits because they are unaware of some simple guidelines.

The following are current priorities for maximally effective aerobic exercise. See Chapter 16 for complete details about each guideline.

(1) Warm up for 3–5 minutes preceding and cool down for 3–5 minutes following each aerobics workout. (2) Exercise rhythmically at a moderate pace. (3) Monitor your heart rate (pulse) to stay within your target heart rate zone (THRZ), which is 65 to 75 percent of your predicted maximum heart rate (PMHR). According to the Institute for Aerobics Research, PMHR for women and unfit men is 220 minus your age; for fit men it's 205 minus half your age. (4) Exercise for a minimum of 20 minutes four times per week or 30 minutes three times per week. For best fat loss results, work into a schedule of 30 to 60 minutes four or five times a week.[56] Another strategy for maximal benefits is to perform 20 to 30 minutes of aerobics twice a day — schedule an early morning session of walking or cycling while you listen to music or an educational tape or watch the morning news, and then one more short session late in the afternoon or early evening. (5) Have fun — and think noncompetitive thoughts such as "calm," "relaxed," "steady." (6) Drink plenty of pure water before and after exercise. (7) Progress gradually and cross train by performing several different aerobic activities each week. This can enhance weight loss.[57]

Outdoor aerobic exercise options include cross-country skiing, cycling, walking, jogging, running, rowing, roller skating, ice skating, canoeing, and kayaking. Indoor choices include cross-country ski machines, aerobic dance, stationary cycles, rowing machines, roller skating, jumping rope, treadmills, and so on.

If your goal is body fat loss, don't choose swimming as your predominant aerobic exercise. From a body fat loss perspective, swimming appears to be less than ideal as a primary aerobic exercise. A recent study at the University of California at Irvine reported that women who swam for exercise had a greater appetite than those who chose other aerobic activities. In addition, they had greater difficulty losing body fat. In fact, some swimmers actually gained fat.[58] It is theorized that cool water can boost appetite or stimulate fat-preserving mechanisms.

Choosing the Right Time to Exercise

When you exercise, not just *how,* is also important for best body fat loss results. "Obese persons should exercise *before* eating," advises Dr. Peter D. Vash, endocrinologist and internist on the faculty of the UCLA Medical Center, "since the exercise will maximize their insulin action."[59] When you exercise affects how many calories you burn and what type of weight you lose. The optimal time for burning maximum calories appears to be *before dinner,* suggests Dr. Kenneth H. Cooper.[60] Physiologist Melanie Roffers agrees: "Exercising at this time of the day elevates the metabolic rate just as it's winding down. Also the elevated body temperature from exercise decreases the appetite right before the largest meal of the day. And the stress reduction effect of exercise reduces stress-induced eating. Before-dinner exercise also burns more fat. . . . But regardless of when people exercise, research has confirmed that exercisers lose more weight than non-exercisers and keep that weight off."[61]

Some studies suggest that people who are overfat but not obese may burn slightly more calories by exercising after the evening meal rather than before.[62] Researchers speculate that this may be related to insulin resistance in overweight and obese people. As already noted, exercise reduces insulin resistance. With less insulin resistance, food can be more effectively metabolized.

Keep an exercise diary. It's a good idea to have a written record of exercise sessions, keeping track of your weekly schedule and entering your comments about which exercise options you enjoy most. Plan when, where, and with whom you'll exercise. These advance arrangements — and simply knowing you have agreed to write down your daily exercises — can make a big difference in long-term success.

Move, Move, Move

Beyond exercise and work, all of us can keep our metabolism higher by simply moving around more — walking, shopping, house cleaning, gardening, and so on. There is evidence from the National Institutes of Health that, in addition to regular aerobic exercise, body fat loss results are enhanced by boosting all kinds of other activities throughout the day.[63] In other words, make extra movement a priority.

How? Walking or bicycling instead of riding in a motor vehicle; parking a block or two farther away from your job or shopping destination; choosing the stairs instead of escalators and elevators; riding a stationary bicycle, rebounding, or rowing while watching favorite television programs or talking on the telephone; spending a little extra "active time" with the family or friends on evenings or weekends; and participating in recreational sports that most people perform at low intensities such as playing catch, shooting baskets, kickball, Ping-Pong, badminton, croquet, and volleyball. To increase your fat-burning success, begin listing — and doing — all kinds of new activities that sound fun.

31 Nutrition Priorities

IT'S QUITE OBVIOUS that nutrition is another key element in the scientific formula for body fat control. But to sort through the maze of contradictory dietary advice, myths, and fads, you need all the accurate information you can get. For every dollar spent in America by research scientists and health professionals to prevent and treat obesity, one hundred dollars is spent by the food industry to lure people into eating more fattening foods.[64]

For decades, the role of food in weight loss regimens has been mathematical. What mattered was caloric content. Most Americans have been led to believe that the equation is simple: eating too much food adds body fat; losing weight requires counting — and decreasing — food calories. But current research shows that not all foods are fat-promoting, and counting calories turns out to be less important than choosing the right kinds of foods and scheduling when, and in what amounts, you eat them throughout the day.

The first dietary guideline is to choose an exceptionally wide variety of wholesome, fresh foods that, overall, are high in complex carbohydrates and fiber, adequate but not excessive in protein, and low in fat, cholesterol, salt, alcohol, and caffeine. Drink plenty of extra water between meals and snacks. Finally, consider choosing recipes that help keep your mind and emotions at their best, as discussed in Chapter 27.

Small, Frequent Meals and Snacks

One of the most powerful strategies for winning the war against excess body fat is eating frequent small meals and light snacks.[65] "Guard against generation of new fat cells by avoiding large intakes of food at one time," says Dr. Peter D. Vash, endocrinologist, eating disorders specialist, and faculty member at the UCLA Medical Center. "Space smaller meals throughout the day. This tactic reduces the hormonal signal that causes fat cells to divide and multiply."[66] Sports medicine authority Dr. Gabe Mirkin adds: *"Five or six small meals a day can keep your brown-fat activity elevated for almost all your waking hours* [emphasis added]."[67]

Small midevening snacks, chosen wisely and consumed several hours after the evening meal and several hours before bedtime, can be a positive step for most of us. It's best to opt for foods high in complex carbohydrates and low in fat and protein — such as frozen fruit sorbet, very-low-fat pasta salad with fruit or vegetables, or a low-fat, whole-grain, high-fiber piece of bread, bagel, muffin, baked pita chips, or crackers with your favorite all-fruit preserve spread on top.

Be aware that a voracious appetite for midevening snacks can be triggered by emotions, social influences, or environmental cues to eat, coming at a time when resistance to poor-quality foods can be down and temptation high.

Another priority: Watch your portion sizes. Study after study has revealed that most of us are very poor estimators of the quantities we eat. First, bypass buffets and smorgasbords. Second, be certain to follow home recipes exactly. Third, invest in a kitchen scale. Use it when you cook, especially for calorie-dense foods such as cheese, fish, poultry, and meat. With practice, you can train your eye to recognize the correct portion size.

Reducing Dietary Fat

"Ninety-seven percent of all fat calories are converted to body fat," says Dr. Robert E. T. Stark, president of the American Society of Bariatric Physicians, a group specializing in treating overweight people.[68] By eliminating excess fat from your diet, you can improve your health and performance and halt unnecessary body fat gain. Furthermore, the fear that *all* carbohydrates can turn quickly into fat is unfounded.

"We don't make fat from carbohydrate," says Dr. Elliot Danforth, director of Clinical Research at the University of Vermont in Burlington. "We make body fat from ingested fat. . . . Researchers have found that when you eat a carbohydrate, it stimulates a greater thermogenic [heat] loss of calories than when you eat fat. In scientific terms, we say carbohydrate is thermogenic; fat is nonthermogenic, that is, it generates much less heat for the same number of calories."[69]

Metabolic efficiency is the key; since dietary fat is already fat, it takes very little energy "cost" — only about 3 calories — to convert 100 calories of fat into new body fat.[70] So gaining new body fat from dietary fat is amazingly easy. In contrast, it "costs" about 23 calories to turn 100 calories of carbohydrate into fat, estimates Jean-Pierre Flatt, professor of biochemistry at the University of Massachusetts Medical Center.[71] In other words, it's *far easier for your body to convert dietary fat into body fat* than it is to convert complex carbohydrates into fat.

Eat Oat Bran and Other Fiber-Rich Foods

Fiber-rich foods such as oat bran, whole grains, legumes, fruits, and vegetables can be included in a variety of recipes in an ideal diet. The body absorbs high-fiber foods more slowly, and this contributes to satiety. Fiber-rich foods also require more energy to digest, which increases the rate at which calories are burned.[72]

Don't Count on Artificial Sweeteners

Don't rely on artificially sweetened foods and beverages to help you lose weight or prevent fat gain.[73] According to an ongoing study by the American Cancer Society involving more than 78,000 women aged fifty to sixty-nine, long-term users of artificial sweeteners are more likely to gain weight than nonusers over the course of one year.[74] In addition, fake sweeteners usually don't satisfy hunger. A recent study on aspartame (marketed under the brand names Nutra Sweet and Equal) conducted at Leeds University in England reported that not only was this sweetener generally ineffective in suppressing appetite, but in some people it actually increased feelings of hunger. In contrast, sugar (glucose) was found to reduce hunger and produce a feeling of fullness.[75]

Dealing with Appetite Pressures

Hunger, appetite, and satiety are often-used terms in dieting circles. *Hunger* refers to the unpleasant sensations experienced when there is an urgent need for food. *Appetite* means a desire for food whether or not you're hungry. Hunger is a *physiological* condition, whereas appetite is primarily a *psychological* state. *Satiety* refers to the genuine biological feeling of fullness when hunger is satisfied.

In other words, when you feel satisfied after a balanced meal or snack, you are no longer physically hungry, although your *appetite* — influenced by environmental cues, habits, emotions, thoughts, social encouragement, or other stimuli — may pressure you to keep eating.

Relax — and Eat More Slowly

One way to reduce your appetite is to slow down the eating pace at mealtimes. A number of hormones are thought to play a role in signaling satiety after we eat a snack or meal. One of these hormones is insulin. When you eat, carbohydrates prompt the release of insulin as blood-sugar levels rise. Insulin travels through the circulation and slowly filters into cerebrospinal fluid (CSF). When the insulin in the CSF reaches a certain level, a satiety or "full" signal is sent to the brain. For most of us, this takes about 20 minutes from the time we eat the first bite of food. Therefore, *fast* eating increases the tendency toward *over*eating.

In sedentary, obese people, insulin generally enters the bloodstream more slowly. It may take longer for the satiety level to be reached, prompting overweight people to eat longer and eat more.[76] One way to slow down your fork is to keep bites small and force longer and longer pauses between them — even as long as a minute or two.

One added point: Most of us neither relax before eating nor ensure a positive mealtime environment — and we suffer because of it. Tension in the abdominal muscles has been linked with enzyme interference and poor digestion.[77] In addition, rapid eaters don't usually chew their food well, and this adds more digestive stress. Make it a priority to choose a pleasant space for eating, eat slowly, and chew each bite thoroughly.

Sensible Variety, with Caution

We humans have an inborn need and love for food variety. While many of us believe we eat an adequately varied diet, research recommends an extraordinarily varied diet. This can improve digestion, increase the availability of essential nutrients, reduce the risk of food allergies, and help fight excess body fat. And a diversified diet also gives a wonderful sense of pleasure in eating.

Replace feelings of food deprivation — real or imagined — with sensory stimuli. Add light, fresh flowers, plants, colors, music, and other environmental brighteners to your dining area. Stimulate your taste buds by using new herbs and spices while cutting back on fat. Bland meals can be transformed into low-fat gourmet cuisine. See Chapters 25 and 26 for ideas.

Here's a cautionary note about our love of variety: Even when your true hunger is satisfied, your appetite may keep pulling you toward eating more, especially if additional food choices *taste* different than the meal or snack you just consumed.

We tend to feel satisfied when our senses tell us the last bites of a meal have the same texture, color, taste, shape, and smell, says Dr. Barbara Rolls, a professor of psychiatry and behavioral sciences at Johns Hopkins School of Medicine in Baltimore.[78] She has completed extensive research on this phenomenon and has labeled it *sensory-specific satiety*. When we introduce a tantalizing series of "extras," such as the chance for dessert, appetite is revived.

Success tactic: Be certain not to fill your refrigerator and cupboards with novel snacks and treats. The temptation to overeat, and eat too much of the wrong foods, is very real. Limit dessert options. Have one or two flavor choices, not dozens.

Psychological Cues Trigger Appetite

Other cues prompt us to overeat or choose poor-quality foods even when we are not hungry: lifestyle habits, emotional upsets, peer pressure, and advertisements on television, radio, billboards, and in newspapers and magazines. By becoming more aware of these cues, we can bring their influence under control.

Begin by identifying and eliminating the reminders that make it easy to eat inappropriately. Keep poor-quality foods out of the house — better yet, don't buy them in the first place. Don't keep snacks visible where they are an ongoing stimulus to eat.

Take command when you are outside the home, too. Anticipate situations that pressure you into inappropriate eating and make specific plans to deal with them. Request that unwanted "extras" (such as high-fat crackers, chips, cheeses, fried appetizers, and dips) not be brought to your table at restaurants. Turn down poor-quality snacks on airline flights and request a better-quality special meal in advance — such as low-fat seafood or vegetarian options. You might also pack your own food for short trips.

Turn up your awareness. Most cravings pass within seconds or a minute or two. With a solid dose of will power at the right moments, you can break through these urges and the more successful you become, the weaker and less frequent the cravings will be.

Some faulty eating is purely a matter of habit. Many of us have become inadvertently conditioned to eat every time we watch television, listen to the radio, or get together in the evening with friends. Food doesn't need to be the central social focus — take steps to break this habit.

To aid in controlling portion sizes, don't eat from serving dishes or containers. Put your portion on your plate and then put the rest away before you begin to eat. And be prepared to refuse suggestions for inappropriate eating that come from family members, friends, co-workers, and others. Most people will support you. Deal assertively with saboteurs (see the next chapter).

Exercise, Water, and Eating Record

Here are several other diet insights. First, remember that aerobic exercise helps ease appetite pressures by promoting hormonal balance, increasing production of fat-burning enzymes, and raising basal metabolism.

Second, don't get trapped by the myth that drinking lots of water will cause bloating or puffiness and you will look fatter. The fact is that by not drinking enough water you slow down fat loss.[79] It is essential to drink plenty of water between meals. This helps you lose excess fat by assisting your body in keeping hunger at bay, preventing dehydration, and aiding biochemical processes.

Third, a written record of what, how much, and when you eat and drink is a very valuable tool.[80] This information helps you become more aware of your eating habits and helps you follow through on *Health & Fitness Excellence* recommendations.

Calorie-Counting Confusion

Calories are a big issue in most popular American diets. Is calorie counting essential? Not necessarily. It is more important to follow the nutritional wellness principles in this book and to eat a wide variety of fresh, wholesome, low-fat foods in frequent small, balanced meals and light snacks. Here's the good news: High-quality, nutrient-dense vegetables, fruits, whole grains, legumes, fish, poultry, and low-fat/nonfat dairy products make it easier to keep the lid on caloric intake.

If you choose to go on a diet that severely restricts total daily calories — to under 1,200 — do so *only* under the guidance of your physician. If you choose to keep your daily caloric intake in the 1,200–1,800 range, be certain that any calorie calculations you make are as accurate as possible. Standards in this field are the United States Department of Agriculture (USDA) Agricultural Handbook No. 8 series and "Calories and Your Weight" (publication number AIB-364), both available from the Superintendent of Documents (U.S. Government Printing Office, Washington, DC 20402).

You might also consider equipping your home or office computer with *Nutrition Wizard* software designed by Dr. Michael F. Jacobson

(Center for Science in the Public Interest, 1501 16th St., N.W., Washington, D.C. 20036; 202-332-9110; 1987). *Nutrition Wizard* gives a standard analysis of dietary needs based on age, body size, and activity level and also features a databank with more than 1,700 food items (which can be expanded by the user) to analyze recipes, meals, and an entire day's diet for 25 nutritional components, including protein, carbohydrate, soluble/insoluble fiber, fat (polyunsaturates, monounsaturates, and saturates), cholesterol, sodium, and many other minerals and vitamins. This program is easy to use, with good, clear instructions.

It's also a good idea to have a favorite recipe book on hand, especially one which follows the basic guidelines of *Health & Fitness Excellence* and in which each snack, meal, and daily menu has a complete nutritional analysis and calorie count. One example is *The Health & Fitness Excellence Cookbook* by Leslie L. Cooper (Advanced Excellence Systems, P.O. Box 1085, Bemidji, MN 56601; 218-854-7300; 1989).

Professional Guidance

People with severe obesity and eating disorders, such as chronic binging and purging or symptoms of anorexia nervosa and related diseases, should be under the care and guidance of a qualified physician. For more information, contact the American Association of Bariatric Physicians (7430 E. Caley Ave., Suite 210, Englewood, CO 80111; 303-779-4833). Information is also available from the National Association of Anorexia Nervosa and Related Disorders (Box 7, Highland Park, IL 60035), the National Anorexic Aid Society, Inc. (5796 Karl Rd., Columbus, OH 43229), and Bulimia, Anorexia Self-Help (BASH, Deaconess Medical Office Center, 6125 Clayton Ave., Suite 215, St. Louis, MO 63139; 800-227-4785; 24-hour crisis hotline: 800-762-3334).

32 The Rest of the Formula

THE BOTTOM LINE in body fat control is to change behavior,[81] learning — and acting on — the whys, hows, and whens of exercise, nutrition, stress management, good posture, mood-thinking patterns, and other areas of *Health & Fitness Excellence*. This chapter looks at three final parts of the basic formula for body fat control.

Part 3: Stress Strategies

Stress *mis*management contributes to failure in most body fat loss programs. Psychological factors such as low self-esteem, anger, anxiety, guilt, worry, frustration, boredom, social pressures, and loneliness can all trigger the urge to eat inappropriately and skip exercise. Hormones produced by stress — including cortisol and epinephrine — make body cells resistant to insulin, and can actually increase the amount of stored body fat.[82]

Taking charge of your weight means taking charge of your thoughts and environment. Choosing appropriate foods, reducing easy opportunities for poor eating, and increasing awareness of psychological cues to eat (television and radio commercials, for example) all help improve results. In addition, it pays to make exercise as fun and convenient as possible — by designating an area of your home for indoor exercise, for instance, or enlisting a friend to work out with you, or joining a health club.

Many people use eating as a way to cope with emotional traumas. It is estimated that nearly one-third of all those involved with body fat control efforts encounter sabotage from family members or close friends.[83] This sabotage can take many forms: other people bringing you food gifts, teasing you by leaving high-fat treats around the house, badgering you to stop at fast-food restaurants that serve only high-fat foods, not supporting your exercise efforts, and so on.

Ultimately, results depend on you, not on other people. Yet in many cases, having a supportive person or group can make the difference between success and failure.

Social Support System

Why do we experience sabotage from others? According to Kelly Brownell, codirector of the Obesity Research Clinic at the University of Pennsylvania School of Medicine, spouses and friends may fear that you will become too attractive or that you'll begin making more physical or emotional demands, start meeting new friends, launch a social life that excludes them, or become more independent or successful.[84] Even when mates and close friends want to help, they often don't know how. They assume the role of body fat police officers, delivering warnings and catching violations. This increases tension and undercuts your self-esteem.

If your spouse or close friends feel threatened by your new weight control program, you may need to reassure them. Then it's time to enlist their true support. First communicate warmly, clearly, and firmly, letting them know you want their help. Be specific, leaving nothing to chance. Refuse offers of inappropriate food without offending. Be ready to increase your assertiveness if necessary — it's *your* health and well-being at stake.

Choose your words carefully (as discussed in Chapter 9) and state requests positively, since this tends to turn saboteurs into supporters, making people feel good and more willing to help. Instead of saying something like "You make it so hard for me to stick to my diet when you eat ice cream in front of me" (a negative, indirect request), say "Please help me by not eating ice cream in front of me" (a positive, direct request).

Instant Calming Sequence

Use the instant calming sequence (ICS) presented in Chapter 7 whenever you want a fast, effective way to handle high-pressure situations. The ICS works by catching the first signal of stress and neutralizing the negative responses that take such a toll on our energy, mood, and state of mind. Examples of stress signals are a critical comment from a friend about your appearance or a glimpse of your physique in a mirror; an upswell of self-doubt or impatience when "final results" are slow in coming; or a sudden urge to eat poor-quality foods, overeat, or snack at the wrong time.

The ICS takes less than one second and uses breathing, facial expression, posture, tension scanning, a "wave of relaxation," and mental focuses to help buffer the onslaught of daily hassles.

Dealing with Plateaus Frustration, boredom, loss of motivation. All of us who work hard to lose excess fat — and keep it off   eventually get stalled by a psychological or physiological plateau. Without a strategy to get unstuck, most of us plunge back into old eating and inactivity patterns.

If you feel you have reached a plateau, it's important to take immediate constructive action. Options include the following:

▶ Choosing a new form of exercise or increasing your amount of activity. This may help boost slowed metabolism.
▶ Adding some excitement to your diet by introducing new foods or recipes.
▶ Changing your pace: expand your social network, make a new friend, become more involved in a project or hobby — or begin a new one.
▶ Zeroing in on short-term goals — one day at a time. Celebrate your accomplishments by giving yourself nonedible rewards: extra time doing some activity you love, a book, a music album, a movie, flowers, a pair of earrings, or a visit to a special event.

If you feel you have cheated on your planned diet, regain control with four quick steps: (1) Forgive yourself. (2) Immediately remove any remaining high-fat, high-calorie foods from the premises. (3) Replace them with good-tasting, better substitutes. (4) Become more active — exercise or take a pleasant walk.

RESOURCES ───────────────────────────────

The following resources provide solid information on managing stresses associated with weight loss:

▶ *The LEARN Program for Weight Control* by Kelly Brownell, Ph.D. (University of Pennsylvania, Department of Psychiatry, 133 S. 36th St., Philadelphia, PA 19104; 1985). A good psychologically oriented plan.
▶ *Maximize Your Body Potential* by Joyce D. Nash, Ph.D. (Bull Publishing, 1986). This book by a psychologist and former director of the Diet and Weight Control Clinic at Stanford University contains many thoughtful recommendations about topics such as "Coping with Social Influences," "Relating to Others," and "Coping with Painful Emotions."

───────────────────────────────

Part 4: Your Mind and Mood

To a surprising extent, your thoughts and mental images determine weight control success. They keep you stuck in old behavior patterns or help you succeed in making changes. First, the pictures in your mind — of how "good" or "bad" you are as a person, for example — set an attitudinal tone for your work and life. Second, the daily stream of self-statements, or "self-talk" that you speak aloud or utter silently, can paralyze — or propel — your progress.

Tactics to Overcome Self-Sabotage

The first step in taking control of your mental imagery and self-talk is to become more aware of your current habits. "If you find that your self-talk, your little voice, is highly critical and judgmental, or self-discounting, or self-indulgent, or emotionally upsetting, you need to retrain the way you are thinking," says psychologist Joyce D. Nash. "You need to teach your little voice to be more objective and supportive — like a coach for a team. When you allow your self-talk to be negative, you allow it to sabotage you, to rob you of motivation, to enmesh you in painful emotions."[85]

One widely used and well-proven method for identifying and changing self-talk habits is the double column technique. Divide a piece of paper down the middle and label the left column "Saboteur" or "Negative self-talk" and the right column "Voice of truth" or "Coach." You enter negative self-statements — "shoulds," put-downs, and so on — in the left column and then replace them in your mind and heart with true statements that you enter in the right column. It is often simplest to make entries in general categories, as suggested in the following examples.

In *goal setting,* an extreme statement such as "I'm *never* going to overeat or eat bad foods again" can be replaced with "I may occasionally overeat or select some 'forbidden food'; the best thing for me to do now is to make healthy food choices and stop overeating whenever I can."

In *anticipating results,* comments such as "I've got so far to go, and I've tried and failed so many times before, why should things be any different now?" can be exchanged for "Maybe the things I tried before were imbalanced or incomplete — or maybe they just weren't right for me. And this time there's more to it than simply losing fat. I'm turning my life around by building up my health and fitness."

In *gauging progress,* appraisals such as "I'm not losing weight fast enough" or "My God! I gained a pound; I might as well quit right now" might be traded for "The most permanent way to lose fat is slowly and steadily" or "I need to stay on track with my program; if I keep making good choices the extra fat will eventually come off. Besides, I'm getting stronger and more toned from exercise — and muscle weighs more than fat. My bathroom scale is probably telling me I'm in better shape, not fatter."

In *daily coping,* statements such as "It isn't fair! I have to do without almost everything I like" may be switched to "I am slowly changing my attitudes and tastes so that healthy choices become easier and more fun for me." Pronouncements like "If I don't lose all this weight by the holidays (or some other target date), I'll never forgive myself" need to be sifted out in favor of "Enjoying my day-to-day life and special occasions doesn't depend on my weight; I am changing my whole lifestyle, and my extra fat will go away a little at a time. I'm not going to make my happiness today dependent on losing a certain amount of fat by a specific date."

"I'll bet my genetics made me fat and I'll always be stuck with this body I don't like" should be cut and replaced with "Even if my genes made it easier for me to put on this extra weight, that's no excuse for staying this way. At the worst, I'll simply have to work a little harder." Weak rationalizations like "I deserve a little treat now and then and this rich dessert looks great — besides, I just finished exercising and I can afford it" need to be released in favor of "Yes, I really do deserve regular rewards for making good choices in my life, but they don't need to be food. Today, I feel like ——— (curling up with a favorite new book later this evening; taking a quiet stroll; buying a new audiotape or some special flowers; snuggling with my spouse, child, or special friend; window shopping or looking through catalogs for ideas on a new piece of clothing; and so on)."

A catastrophic statement such as "Well, I blew it this time — there goes my diet" or "Like the irresponsible person I am, I didn't even take the time to exercise today. I might as well give up right now" should be cast off in favor of "Temporary setbacks don't mean I have to dive into a tailspin. What I am doing *most* of the time will build progress and carry me through. I am going to keep learning new ways to make better choices."

RESOURCES

In addition to Chapters 6 and 44, the following resources give recommendations for overcoming self-sabotage by taking charge of your mind and mood.

- ▶ *Imagine Yourself Slim* by Emmett E. Miller, M.D. (Source, P.O. Box W, Stanford, CA 94309; 415-328-7171). A warm, supportive audiotape focusing on clarifying goals and modifying eating behaviors for body fat control.
- ▶ *Maximize Your Body Potential* by Joyce D. Nash, Ph.D. (Bull Publishing, 1986). Sections entitled "Talking Yourself into Success" and "Thinking Smart" offer helpful suggestions.
- ▶ *Rapid Relief from Emotional Distress* by Gary Emery, Ph.D., and James Campbell, M.D. (Fawcett, 1986). A book on rapid cognitive therapy, with quick, practical ways to overcome anxiety. A corresponding audiotape series is available from Los Angeles Center for Cognitive Therapy (630 S. Wilton Pl., Los Angeles, CA 90005; 213-387-4737).

Part 5: Postural Vitality

Posture is a frequently overlooked consideration in body fat control. Balanced posture gives you an exhilarating sense of no effort in action, of floating buoyantly, comfortably in space. In contrast, poor posture places the body in a state of tension and effort, which contribute to fatigue, pain, lowered self-esteem, and aversion to vigorous activity, and may even *cause* depression.

By performing some simple exercises, using mental imagery, and increasing your awareness of where you tend to hold unnecessary muscular tension, you can improve your posture, often dramatically. The next two chapters tell you how.

Buoyant posture promotes self-confidence and control over your mind and mood. In addition, your body doesn't suffer from "pelvic tilt," a common condition in which the lower back sways in and the lower abdomen distends forward, giving the appearance of a "pot belly." This is a tiring position that leads to chronic tension and pain. Eliminating pelvic tilt is perhaps the fastest way to look like you've lost ten pounds. You immediately appear and feel slimmer and more fit. You'll also find it easier to exercise and perform daily activities.

The five integrated steps to body fat control presented in this section of *Health & Fitness Excellence* provide a myth-free plan for lasting success. Which parts of the formula have you been missing?

Step 5

POSTURAL VITALITY

33 Introduction

MYTH: "Good posture" simply means sitting and standing up straight.

FACT: Of the 680 muscles in your body, only a few — including the rectus capitus, semispinalis, and serratus — are specially designed to hold your body upright and relaxed. Yet most of us tense dozens — sometimes hundreds — of the wrong muscles when we sit, stand, and move. The result is reduced lung capacity (sometimes by one-third or more), fatigue, muscular pain, headaches, eyestrain, decreased blood and oxygen to the brain, and diminished productivity. Solution: Learning fast, simple ways to create buoyant, balanced posture.

MYTH: As long as you have a good mental attitude and do aerobic exercise, your posture will take care of itself.

FACT: Great posture doesn't happen by accident. It takes a willingness to become more aware of the way you stand, sit, and move. And it requires finding the places where you are tense or misaligned and then making changes — in your movements and muscular balance — until tension in those trouble spots is gone.

MYTH: You develop good posture through exercises — like sit-ups, leg-lifts, toe touches, back arches, and hurtler's stretches.

FACT: Exercise alone isn't enough. In fact, the exercises mentioned in this myth actually make posture *worse*. Guided mental imagery, sensory awareness, environmental supports, and some little-known trauma-free exercises are the key.

MYTH: There's really no way to sit on most sofas or chairs without feeling uncomfortable before long. Pretty soon, your back, neck, or shoulders get tight.

FACT: You can stop accumulating tension and pain from standing or sitting by learning new ways to take pressure *off* your back, neck, and shoulders during the day.

MYTH: Gravity pushes us down all the time. By the end of every day, we're bound to be an inch or two shorter than we were in the morning. No wonder everyone gets so tired!

FACT: Gravity holds us on the earth but can collapse your posture only when it's imbalanced: neck too far forward, chin out, shoulders rounded, back swayed, chest in, or pelvis tilted. By learning to choose your own best posture, you can greatly reduce fatigue and tension.

Posture is one of the most overlooked keys to best health and performance. Good posture not only improves fitness, thinking ability, emotional state, and general vitality, *it can actually help reverse the aging process* — not just cosmetically but functionally.[1] That's the finding of some leading scientists, including Dr. Rene Cailliet, director of physical medicine and rehabilitation at Santa Monica Hospital Medical Center in California and clinical professor at the University of Southern California School of Medicine. This fifth step to *Health & Fitness Excellence* focuses on postural vitality: what it is, how to achieve it, and how to maintain it.

The Golden Circle

Posture is affected by, and affects, every aspect of our lives. It is one of the seven primary threads in the golden circle of *Health & Fitness Excellence*. You can begin anywhere in the next two chapters, with the simplest idea or technique. Your state of nutrition, exercise, stress management, body fat control, and mental development depend to a significant degree on your posture. With good posture, nearly everything happens more smoothly, with greater ease. Exercise is more enjoyable, digestion improves, the mind is clearer, senses sharper, and problems seem more manageable. In contrast, poor postures — tense, slumped, struggling positions — sabotage your every thought and movement.

"There is a relationship between good posture and physical fitness — one helps the other," writes exercise physiologist Dr. Per Olof-Åstrand. "Good posture acts to avoid cramping of internal organs, permits better circulation, prevents undue tensing of some muscles and lengthening of others. It contributes to fitness."[2]

How Poor Posture Affects the Body and Mind

Poor posture distorts the alignment of bones, chronically tenses muscles, and contributes to stressful conditions such as the following:

Loss of vital lung capacity (by as much as 30 percent or more)[3]
Reduced blood and oxygen to the brain and senses[4]
Reduced range of motion, stiffness of joints, and pain syndromes (headaches, jaw pain, muscular aches)[5]
Premature aging of body tissues[6]
Faulty digestion[7] and constipation[8]
Back pain (perhaps 80 percent of all cases)[9]
Tendency toward cynicism, pessimism, drowsiness, and poor concentration[10]

Poor posture also slows reaction time, magnifies feelings of panic and helplessness, and may even *cause* depression.[11]
Tense muscles in the neck, chest, shoulders, or upper back can diminish blood flow to the brain and cause impairments in thinking and emotional control.[12] Moreover, some poor sleep postures add to physical tension all night long rather than diminish it.[13] A University of Colorado study suggested that chronic pain may be due to brain stress caused by prolonged, unnecessary muscle tension.[14] This, in turn, throws the body's movement patterns out of synchrony.

Optimal Posture Is Within Everyone's Reach

In addition to helping prevent or reverse the above conditions, optimal posture brings a wondrous sense of ease and elegance to even the simplest of movements; enhanced pleasure and safety in exercise; a boost in self-image and thinking abilities; greater emotional control in stressful situations; a slimmer abdomen; and more.

By definition, *posture* is the relative position and alignment of the various masses of the human body. But what comes to mind when most Americans think of "good posture"? A stiff, military-like, square-shouldered stance. But that's not at all the focus of this chapter.

With optimal posture — what I refer to as *postural vitality* — you have an exhilarating sense of no effort in action, of moving buoyantly, fluidly, comfortably in space. The chest is open and "floats" upward; the head is up, with neck long and chin slightly in; jaw and tongue are relaxed; shoulders are broad and loose; pelvis and hips are level; back is comfortably straight; and the abdomen is free of tension. You are "resting in motion" — an imaginary sky hook is gently lifting your whole spinal column upward from a central point on top of your head.

Every movement you make depends on the split-second tensing and relaxing of muscles that keep the bones of the body aligned. *How* you use those muscles in your body can make the difference between feeling stiff, irritable, and out of balance or fluid, energized, and productive.

How Does Posture Get Imbalanced?

The antecedents of postural imbalance reach back to childhood. During our most formative years, we imitate those around us. We become a mirror image of the people we look at most of the time.

Posture is also shaped by our physical environment: our beds, shoes (from sneakers to sandals; stiff dress shoes to launching-pad high heels), backpacks, purses, briefcases and bookbags, soft chairs, vehicle seats, desks, work stances, television viewing positions, and related factors, all contribute to our postural state.

Our physical movements operate out of habit most of the time. Here is an example: Cross your arms. Now cross them the opposite way. Was it more difficult to carry out the second assignment? It's interesting to note that there is no anatomical reason why one arm-crossing position should be less comfortable than the other. It's simply a *learned preference*. Similarly, the way you sit, stand, sleep, bend, and move also come from repetition and habit.

By nature, we are designed to stand upright with almost no effort. But once out of balance, we must strain against gravity to resist its pull.

The slightest shift from our natural alignment — head or neck forward, a shoulder rolled down, lower back swayed, pelvis tipped, or abdomen distended — lets gravity seize the displaced area. Without a streamlined bone-through-bone flow to distribute the force of gravity, we get slowly, steadily pushed down. Slouching at home or work begins to determine your posture the rest of the time, says Howard Hunt, chairman of the physical education department at the University of California at San Diego.[15] At some point, a slump becomes your *only* option.

For each comfortable position and fluid movement of the body, a very small number of key muscles provide support. Tightness and strain often come from using extra muscles — or the wrong muscles — to prop the body up or propel it.[16] Instead of first relaxing tense or injured areas of the body, we tend to correct our imbalances by adding counterbalancing muscle tension to tensions that are already there.

Example: Stand up and try this experiment. Pretend you have just strained your right knee. The natural thing to do is to compensate by transferring weight off the right leg and onto the healthier left side of the body. Do you notice the pressure this adds to your left foot, knee, and hip and the increased tightness in the left leg? Are you aware of the line of tension that shifts up the spine to the neck? Now walk a few steps in this adjusted position. How has it thrown off the timing of your gait?

Now project ahead in your mind. As you use this altered position over the upcoming days, you adapt — tensing dozens of extra muscles to keep from feeling (and looking) like you're leaning too far to your left and to keep the pressure off the right knee. You learn to tolerate the new position and to a certain extent unconsciously accept it. Finally, even when the right knee is healed, you may fail to *fully release the tense, unnatural position* as you resume normal activities. Unknowingly, you end up with tension on top of tension.

If you happened to be frightened or injured from falling as a child, you may have picked up the habit of holding your shoulders back, weight on the heels, neck forward, and eyes down to better see what's in front of you and make it harder to fall forward again. This has put unnecessary strain on your spine, neck, and pelvis. Soon the habit became ingrained, automatic. If you have been physically threatened or assaulted, you may have hunched your shoulders up and forward and tensed your arms for a sense of protection. Years later, you may still be holding this unnatural position and causing headaches, shallow breathing, and fatigue.

Year after year, we unwittingly turn life's bumps, bruises, and emotional traumas into ever-greater tension for the body. Ease turns into effort. Eventually, the simple act of standing, turning, or bending becomes a herculean task. We start looking at life through the eyes of chronic fatigue. What started as a series of minor discrepancies has now turned into a major stress.

Turning Things Around — Good Posture Begins with Awareness

Many people assume that good posture is instinctive or automatic. It isn't. "We're not born knowing how to do it right," says Dr. Wilfred Barlow, medical director of the Alexander Institute in Great Britain and author of *The Alexander Technique*. "No reflex system sets that up. We have to learn it."[17]

"Use," adds Dr. Barlow, "means the way we use our bodies as we live from moment to moment. Not only when we are moving, but when we are keeping still. Not only when we are speaking, but when we are thinking. Not only when we are making love, but when we are feeling or refusing pleasure. Not only when we are communicating by gestures and attitudes, but when, unknown to ourselves, our bodily mood and disposition tell people what we are like and keep us that way whether we like it or not."[18]

Right now, you are sitting somewhere reading this book. Exactly *how* are you sitting? Direct your attention to various areas of your body as you read these pages. Are your knees open or crossed? Is one shoulder higher or more forward than the other? Where are your shoulder blades? Is the weight of your body more on one buttock than the other? Where is your neck positioned? Do you feel any tightness in the muscles there? Where are your elbows? Which of your upper arms is more relaxed? Is your chest "open" or collapsed? How does your lower back feel — is it straight or swayed forward or backward? Ankles and feet relaxed or cramped? Is your abdomen tight or knotted up? How about your jaw and tongue?

It is easy to keep these areas needlessly tense. Are you aware of how each of your hands is holding the book? Direct your attention to your wrists, palms, and fingers for a moment. Notice the pressure on your palm or fingers where they take the weight of the book. As you run your eyes over the page, does your head move from side to side to shift your eye position or do just your eyes move?

If you expand your awareness, you can lift your posture. The next chapter teaches you how.

Postural State, Mental State

"Posture is not solely the manifestation of physical balance," writes rehabilitative medicine specialist Dr. David Imrie. "It's also an expression of mental balance. Think about the way you stand when you are depressed or tired: you stand with your shoulders rounded and drooping. Your body represents your emotions by giving up the fight against gravity,

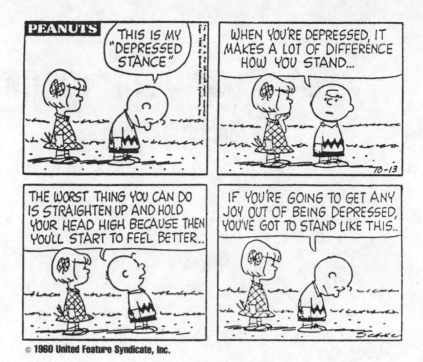

© 1960 United Feature Syndicate, Inc.

sagging just as low as you feel. . . . It's also notable that the term 'well-balanced' is used to describe someone who 'won't go over the edge' and whose emotions are 'on an even keel.' "[19]

"Our conception of ourselves is derived from our feeling of the way in which our body is oriented in space," writes Moshe Feldenkrais, a leading postural researcher. "This self-image is of the contours of the body . . . [and all of our sensory signals]. Each of us acts in accordance with this self-image: he eats, walks, sits, speaks, thinks, loves, and so on, in his own particular way; and he identifies himself with this image."[20] A recent series of university studies reported that, compared with subjects in a good postural position, subjects with a slumped posture had a greater tendency toward feelings of helplessness and frustration during work tasks and perceived themselves to be under greater stress.[21]

Here is another important discovery: Your "facial posture" is linked to mental attitude, mood, and performance. A positive facial expression — even if it's only a slight smile and even if you don't *feel* like smiling — increases blood flow to the brain and predisposes neurochemistry toward favorable emotions.[22] Studies also reveal that posture influences your voice quality and ease of speaking: good posture contributes to a "compelling, natural voice image."[23]

Now let's learn some specific ways to increase postural vitality.

34 Posture Improvement Techniques

BEST POSTURE ARISES from five interconnected factors:

1 Sensory awareness
2 Guided mental imagery
3 Key posture muscle exercises
4 Environmental supports
5 Massage therapies

Sensory Awareness

We discussed sensory awareness techniques in Chapter 4. One scientific postulate, the Weber-Fechner law, states that "the difference in stimulus that produces the least detectable difference in sensation is always in the same ratio to the whole stimulus."[24]

Here's the translation: If you are exerting a lot of muscle tension in a certain part of your body, it's very difficult for your senses to detect small reductions in that tightness. In essence, the tension numbs your awareness. To become more alert to the tension level of certain muscles — in your neck, back, or shoulders, for example — first relax the area as completely as possible so that your senses can "become more sensitive." This enables you to detect and release unnecessary tension.

Increasing your awareness takes practice. Set aside 10 minutes a day over the next several weeks to relax your body fully (see the instructions in Chapter 4) and increase your sensory awareness. Mental imagery techniques are a simple, powerful way to sharpen your senses.

Guided Mental Imagery

The ability to fully focus your attention is, overall, the most important factor in making lasting postural improvements. Neuroscience literature is filled with evidence that the mind's internal gaze can be harnessed to change attitudes, emotions, and physical posture.

Ideokinetic and Kinesthetic Imagery

Two imagery methods are often used in postural therapy. The first is *ideokinetic imagery,* which relies on the movie screen of your mind. By creating a vivid mental picture of movement — without actually moving your physical body — you pattern the imagined motion into your subcortical brain and nervous system.[25] "Only by *changing the coordination* of muscles toward patterns of balanced action . . . can the structure simultaneously be brought into better alignment and . . . mechanical balance," says Dr. L. E. Sweigard in *Human Movement Potential: Its Ideokinetic Facilitation.*[26]

"Your first step will be to be able to feel your whole body," adds movement authority Gerda Alexander, founder of the European technique called Eutony, "beginning with the surface, inch by inch, always keeping aware — not only intellectually — of your sensations and the direction in space. . . . While you are reading this, let us work with your legs just where you are sitting on a chair, or lying on your bed. Try to become aware of where your right foot is placed, without looking, just through the sensation of your skin. Find your heel through its touch to the floor or to the mattress. Feel the entire foot sole, the arch, the bones and muscles covering the whole area. Add the toes, one by one."[27]

The basic idea is to let all the sensations from each area of your body come forward "like many voices" telling you precisely what you feel in that area. Here is another Eutony example: Lying on your back on a mattress or a padded floor surface, "let the arms lie along your trunk with the palms turned to the floor. Then — without making any movement — *pretend* to stretch the fingers of one hand, one after the other. Pretend to stretch them as far as possible, rest, and do it again with all fingers together. Now lift the whole arm from the fingertips, lift the other arm on which you have not been working, and compare the sensations of both. Although you have only pretended to move, there will be a difference because muscle tonus and circulation are influenced by the intention to move in the same way as if you had carried out the movement."[28]

The second type of mental visioning is called *kinesthetic imagery*. It combines sensory-rich images with actual physical movements, as illustrated in the following examples.

Head and Neck Position

Poor posture often causes headaches and jaw pain. "It's extremely difficult to work in a technological society and not develop a forward head," says rehabilitative medicine authority Dr. Rene Cailliet in *The Rejuvenation Strategy*. "If you're sitting at a typewriter or a computer, or working on an assembly line, chances are that you have one. Even cooking and cleaning can produce one. Any activity that requires you to look down for protracted periods, even reading or simple desk work, can produce a chronic forward head position."[29] And this postural stress causes or contributes to tension headaches, vision problems, and jaw and neck pain.[30]

"Jaw joint pain is so widespread today," says Dr. Cailliet, "that a majority of adults have experienced it. This type of discomfort was once considered to be exclusively a dental problem. . . . We now know that it is just as often caused or aggravated by faulty posture."[31]

Rounded shoulders are another prime source of pain — straining the muscles that attach the upper border of the shoulder blades to the base of the skull. This contributes to a humped upper back and swayed lower back.

Unless you develop a keen awareness of postural balance, backed by proper exercises, your spinal column will slowly compress and deteriorate — you can literally become shorter in height as you age. The four natural curves of the spine deepen. Stress to surrounding tissues increases, causing tightness, tiredness, and pain. Fortunately, there is no need for this to happen.

For years, physical education instructors have admonished Americans to "stand up straight" — shoulders broad and pulled back, buttocks tucked, back ramrod straight, stomach sucked in. Pure military. The advice is well intended, but it doesn't work. The muscular bracing looks artificial, feels horrible, and causes fatigue. Even worse, you need to keep reminding yourself to maintain this stiff, unnatural position. What happens when it slips from your awareness? Your body gratefully collapses into old patterns.

Postural vitality isn't forced; it's unlocked. The most important part of the change comes in your head and neck position. Your head weighs between 10 and 15 pounds. To avoid stress on the neck, shoulders, and spine, the head must be poised precisely at the crest of the spine. The best way to ease strain in the spine is to lengthen your neck and let your head move upward, chin slightly in, shoulders broadening, lower back flattening. Now gently lean your head to the left and then to the right, coming back to the most central, most balanced spot you can sense.

Next, move slightly forward and then back, finding the precise center once again.

Here's another picture: "If you put a five-pound weight on your head, and you do nothing more than push up against the resistance, you will straighten out your spinal curves without so much as a thought," says Dr. Cailliet. "It is the weight that's doing the work by giving you feedback, telling you to push up toward the ceiling, and to stand tall. To your body, any other response is intolerable."[32]

Begin right now to think tall, to encourage your head to float upward. Don't push or strain your neck; simply bring your head back over your shoulders, with your chin slightly in. You'll sense the difference — and see it in the mirror.

It is important to realize that the head does more than simply rest atop your neck. Your head should lead nearly all body movements. The Alexander technique, a successful guided imagery approach to postural balance, summarizes it this way: *"As you begin any movement or act, move your whole head upward and away from your whole body, and let your whole body lengthen by following that upward direction."*[33] The process is based on learning a new way to use your body, with smoothness and ease. Nothing is forced.

Two special notes: First, practice smiling. As explained in the previous chapter, a positive facial expression increases blood flow to the brain and helps make you less reactive to negative stress.

Second, don't let your shirt collars or ties get too tight. Cornell University researchers found that a collar snugged a mere 1.27 centimeters smaller than your relaxed neck size restricts blood flow in the pulsing veins in the back of the eyes.[34] This appears to harm visual perception, substantially slowing the ability of the brain to process visual information and convert it into a physical response. Among businessmen tested, two thirds wore collars and ties that were too tight, and nearly one in seven had a tightness of at least 1.27 centimeters. This finding has particularly important implications for people in occupations where eye-body coordination is critical — airline pilots, computer operators, athletes, artists, motor vehicle drivers of all kinds, accountants, and so on.

Breathing into the Lower Back

Here is an exercise to gently flatten the lower back while you are sitting or lying down. It complements postural exercises such as the pelvic leveler and pelvic lift (presented in Chapter 15). Sit comfortably in a straight-back chair or on the floor with a back sling (see "Resources" at the end of this chapter), or lie down on your back on a padded surface. Inhale a slow deep breath, feeling the air expand your ribs, and then gently push from the inside out against the lower spine, flattening your back. Exhale, imagining all tension floating away with your breath while leaving your back as flat as is comfortable. Repeat several times, feeling the air massage your posture into a better position.

Standing

Most people find it difficult to stand for an extended period of time. Standing fatigue occurs when you remain in a stiff, motionless position, wasting energy from tension and blocked circulation in the legs. In contrast, the person with efficient, dynamic posture expends very little muscular energy and has minimal sagging against ligaments and only slight, intermittent pressure on veins.

First, stand in a relaxed manner, with your feet side by side about shoulder width apart. Slowly shift your weight left and right from your ankles. Notice the precise point where your weight feels perfectly, evenly balanced between the ball and heel of each foot — carried through the center of your ankles. Once you have found that comfortable, stable position, bend your knees (just enough so that they are slightly unlocked).

Some experts recommend standing in a slight step position, with one foot several inches ahead of the other.[35] Then slowly, gently shift some of your weight from foot to foot, keeping your pelvis level. This keeps leg circulation moving and reduces standing fatigue.

The image of a sky hook helps you keep your chin from pointing forward and thereby retracting your head and tensing the neck. Imagine that the crown of your head is attached to a strong cord extending up in the air to a large balloon. By releasing tension — rather than using force — your head can gently float upward at the crown, with your neck lengthening.

"Since the weight-supporting bones of the body are Class I levers stacked from foot to head," explains Dr. Sweigard, "their balance depends on the centering of weight through their fulcrums [joints]."[36]

Here are some basic standing position guidelines:

1 Let your neck lengthen and become vertical, head floating on top (gently buoyed up by an imaginary sky hook), chin slightly in.
2 Breathe diaphragmatically — with the lower ribs expanding outward to the sides on each inhalation.
3 Feel your spine lengthening, your back widening and flattening, abdomen trim, buttocks tucked in slightly, upper body floating upward from a level pelvis, not tipped forward (with pot belly and sway back) or backward (with too much buttocks tuck, which keeps the legs off balance).
4 Keep your knees slightly unlocked, floating your weight over the center of your ankles and evenly between toes and heels.
5 Vary your stance regularly.

Certain working positions require special attention. For example, whenever you are working at a counter or sink for a long period of time, bend one knee and place that foot up on a short stool or box. This relieves strain to the lower-back area.[37]

Don't try to *force* your body into a better postural position — this overtaxes muscles and quickly tires you out. Instead, use awareness and mental imagery suggestions.

Sitting

The way you sit — your sitting posture — has a dramatic influence on energy and productivity. Most chairs can create excessive stress on the spine, back, and neck. Especially during prolonged hours of work, choose chairs that are fully adjustable. For best support and comfort, your chair must fit the length, size, and contours of your body. If you sit in various chairs in the course of the day or if another person uses your chair, adjust it each time you use it, just as you would adjust your car seat, steering wheel, and mirrors after someone else has driven your car.

The height of the seat should be adjusted to precisely match the position of the desk, drafting table, or countertop where you work. This enables you to sit with your feet flat on the floor, thighs approximately parallel to the floor, knees slightly higher than hips and to work at about elbow height. The chair should be lightly padded and provide firm back support, especially for the lower back. The best backrests arch forward to support the natural curve of the lower back. If your backrest doesn't arch forward, and you can't replace the chair, try a small pillow or back sling to boost support (see "Resources" at the end of this chapter). Some people may need a chair with a full back, providing support all the way up to the shoulders. Cushions with fabric upholstery help prevent slipping and sliding.

There are nine common faults with most chairs, writes rehabilitative medicine authority Dr. Janet G. Travell: "No support for your low back; armrests too low or too high; too scooped a backrest in its upper-portion; backrest nearly vertical; backrest short, failing to support your upper back, jackknifing effect at hips and knees; high front edge of the seat, shutting down the circulation in your legs; seat bottom soft in the center, creating a bucket effect which places the load on the outer side of your thighs, rather than on the bony points in the buttocks; an excellent chair may be the wrong size for you."[38]

Your type of work determines the best way to adjust your chair. If your job requires reading, telephoning, using a calculator, or writing at a desk, it's important to lean forward — so the "seat pan" of your chair should be tilted forward 10 to 15 degrees so that the thighs can be directed downward to minimize back strain. Your elbows or forearms should be able to rest comfortably on your work surface.

If you operate a computer video display terminal (VDT) with a keyboard, the seat pan can be tilted backward so that you assume a position much like a car driver's. Your forearms should be held at a 70-to-90-degree angle to your upper arms. If you are using a typewriter, the forearms may be angled even higher (50 to 60 degrees).

If your work necessitates leaning forward a lot, you may want to use a chair with a spring-loaded back support to move as you move. A 10 percent rearward incline of the chair back is ideal, says Dr. Cailliet,[39] and a short, stable footrest (a stool or hassock that is angled 5 to 15 degrees upward toward the toes and is comfortably wide with a nonskid surface) will help keep your thighs slightly elevated.

Be certain you have good lighting (see Chapter 37) to minimize eye-strain, and keep your work between mid-chest and face height whenever possible. This can be accomplished by using an adjustable work surface like a drafting table or slanting desktop.

Seat yourself squarely on your "sit bones," the ischial tuberosities; don't slump. Slouching creates *10 to 15 times* as much pressure on your lower back as does sitting up straight.[40] Leaning to one side or becoming off-center in any other way shifts the line of gravity and causes problems if you stay in that unbalanced position for very long. Armrests on a chair can relieve about 25 percent of the load on the lower back[41] and help provide stability and support when you are adjusting positions during work time. A back sling (see "Resources") can support the lower back when you are forced to sit on a backless bench, stool, or short-backed chair.

Several years ago, the *New England Journal of Medicine* published a study showing that chronic back pain was alleviated for many men once they stopped carrying fat wallets in their back pockets![42]

After your buttocks and upper legs are centered on the seat, simply let your buoyant upper body bend at the thigh/hip joints (*not* the lower spine) as you settle your properly aligned back (and neck if the chair is tall enough) against the seat back. If you must cross your legs, do it at the ankles. Crossing at the knees misaligns the pelvis and can lead to back tension and pain if you don't change positions frequently enough. Whenever possible, place your feet flat on the floor. Another good option is keeping one foot elevated on a chair rung or placing it slightly forward of the other foot on a small stool.[43]

To find your most centered, unstressed sitting position, first repeat the instructions for balancing the neck: gently lean your head to the left and then to the right; then return to center. Next, lean slightly forward and then back, returning to the spot you sense as the exact center. To center the torso, repeat these instructions bending at the hips/thighs.

Perhaps most important of all: *Once you've found a chair you really love, leave it. Often.* If you work at a desk, put some items you need during the course of the day on a countertop, shelf, or file across the room. This makes certain that you regularly walk the dozen steps or so to reach them. Get up at least once every 15 to 30 minutes. And take rejuvenation-in-motion breaks (Chapter 10) every hour or so throughout the day.

Reading, Writing, and Telephoning

Select your reading position carefully. Do you like to curl up like a pretzel, buried deep in your favorite chair? Watch out for a retracted or extended head position, protruding or dipped chin, distended neck, drooping shoulders, and sunken chest. These imbalances create tension, cut circulation to the eyes and brain, and decrease reading speed and comprehension.

Heighten your sensory awareness to find your own best postures. By adjusting your seating arrangements, you may be able to bring reading material up to your field of vision and avoid the strain of dropping your head down to it. Try a bookstand to hold books at a comfortable slant, and consider buying a small reading light that clips onto the book (available at many bookstores).

When talking on the telephone, bring the handset up to your ear and mouth; *don't* bend your head and neck down to the phone or cradle it between your ear and shoulder by forcing your neck to the side. Use an adjustable shoulder support, hands-free headset, or desktop speakerphone when you want best posture or need both hands free for desk work during conversations.

Reaching, Bending, and Turning

Here is a cardinal rule for everyday movements: Whenever you turn to reach for something, take a step in that direction. This helps coordinate and focus your power, integrating the body as it moves and taking strain off back muscles by better using the legs and trunk. When reaching, bending, or turning, remember to lead the movement with your head floating upward, followed by your whole body.

In the Car

Although they feel comfortable when you slide behind the wheel in the auto dealer's showroom, most car seats force the driver and passengers into a pressured, flexed position without adequate back support. In fact, seating is so important that the type of car you drive correlates to back pain, says Dr. Jennifer Kelsey, professor of Public Health at Columbia University.[44] Motorists driving cars with poor-quality seats faced three times the risk of developing lower-back problems over drivers of many Swedish and Japanese cars. A number of foreign cars and a growing number of domestic ones offer seats with dozens of easy adjustments for supporting all areas of the back. In terms of health and reaction speed when driving, this is a vital factor.

Of course, it's rarely worth selling your car just because the seats aren't ideal. In many cases, a small pillow or two can help back support. During long trips, you can incorporate a variety of techniques to avoid postural distress.

First, adjust the seat and pillows so that you have the best visibility and easiest access to gauges, mirrors, and controls. For many people it is helpful to move the car seat forward so that the knees are moderately bent. Develop the ability to tense only those muscles necessary for driving control, leaving your shoulders, neck, and back relaxed. Make frequent stops for rejuvenation-in-motion breaks that take as little as 30 seconds (Chapter 10).

Pushing, Pulling, Lifting, Carrying

Ease in pushing, pulling, lifting, and carrying objects depends on the alignment of your bones so that force can be applied in a balanced way. In pushing and pulling, the center of the height and weight of an object determines how much bend in the hip, knee, and ankle joints is necessary. If you apply power too high or low on the object, the lower back is strained. When lifting objects you can comfortably manage, avoid unnecessary tension, especially in the neck and jaw, and don't hold your breath. Grasp the object securely, keeping it close to your body's center of gravity, with your feet on either side of it when possible. Keep your back straight and lift with your legs.

When carrying objects for a distance, it is also best to hold them near your center of gravity. Keep purses, briefcases, and luggage as light as possible. When scurrying through airport terminals, consider a well-designed backpack or a cart on wheels to move your travel bags. When carrying or pulling an item on one side of the body, be sure to switch sides periodically to ease stress.

Walking

Walking with relaxed, buoyant posture requires practice. Take a walk around the room right now and observe how the weight of your body shifts through each foot as you move. After the middle of your heel touches the ground, your weight should generally flow ahead to the center-forward part of the foot at the second or third toe. Ideally, your foot will be pointed straight ahead, not turned out or in. Do your heels strike the ground hard? Does your torso sway or do your hips move side to side to keep you upright? Do you feel tension in the neck, lower back, abdomen, hips, knees, shins, or ankles? Are your strides short and hesitant? Midlength and comfortable? Or long and strained?

With practice, graceful, nearly effortless walking can become a matter of habit. First use the guidelines for standing (presented earlier in this chapter). Pay special attention to your head alignment over your shoulders — using the sky hook image — and keeping the chin slightly in. Your shoulders, arms, spine, back, hips, and knees should be centered and free of unnecessary tension. Let your whole body shift several degrees in the direction you have decided to walk, as one knee bends and swings easily forward leading the movement. At no time should your knees be locked. Let the arches of your feet feel relaxed and resilient, springing up slightly with each step. Your pelvis remains level — a bit like balancing a bowl of water — as you move.

Your arms should stay relaxed and swing straight ahead, not across your chest or out to the sides since this throws off your gait and wastes energy. Use a heterolateral rhythm; that is, move your left arm forward as your right leg advances, then right arm forward with left leg, and so on. The uplifted direction of your head and torso will help move you forward.

Proper Posture Enhances Sleep, Exercise, and Sports
As noted in Chapter 8, your sleep posture makes a difference in the quality of your nightly rest. When performing exercises or participating in sports or recreational activities, don't forget to learn the best postural patterns, or biomechanics, to avoid injuries and receive greatest fitness benefits. See Chapters 11–19 for recommendations.

Key Posture Muscle Exercises

Without first increasing your awareness and learning mental imagery guidelines for best posture, exercises to strengthen posture muscles generally aren't very effective. But once the sensory and mental aspects are coming under your control, Chapters 13–15 and 18 offer a series of exercises that help tone and balance postural muscles.

Environmental Supports

The design of your chairs, shoes, desks, bed, telephones, and other environmental factors makes life easier — or more difficult. We have already discussed chairs, desks, and telephones. Chapter 8 reviews sleep and rest, including beds. What about shoes? Correct footwear makes a difference in postural alignment and ease of movement.

High-heel shoes aren't recommended — they put far too much weight on the front of the foot and force the legs, pelvis, and back to compensate. Stiff, flat, hard-soled shoes or sandals are another poor choice — they make it very difficult for the twenty-six bones in your feet to adjust to the ground surface and distribute your weight. Side-to-side imbalances from uncomfortable shoes tend to flow upward and twist the rest of the body. Better-quality dress shoes and sandals are often well designed and flexible. Insoles help buffer ground shock waves and increase comfort.

Negative-heeled shoes, in which the heel is lower than the toe area, can be temporarily helpful for people with the habit of tilting the pelvis forward. However, once you learn to balance your posture, these shoes start to cause stress, throwing your weight too far back over your heels.

A new generation of scientifically designed shoes for walking, running, aerobic dance, and other activities provide a much needed combination of comfort and support. Select footwear carefully, matching it to your exact foot size and shape and sports requirements. If necessary, consult an orthopedic physician or podiatrist for professional guidance. And spend some time each day going barefoot. It's a great way to become more aware of foot positioning and weight distribution as you stand and walk.

Massage Therapies

Human touch can be wonderfully nurturing and therapeutic. Massage is a well-proven way to release tensions, increase sensory awareness, and aid in choosing better posture. Chapter 36 reviews massage therapies, both those given by professionals and those you can do yourself at home.

Professional Posture Therapies

A growing number of professionals in the United States specialize in various forms of massage therapy, posture alignment, and movement education. Could professional help benefit you?

First, decide what your specific posture-related goals are. Are you already using sensory awareness and mental imagery and simply want help balancing and relaxing tight areas of your body? Or do you feel you have a relaxed, responsive body but need help learning how to use it with greater coordination and ease? Or are you looking for a comprehensive posture education program?

Some posture therapists specialize in deep massage therapies without movement education — in other words, the therapy is done *to* you, not *with* you. As should be obvious by now, this incomplete approach at best gives incomplete results. Your body's structure may be relaxed and loosened by the therapist, but you end up with no idea of how to use your body with peak efficiency. So it's easy to fall back into old patterns and to regress.

Other therapists specialize in movement education without any massage therapies. In this case, the client is integrally involved in the therapy experience but must often commit to a major time investment (in some cases years, not months) and expense.

Usually the fastest, most lasting results come from a combination of movement education and personalized massage therapies.

When considering any posture therapist, be certain to check his or her credentials and get a list of past clients you can talk to about the therapy. Massage therapists who have graduated from a bona fide program and adhere to stringent professional standards are often members of the American Massage Therapy Association (AMTA). This professional organization has established official national standards. For information, contact the AMTA (National Department of Information, 1130 W. North Shore Ave., Chicago, IL 60626; 312-761-AMTA).

In addition to chiropractic and rehabilitative medicine educational programs, major schools of posture therapy in America include the Alexander Technique (508 W. Washington, Urbana, IL 61801; 129 W. 67th St., New York, NY 10023; 1913 Thayer Ave., Los Angeles, CA 90025; or 931 Elizabeth St., San Francisco, CA 94114); Aston-Patterning (P.O. Box 544, Mill Valley, CA 94941); the Feldenkrais Method (P.O. Box 1145, San Francisco, CA 94101); Hellerwork (147 Lomita Dr., Suite H, Mill Valley, CA 94941); Lomi Work (Lomi School Foundation, Box 318, Tomales, CA 94971); Rolfing (P.O. Box 1868, Boulder, CO 80306); and the Trager Approach (10 Old Mill St., Mill Valley, CA 94941).

There are also a number of effective, lesser-known approaches to posture therapy. You can best learn about them through your local network of health professionals and health-conscious friends.

RESOURCES

Several posture-related products are of particular interest.

▶ Aston Line (P.O. Box 544, Mill Valley, CA 94941; 415-381-6683). Judith Aston, a well-known movement therapist, has designed several useful back support devices, including some lightweight wedges and cushions.

▶ Lehrman Back Center (1680 Michigan Ave., Suite 1000, Miami Beach, FL 33139; 305-538-1130). Dr. David Lehrman, founder and director of this medical center, has designed a portable plastic back support that can be carried in your pocket and inflated for travel.

▶ Nada Chair (842 22nd Ave., S.E., Minneapolis, MN 55414; 612-623-4436). The Nada (Spanish for "nothing") Chair is a portable legless chair, or sling, that weighs less than a pound and consists of two loops of webbing attached to a padded backrest. When the loops are slipped around the knees and adjusted, the reverse pressure gently holds the back erect while you are sitting. It can be used in conjunction with conventional seats such as office chairs, desk chairs, or couches, or passenger seats in cars, buses, airplanes, or trains. It can also be used for lower-back support where none is provided — in bleachers, on a stool, in a canoe or fishing boat, or in a meditation position on the floor. The chair helps stabilize the pelvis and relieve muscular stress and has been used by physicians at the Mayo Clinic to help back pain sufferers learn better posture.

Posture can be seen as a metaphor for your body's response to life's challenges. With postural vitality, events seem to happen more smoothly and you feel less separated from the world. Exercise is more pleasurable, thinking becomes clearer, smiles come more easily, and problems seem more manageable. No matter how you view it, postural vitality is an essential step to *Health & Fitness Excellence*.

Step 6

REJUVENATION AND LIVING ENVIRONMENTS DESIGN

35 Introduction

MYTH: Our senses — vision, hearing, touch — function at their peak by the time we reach adulthood.

FACT: Few of us ever come close to fully developing our senses. Researchers have discovered a little-known way to build brain power and slow — even reverse — many effects of aging: it's called sensory wellness. By learning to expand and enhance your vision, hearing, touch, and other senses, you can increase blood flow and metabolism within the brain, boost mental sharpness and memory, and promote longevity. (*See Chapters 36 and 37.*)

MYTH: The biggest pollution threats come from heavily industrialized areas and the outdoor environment.

FACT: New studies by the Environmental Protection Agency show that *indoor* pollution in homes and offices is up to 100 times greater than outdoor pollution levels, even in smog-filled industrial areas. Learn eight of the most serious indoor pollution problems and the simplest ways to solve them. (*See Chapters 39–41.*)

MYTH: Massage is for athletes and rich or famous people who have lots of spare time.

FACT: Scientific research has brought massage into mainstream health care programs throughout the world — and for good reasons. It can be a fast, effective way to release muscle tension, increase circulation, relieve pain, and improve posture. You can easily learn at-home skills for a 10-minute seated massage or a 30-minute full-body massage. (*See Chapter 36.*)

MYTH: Getting tangled up in sexual problems or feeling sexually unfulfilled is nearly inevitable. It's difficult to talk with a loved one about sex because men and women see things differently.

FACT: According to scientific research, sex can be as warm, intimate, and fulfilling at age seventy-five — and beyond — as at twenty-five. Most sexual difficulties arise from four basic causes: lack of communication (both the failure to communicate and the lack of a shared vocabulary about sex), feelings of vulnerability, lack of practice, and "cultural scripting," the myths about how men and women are supposed to feel and act sexually. Learn simple, specific ways to improve intimate relationships. (*See Chapter 38.*)

MYTH: Dental hygiene is easy — you just brush and floss your teeth every day and use a good-tasting mouthwash.

FACT: New discoveries suggest that best dental hygiene involves brushing, gentle flossing, frequent replacement of toothbrushes, especially when you're sick, and *not* using mouthwash. (*See Chapter 38.*)

MYTH: Without becoming paranoid, there is little you can really do about toxic indoor chemicals — cleaning products, building materials, radon gas, insecticides, and all the rest.	**FACT:** In general, the more "tight" and energy-efficient a building, the greater the indoor pollution problems. This is now called "sick building syndrome" by European scientists. Learn how to cut your risks and save money in the process. (*See Chapter 41.*)

Rejuvenation: Introduction

"Making young or youthful again; causing or undergoing rejuvenescence." That's the dictionary definition of *rejuvenation*. It is one of humankind's oldest, most cherished dreams. Modern science suggests that, to a surprising extent, it can be a reality.

First of all, rejuvenation — step-by-step *scientifically based* rejuvenation — won't undo years of health-destructive habits. In the course of my study trips to research and medical centers in Switzerland, Austria, and Germany, I interviewed staff physicians and talked with patients seeking "quick cure" rejuvenation or "fountain of youth" results. They never found either one. True rejuvenation isn't magic, isn't instantaneous, and isn't easy. But it *is* possible to make the body, emotions, and mind more youthful, to maximize vitality at every age. In its fullest sense, rejuvenation cannot be achieved with a fragmented, piecemeal approach; it requires a comprehensive program such as *Health & Fitness Excellence*.

Scientists have discovered that rejuvenation depends to a basic degree on sensory wellness, the focus of the next several chapters. It would be easy to charge off performing regular exercise, managing stress, and eating well — and overlook the priorities presented here. Nearly all health and fitness books do. But that's a mistake. The inherent vitality of our bodies and minds can be reawakened each day using simple, proven methods. Over time, these small choices pay large dividends.

Becoming More Sensational

The unity of the perceptual field . . . must be a unity of bodily experience. Your perception takes place where you are and is entirely dependent on how your body is functioning.

— *ALFRED NORTH WHITEHEAD,*
MODES OF THOUGHT

The full development and continued use of our senses goes far to keep our brain healthy and sharp, our emotions manageable, and our body energized and aware.[1] In addition to the traditional five senses — touch, sight, hearing, taste, and smell — scientists have now identified at least a dozen other sensory systems in the human body.[2]

"If we learn to modulate our senses," says neuroscientist Dr. Arthur Winter in *Build Your Brain Power,* "and develop them even in advanced years, we increase our pleasure in living and we maintain normal function in the cells that receive and respond to sensual input. A decrease in sensory input due to changes in the sense organs or to social isolation is reflected in reduced metabolism and blood flow within the brain."[3] This is confirmed by research presented at the National Institutes of Health.[4]

When we view our environments as enriching and interesting, the nerve cells in the brain's cortex apparently grow larger.[5] When we feel sensorily stimulated by our lives and the world around us, we are likely to increase our mental sharpness and longevity.[6]

"The remarkable ability of the brain to undergo actual physical changes in response to our perceived environments is providing new insights . . . into memory and learning," says Blair Justice, professor in the School of Public Health at the University of Texas Health Sciences Center. "The synapses [junctions] that connect each of our 100 billion neurons with as many as 50,000 other brain cells can be deactivated or enhanced based on our experiences. If we see ourselves trapped in a never-changing, gray environment, the synaptic connections may shut down and the release of neurotransmitters may diminish. Conversely, an experience of stimulation increases transmitter release and brings positive changes not only on the molecular but genetic level."[7]

The following three chapters discuss rejuvenation discoveries and recommendations. Living Environments Design is introduced in Chapter 39 and is discussed in detail in Chapters 40–42.

36 Sensory Wellness: Touch and Massage

The Science of Touch

Without the language of touch, life would be cold, distant, and stilted. Our human skin is rich with nearly a million sensory receptors that detect touch, temperature, pressure, and pain. This information is fed to the brain, which has a very large area reserved to receive sensory messages. Nerve fibers conducting tactile (touch) information are generally larger than those associated with other senses.

The National Institutes of Health have gathered scientific data demonstrating the remarkable therapeutic benefits of human touch. The biomagnetic fields emanating from loving, caring touch can reportedly alter membrane permeability, speed the healing of ulcers and bone fractures, and reduce anxiety. Experiments include treating cardiac patients, babies in respiratory distress, and wounds in laboratory mice.[8]

Touch is our swiftest form of communication, yet it has been woefully neglected in Western societies compared with other kinds of human expression. Babies and older people who are not touched suffer not only emotional but physical decline.[9]

Touch expresses our feelings and describes our perception of other sensations. A recent survey of nearly four thousand undergraduate students at San Diego State University revealed that, regardless of gender, people who were less comfortable about touching were also more apprehensive about communicating and had lower self-esteem.[10] Other studies have reported that those who are more comfortable with touch have less anxiety and tension in their everyday lives.[11] Psychologist Richard Heslin at Purdue University has analyzed the spectrum of human contact and proposed five categories of touch based on people's various roles and relationships: functional-professional; social-polite; friendship-warmth; love-intimacy; and sexual-arousal.[12]

For a guided tour of the latest research on touch, see *Touching: The Human Significance of the Skin,* 3rd edition, by Ashley Montagu, Ph.D. (Perennial Library, 1986). This extensively referenced book examines the importance of tactile interaction — touching — on all facets of human development. Subjects include the relation of the skin to mental and physical health; the discovery of the immunological functions of the skin; the importance of touching, especially for infants and older people; gender differences; and the relationship between touching and imaging.

Touching Exercises

You can enhance your sense of touch by massage, hugging, holding, giving pats on the back, and spending as little as several minutes a week fine-tuning your touch on a variety of objects and materials. Assemble a collection of different types of cloth, leaves, containers, office items, figurines, yarn or string, and so forth. Close your eyes and select an item. Concentrate fully on its many unique features. Could you describe it in great detail to a friend who'd never seen or felt anything like it?

Massage — Professional Endorsements Growing

Nearly everyone has had a massage. It might have been performed by a professional therapist or under the hands of a caring relative or friend. It could have been a relaxing full-body routine; a specific professional technique for shoulder, neck, arm, or leg; or a simple back rub. In all probability you felt better and happier as a result. For some people, massage releases pent-up tensions and helps bring their lives into focus.

Massage is a traditional touch therapy for the body, emotions, and mind. In recent years, it has achieved long-overdue professional status as a beneficial health care option. Massage is no longer linked to red-light districts or thumping rubdowns in athletic locker rooms.

Massage therapy has entered mainstream health care programs throughout the world — and for good reasons.[13] It can be a fast, effective way to release muscle tension, increase circulation, relieve pain, and improve posture. Some neuroscientists suggest that massage may even help the brain as much as the body.[14]

Regular massage can also increase the elasticity of muscles and tendons, promoting flexibility and making athletes less susceptible to injury, says Dr. Willibald Nagler, chief of rehabilitative medicine at New York Hospital–Cornell Medical Center.[15]

"Americans are rediscovering the value of the ancient healing art of massage," writes *New York Times* health columnist Jane E. Brody. "Once considered a luxury item for the elite — [it] is fast becoming a necessity for people trying to cope with fast-paced lives."[16]

Top-level professionals aren't called masseurs and masseuses anymore — they're "massage therapists." Professional services include traditional full-body Swedish massage; specialized therapies (neuromuscular technique, acupressure, sports massage, shiatsu, myofascial therapies, and dozens of variations); and 10-to-15-minute "on-site massage," where clients are fully clothed and receive a massage while seated comfortably on padded therapy chairs. These "stress break" treatments are now being offered at corporate offices, industrial plants, schools, government buildings, neighborhood community centers, and shopping malls.[17]

It's a great idea to begin having some kind of massage at least once a week, more often if you are struggling with a heavy stress load. If a family member or close friend agrees to give you a massage, you can switch roles and return the favor.

While it's ideal to learn massage techniques from a qualified professional, you can create a good basic routine on your own. This is especially true if you work with a partner who is sensitive and willing to give you verbal feedback to improve your strokes. Massage can be a wonderful shared experience for family members and friends, even if it's simply a minute or two directed toward melting away tension in the hands, arms, back, neck, or shoulders.

Seated Massage

Whereas many couples prefer full-body traditional massage, seated massage is a fast, effective technique for business settings, travel, and family time. Seated massage can be performed using a specially designed massage chair or simply having the recipient sit backward straddling a straight-back armless chair. You want to establish a comfortable, supported position with no back sway, so you might need a pillow or two to place between the front of the recipient's torso and the chair.

Here is a simple method for performing a 10-to-15-minute seated massage. First, be certain your hands are warm and relaxed. Clear your mind of all unnecessary thoughts — there's nothing else you have to do right now but provide an effective massage, no place you have to go, no problems you have to solve. Be aware that your state of mind and emotions is communicated through your touch. Stand slightly less than one arm's length away from your partner's back.

Step into a balanced, martial-arts-like stance with one leg forward, knee bent, rear leg straight but not locked, torso erect, neck and head buoyantly suspended on top of your straight back. Arms and shoulders should be relaxed. Your pressure can be increased or decreased by shifting your stance forward or backward rather than tensing or de-tensing your arm muscles. The massage recipient's feedback about your pressure — too light, feels great, too hard — is essential. Pay attention. If you find any areas that the recipient says are particularly uncomfortable or painful, immediately ease off the pressure.

It's time to begin a short routine. Stand behind your partner and place your hands, palms down, on the shoulders, fingers over the top, thumbs on the back side. Always use light to moderate (never heavy) pressure. Loosen the muscles by slowly, smoothly kneading them. Keep in mind that your touch is inviting — rather than forcing — the muscles to release accumulated tension.

Continue up from the shoulders to the neck, working your way across the upper-back muscles. You will end up at the sides of the neck. Use your finger pads or thumb pads to gently massage the back of the neck right up to the base of the skull. If you find sensitive points, you may hold them with light pressure for 5–10 seconds and then release. This technique is a very simplified form of neuromuscular therapy or acupressure.

Next, begin working your way down the back, using your whole palm or thumb pads to apply light to moderate pressure. Once again, if you find sensitive points, hold for 5–10 seconds and release. Slowly move down between the shoulder blades on either side of the spinal vertebrae until you reach the lower back and feel the top of the pelvic bone. If you and the recipient feel comfortable with it, consider using thumb pressure to massage the upper and outer buttocks area. You might also massage the upper and outer thighs.

Return to the shoulder blade areas now and work your way down again, staying a little farther out to the sides from the spinal column this time. Finally, move to the back of the shoulders and the upper arms, massaging with gentle cupping strokes and thumb pad pressure. Step to either side of the chair and massage the forearms and hands. Then give a light, smooth-stroke massage (with fingertip pads, thumb pads, or palms) to the scalp, forehead, and outside jaw, especially the temporomandibular joint area — the hinge of the jaw — to release accumulated tension there. You might also have the recipient turn around in the chair so you can reach over from the back to release tightness in the upper chest (above the breast area) and shoulder fronts.

Full-Body Swedish Massage

Here's how to give a basic full-body Swedish massage. Select a warm, quiet room and a padded massage table, level sofa, or firm bed. Cover the massage surface with a clean sheet. Use a large towel to keep the recipient's body covered and warm in all areas not being directly massaged. Bring a bottle of natural oil (apricot kernel, avocado, and sweet almond are favorites; sometimes natural flower or plant essences are added). Soft, positive background music can enhance the relaxation.

Have the recipient lie face down on the therapy surface while you wash your hands. Become present-moment aware and assume a good balanced stance (legs bent, torso upright, arms and shoulders relaxed). Apply some warm oil to the skin of the recipient's upper-back area. Begin with the back or shoulders and use slow, flowing strokes with moderate pressure, always going toward the heart (this aids venous blood flow near the surface of the body). You should use enough oil so that you are not pulling on the skin or body hair, but not so much that you lose body contact because your hands are too slippery.

Move your arms and relaxed hands as extensions of your whole body, bending your knees and using your legs and torso to move your arms forward and back. Ease off the pressure as you go over joints. Don't bend any part of the body in a manner that's uncomfortable. Work your way down each arm and out to the fingertips.

Then, applying oil to each new area as you proceed, gently massage the back of the neck and work your way out onto the shoulders. Now, firmly, smoothly go down the whole back using the same technique as for the seated massage. Massage feels wonderful — it shouldn't hurt. Learn to be sensitive with your hands and to control the amount of pressure you give to each area of the body. Ease off at the first sign of pain.

Move on to the backs of the legs, ankles, and feet. Next, have the recipient roll over so you can massage the upper chest (above the breast area) and shoulder fronts and the front of both legs. You may wish to have the recipient roll over one final time so you can end with several more strokes down the back.

Massage tables and chairs.   If you begin to take regular advantage of at-home massage, you may reach a point where you are interested in purchasing your own therapy table or massage chair. One reliable source — with models for families and professionals — is Living Earth Crafts (600 East Todd Rd., Santa Rosa, CA 95407; 800-358-8292).

Professional Massage Therapies

The leading national organization for professional therapists is the American Massage Therapy Association (AMTA). AMTA members are graduates of nationally approved massage therapy programs (usually requiring a minimum 1,000-hour course of study) and adhere to stringent ethical and professional standards. For more information, contact AMTA National Department of Information (1130 W. North Shore Ave., Chicago, IL 60626; 312-761-AMTA). AMTA is also the best source for professional recommendations on massage books and videotapes for personal instruction.

One final note on massage and touch: Hugging our children is vital to their lifelong good health, and family "massage breaks" are a great way to strengthen relationships. Parent-child bonding happens to a great extent through touch, and regular massages can begin in infancy. Two good books on this subject are *Baby Massage: Parent-Child Bonding Through Touching* by Amelia D. Auckett (Newmarket Press, 1981) and *Infant Massage: A Handbook for Loving Parents* by Vimala Schneider (Bantam, 1982). To help break down the barriers to nonsexual, nurturing human touch for people of all ages, and for a light-hearted look at hugging, see *The Hug Therapy Book* (CompCare, 1983) and *Hug Therapy 2: The Wonderful Language of Hugs* (CompCare, 1987), both by Kathleen Keating, R.N., M.A.

37 Sensory Wellness: Vision, Light, and Hearing

Vision

Eyesight is our predominant gateway to the external world. It's a complex sensory system that is rarely developed to its fullest potential. Under repeated strain, vision deteriorates, creating the illusion that failing eyesight is "normal" at younger and younger ages.

So-called refractive errors of the eye — interferences with your ability to see clearly — are the principal reason that 120 million Americans wear glasses or contact lenses.[18] Today, more than 33 percent of all Americans are myopic, or nearsighted — up from only 14 percent in 1930.[19]

Stress from extended periods of close work at school may partly account for the fact that while only 3 percent of kindergarteners are nearsighted, more than 17 percent of teenagers are.[20] Dr. Tosten Wiesel, 1981 Nobel laureate, has shown that both environmental and genetic factors play a role in nearsightedness, concluding that the condition is primarily inherited, although "too much close work can disrupt eye growth."[21]

Eyes work best for distant seeing and must exert extra effort to focus on close work, which, without frequent breaks to rest and change eye focus to more distant objects, strains the eyes. "Some architects use the phrase 'designed for visual release,'" says Calvin W. Taylor of the University of Utah. "Physiologically, our eye muscles relax if we are looking at a far-distant view, and this effect can lead to a more generally relaxed state of the person. The physiological release or relaxation of the eye muscles often has a concomitant mental release, which can free the mind to think."[22]

One Connecticut public school study reported that nearsightedness was reduced by 50 percent when test anxiety was abated and teaching was conducted in a more multisensory environment — that is, in an area with bright colors and natural scenes.[23]

Lifetime exposure to sunlight is a major factor in blindness, reports Dr. Richard Young of UCLA's Jules Stein Eye Institute.[24] Ultraviolet (UV) light can damage the eye's transparent coating, the cornea, as well as the lens. Long-term exposure to the sun's violet and blue wavelengths also appears to damage the retina of the eye. Called age-related macular degeneration, this condition affects perhaps 30 percent of elderly Americans and is a major cause of blindness. Yet it's preventable if your eyes are protected when you are outside in bright light.

For seeing distant objects most clearly *and* protecting your eyes, many ophthalmologists recommend sunglasses that filter out all ultraviolet rays plus most or all of the blue and violet wavelengths. Most sunglasses don't do a good enough job and may even be hazardous. That's because faulty sunglasses reduce the amount of light entering the eye but do not filter out the ultraviolet rays, and therefore the pupils remain dilated, allowing the harmful unfiltered UV rays to reach the lens and retina.

Since excess light can damage the retina, it's important that lenses are tinted enough to block 75 to 90 percent of visible and infrared light. Some sunglass brands bear labels calling this blocking property the "transmission factor." If this isn't noted on the label, check with your optical expert or the manufacturer. You might also try the glasses on and look in the mirror — if the tint is dark enough you shouldn't be able to see your eyes.

Plastic-lens glasses that block UV rays may also provide important protection from lifelong damage contributing to cataracts.[25] Consult your eye care professional for current recommendations.

For information about specific brands — a list of the most protective sunglasses, complete with sources and prices — send a stamped, self-addressed envelope to Dr. Richard Young (Department of Anatomy, UCLA Medical School, Los Angeles, CA 90024-1763).

Here is a summary of some important guidelines:

1 Wear good-quality, good-fitting sunglasses when out in the sun.
2 Use bright lighting when reading.
3 Maintain good posture — with relaxed muscles in the shoulders, neck, and face — for best blood flow to the brain and eyes.

4 Hold reading material at an angle, not horizontal. Use a clipboard, lap desk, or secretary's adjustable bookholder device to make reading easiest.

5 Avoid glare — high-gloss paper increases the strain in focusing.

6 If you are nearsighted, don't wear your distance glasses for reading unless advised to do so by your ophthalmologist or optometrist.

7 Take frequent breaks (every 10–15 minutes) and look at distant objects to change your visual focus and relax the eyes.

Nerve cells in some of the cortical areas of the brain can be activated only by specific features of what the eyes see, according to Nobel laureates David Hubel and Torsten Wiesel.[26] This discovery points out the need to provide your eyes with a wide variety of stimulation and regular periods of relaxing rest. By expanding your light perception and various aspects of vision, you can stimulate and enhance brain function.[27] Here are some simple exercises you can perform several times a week:

Expanding Peripheral Vision

Prepare a collection of 8½-by-11 pieces of paper and 3-by-5 index cards with a single full-sized digit (0 to 9) or letter of the alphabet on each page or card. Use bright markers for visibility.

Shuffle the large papers and place them on a table just outside your field of vision when you sit in a comfortable chair. Once seated and relaxed, with your eyes looking straight ahead at a point about eye level on the opposite wall, reach over and bring the top page slowly into your peripheral field of view from the side. With practice on both the left and right sides, you should be able to identify the letters and numbers at an angle of about 70 to 78 degrees from straight ahead. Once this is comfortable, switch to the smaller cards. Over time, you may even be able to read a book or admire the details of small pictures using your peripheral vision. Blink your eyes often to reduce fatigue. Performing this exercise for one or two minutes several times a week can often produce significant improvements.

Light Perception Exercise

This exercise stimulates various areas of the brain involved with light perception.[28] Standing with a penlight in your right hand, extend the light overhead while keeping your eyes looking straight ahead. Look up at the light without moving your head — look with your eyes only. After several seconds, return your gaze straight ahead and lower the light below, and slightly forward of, your chin. Look at the light without shifting your head. After several seconds, return your gaze to the front. Now move the light about 6 inches out to the right of your right ear. With your head still, shift your gaze to the light for several seconds. Then move the light to a spot about 6 inches out to the left of your left ear and move your gaze, not your head, there for several seconds more.

Now expand the exercise: Follow the light beam with your eyes, head remaining still, as you move the light in a circle over your head, past your ear, below your chin, and returning above your head. Then track with your eyes as you extend the light out to full arm's length in front of your face and return it to a point about 6 inches in front of your nose. Finally, follow the light with your eyes as you move it from arm's length out to the side of one shoulder in an arc across in front of your face and around toward the opposite shoulder.

Repeat these exercises while holding the penlight in the other hand.

Shifting Focus Exercise

The eyes register the most information in the first several seconds of looking at an object or person. When your gaze remains fixed, your eyes become strained and good vision diminishes. In most situations, it's best to keep fluidly shifting your gaze to help your eyes stay relaxed *and* take in more information from the scenes around you. Perform a simple focus shifting exercise by looking at a person or object and moving your gaze every second or two, blinking your eyes often to lessen fatigue, smoothly guiding your vision from one feature to another.

Tracking Moving Objects

Many people steadily, needlessly, lose their perception of moving objects, called visual tracking. One exercise to prevent this loss is tracking moving objects — for example, watching a tennis match from the sidelines. Another technique is to hang a small ball or other object on a 4-to-6-foot string. Swing the ball, sit down close by, and for a minute or so follow the movement of the ball with your eyes, keeping the head and body still. Next, move your seat to a different position and repeat.

Taking In More Detail

You can train your eyes and brain to take in greater detail each time you look quickly and closely at a person, place, or object. This exercise takes less than a minute. Pick up a small object — a pen, pencil, key, watch, small book, or anything else you have nearby. Look at it from all angles, really concentrating on every detail. As you look describe its features — colors, textures, size, shape, usefulness, imprinting, and so on. After 10 to 20 seconds, put this object down and pick up another.

Second idea: Create a set of small flashcards with symbols, words, phrases, or numbers on them. Have a friend quickly flash one card at a time in front of you. Your task is to accurately identify what's on each card. With some practice, you'll be able to discern the inscription no matter how fast your helper's hand moves. Then have your friend move farther away and continue the exercise.

Visual Scanning Exercises

Scanning is another valuable sensory skill for driving a car, working with appliances and machinery, and other common tasks. Crossword and jigsaw puzzles are excellent for stimulating your scanning ability. Another fun exercise is to take a newspaper or magazine article and cross out all of any single letter of the alphabet you find on the page. For example, find and cross out the letter *A* wherever you find it. Time yourself so that you go as rapidly as possible.

Bringing More Beauty into Your Life

Years ago psychologist Abraham Maslow suggested that beauty promotes health.[29] A variety of scientific studies have now verified that when we view beautiful nature scenes — of water, sky, and plants — we reduce anxiety, feel more positive, and can relax more easily.[30] We are also less likely to have negative thoughts or experience stressful symptoms in the body.[31]

Schedule some time each week to take a walk in a beautiful neighborhood park or a community arboretum or to cultivate a small window box of flowers or back yard garden. At the very least, you can bring some beautiful flowering plants into your home and office. You might also set aside some time every once in a while to view nature scenes on videotape accompanied by relaxing music. Two good sources for tapes are Windham Hill Productions, Inc. (Box 9388, Stanford, CA 94309) and Emmett E. Miller, M.D. (Source, P.O. Box W, Stanford, CA 94309; 415-328-7171).

Light

Light affects mood, metabolism, health, and behavior. There is something very exhilarating about spending some time outside on a bright day. Many of us feel increased vitality and relaxation — a wonderful combination. Over the years, experts have attributed this feeling to psychological factors. Yet there is some evidence that our need for regular, very brief exposures to sunlight — avoiding the 10 A.M. to 2 P.M. peak time period when the sun's rays are most damaging — is also physiological.[32]

Cautious exposure to sunlight during nonpeak hours can be an excellent source of vitamin D for the body, says Dr. Michael F. Holick, director of the Vitamin D and Bone Metabolism Laboratory at the USDA Human Nutrition Research Center on Aging at Tufts University.[33] Scientists have also reported other benefits from brief exposures to sunlight (the best times to be outside are early morning, late afternoon, or early evening).[34]

There is also unequivocal evidence that without skin and eye protection, the sun's rays are damaging, causing burns, premature skin aging, and skin cancer. To learn more about sunlight research, send a stamped, self-addressed envelope for a free copy of the Skin Cancer Foundation's newsletter *Sun and Skin News* (Skin Cancer Foundation, P.O. Box 561, New York, NY 10156).

Preventing Skin
Cancer and
Premature Skin
Aging

Here is the negative side of the sunlight issue. An estimated 400,000 new cases of skin cancer develop every year in this country. Most are preventable, according to researchers from the National Cancer Institute, the American Cancer Society, and the Skin and Cancer Hospital in Philadelphia. The sun's damage is cumulative. In addition, sun exposure is the primary cause of premature aging and wrinkling of the skin.

"*Suntan* really means *skin damage*," says Dr. Nelson Lee Novick, assistant clinical professor of dermatology at Mount Sinai Medical Center in New York. "If you want 'just a little tan,' it means that you will have just a little damage."[35]

The Skin Cancer Foundation reports that one of every seven Americans will develop skin cancer.[36] Within the last sixty years the incidence of malignant melanoma, by far the deadliest form of skin cancer, has gone from 1 in 1,500 white Americans to 1 in 138. By the year 2000, it could be 1 in less than 100.[37] At least 95 percent of the risk is related to the sun. In a statistical study at Harvard University, Dr. Robert S. Stern and colleagues concluded that regular use of an effective sunscreen during the first eighteen years of life would reduce the risk of developing the most common skin cancers by nearly 80 percent.[38]

About fifteen years ago, scientists discovered that the ozone layer — the part of the atmosphere that shields the earth from the sun's rays — was losing some of its filtration effect, allowing too much harmful ultraviolet light to pass through. Manmade gaseous chemicals — chlorofluorocarbons — that rise up in huge quantities and destroy the ozone layer are being blamed. This is a very serious environmental issue.

The risk of skin damage from the sun is now considered so great that it is imperative to wear an effective sunscreen on all exposed skin surfaces *at all times* when outside during peak exposure period — 10 A.M. to 2 P.M. standard time (11 A.M. to 3 P.M. daylight saving time). And it's also wise to don a sunscreen if you're outside for more than 5 minutes or so at nonpeak times. And beware of overcast days — the sun's rays are almost as damaging as on bright days. In fact, as much as 85 percent of UV rays can penetrate clouds.

The advice applies equally to children, adults, people with fair skin, and those whose skin is naturally dark. Contrary to popular opinion, every tan comes with some risk of cancer. Tanning does give skin cells some protection from UV rays, but more cellular damage is caused by the rays than the tan eventually protects.

There's a double payoff to skin protection. Not only are you cutting your chances of developing skin cancer, but you also help preserve the skin's youthful elasticity and beauty. Excessive tanning makes blood vessels more prominent and turns the skin stiff, dry, yellow, and mottled and promotes wrinkling.

Sunscreens are rated according to an SPF (sun protection factor) scale, ranging from 2 to over 30; the higher the number, the greater the protection. Sunscreens with an SPF of 15 or above are most universally recommended by dermatologists. Some sunscreens must be reapplied every hour or two, since they lose their potency. They may also wash off in the water or be diluted by heavy perspiration. Follow product directions.

For a sunscreen to offer full skin protection, it must block the two predominant ultraviolet rays, UVA and UVB. Since no single sunscreen ingredient can shield against both types of UV rays, the best sunscreens combine several active ingredients. Para-aminobenzoic acid (PABA) and its esters (glycerol, padimate O, padimate A) are considered the most effective for screening UVB, but they don't block UVA. Benzophenones (methoxybenzone, oxybenzone, and sulfisobenzone) provide excellent protection against UVA but much less against UVB.

Children need special attention to prevent sun damage. The Skin Cancer Foundation recommends shielding infants from all exposure to the sun during peak daylight hours.[39] Use a carriage with a hood or a stroller with a canopy or umbrella attachment. Do your best to schedule your kids' outdoor activities in the early to midmorning and mid- to late afternoon to avoid intense sunshine. See that older children adopt the habit of covering their skin with long pants, a long-sleeved shirt, and hat, especially if they have fair skin, blond or red hair, and light-colored eyes. For more advice on how to teach children good sun protection habits, write for a free copy of *For Every Child Under the Sun* by enclosing a stamped, self-addressed business-size envelope to the Skin Cancer Foundation (P.O. Box 561, New York, NY 10156).

The dangers of ultraviolet radiation from the sun apply equally to tanning lamps, parlors, salons, and booths that have become popular in America in recent years.[40] Avoid them.

Indoor Light

In general, the brighter the room light, the better the performance. "There seem to be increases in activity and productivity right until you reach the level of glare," says Jean Wineman, professor of architecture at Georgia Institute of Technology in Atlanta.[41] There is "a great preference for natural lighting, far beyond the contribution made by that light." The presence of a window helps people feel and perform better.

"At last count there were 56 cities in this country investigating laws that would guarantee a person's right to [windows and] sunlight in places of residence," says Ralph Knowles, professor of architecture at UCLA. "A 'solar envelope' is important in maintaining both the comfort and joy that derive from seeing the rhythmic variability of nature."[42]

Very bright light in the morning and evening can provide dramatic relief for people who suffer severe winter-long depressions known as "seasonal affective disorders," reports Dr. Albert Lewy, director of the Sleep and Mood Disorders Laboratory at the University of Oregon

Health Sciences Center.[43] Light can be used to improve emotional state, mental outlook, and visual perceptions.

Here are some important recommendations:

1 Avoid indoor tanning salons.
2 Wear a sunscreen with a Skin Protection Factor (SPF) of 15 or greater during all sunlight exposure (and have your children do the same).
3 Wear dark-tinted, good-fitting sunglasses (which block all UV rays, most or all violet and blue light, and 75 to 90 percent of visible and infrared light) whenever you are outdoors during bright, sunny daylight hours, especially during the 10 A.M. to 2 P.M. time period.
4 Whenever possible, use natural window light for reading. When this isn't feasible, sit close to a bright indoor light source, generally within two feet.

Hearing

Loud noise is the most prevalent pollution in America. It not only damages our ears but alters moods, reduces learning abilities, and may increase blood pressure.[44]

Pleasant auditory stimulation such as music can calm or excite emotions, raise or lower heart rate and blood pressure, change breathing patterns, and affect our brain cells.[45] If played too loudly it can also destroy hearing.

The auditory system influences the frontal lobe of the brain, which plays a primary role in personality and intellectual functions. Loud noise (above 80 decibels — which includes the roar of traffic or factory machinery) and noise that may be soft but irritating can produce harmful physical and mental effects.[46] The sustained low-level din of urban life — moderately loud rush hour traffic, for example — can gradually destroy your hearing. This "hidden noise" has an insidious cumulative effect. One interesting discovery by researchers at the University of North Carolina School of Medicine is that high blood pressure and high-fat diets seem to make hearing loss even worse.[47]

The American Speech and Hearing Association estimates that 40 million Americans live, work, or play every day around noise that is dangerously loud. According to the EPA booklet *Noise Around Our Home* (Government Printing Office, 1980), nearly half of all Americans are regularly exposed to levels of noise that interfere with speaking, listening, or performing tasks.

High levels of noise from radios, televisions, stereo music systems, and other sources have been shown to disrupt the sensory and motor skills of children, especially during the first two years of life.

And noise cuts deeply into quality of sleep. Stanford University studies reveal that even when people don't think that noise has affected them while sleeping, their energy level and work efficiency the following day are markedly reduced. French researchers at the Bioclimatic Study Center report that even when people who slept in a noisy environment claimed they were no longer disturbed by the noise, their bodies failed to adjust to it.[48]

Noises from common household appliances — food processors, electric shavers, vent fans, garbage disposals, dishwashers, electric mixers, knife sharpeners, vacuum cleaners — produce heightened body arousal and general nervous tension, according to a University of Wisconsin study.[49] Home noise can reportedly contribute not only to noise-related health damage but to conflicts between household members.[50]

Half of all Americans over sixty-five and two-thirds of those over eighty suffer some form of hearing impairment. This hearing loss is not an inevitable part of aging, because in less industrialized, quieter societies, hearing "is as keen at 75 years as at 17 years."[51]

Here are several guidelines for reducing noise in your environment:

1 Become sound-conscious, reducing or eliminating noise whenever and wherever it is reasonable to do so.

2 Before buying new appliances and electronic equipment, compare noise levels and select a quiet model.

3 Avoid children's toys that make loud, sharp, or irritating sounds.

4 When looking for your next home or apartment do some detailed "sound" research before making your decision.

5 Remember that carpeting, rugs, and extra wall insulation help reduce noise levels.

6 Put foam pads under small kitchen appliances and office machines such as typewriters and computer printers.

7 Use noise-absorbing insulation and vibration mounts for dishwashers, garbage disposals, and other home appliances.

8 Wear hearing protection whenever it's necessary to be near loud or even moderately loud noises.

Exercises to Help Improve Your Hearing

Auditory sharpness can often be improved through training. Here are several simple exercises.

Extend Your Hearing Exercise

First, relax in a comfortable position. Sit quietly with your eyes closed, listening to the sounds all around you for several minutes. Extend your hearing radius outward from your body (where you can hear your breathing) to as far away as you can stretch it — perhaps to a car horn honking or a dog barking several blocks away.

Pierce Exercises

Alexandra Pierce, professor of music at the University of Redlands in California, has taught courses in listening for nearly two decades. She recommends the following:[52] "(1) Notice that you are surrounded by subtle sounds: breathing, coughing, doors closing, distant passing cars, birdsong, hum of fluorescent lights; (2) Put your attention on in and out breaths. As the body feels quieted, subtle hearing becomes second nature; (3) Limit other sensory modes. That is, close your eyes or avoid touching, to heighten your awareness of sound; (4) Listen to sounds in parts: *Bend* — the line a sound makes. Does it go up and down, as in the voice of a singer, or straight, like a motor. The *bend* itself has a bend; *Height* — tops and bottoms of bends; *Grain* — roughness and smoothness of sound. Grain of a rotating concrete mixer: rough. Grain of flute music: smooth; and *Volume* — loudness or softness."

Lower the Volume Exercise

For this exercise, locate a news program or talk show on television or radio and turn the volume down so that you can barely hear it. After about 15 seconds, turn it down even more. Make yourself work to hear the conversation for about half a minute. Repeat the procedure the next day with the volume a bit lower. This exercise sharpens both hearing and concentration.

Selective Awareness Exercise

This exercise helps you develop selective awareness, zeroing in on a certain sound while diminishing your attention to others. Put on your favorite music — ensembles first and then working up to songs which feature or include a full orchestra. Focus your attention for 30 seconds or so on the music line of only one instrument or voice rather than the total sound. Then switch to another performer. Then another. Once this becomes reasonably comfortable, you might try tracking two voices or instruments at the same time while blocking out the rest. Then switch to other voices or instruments. And so on.

Music

Researchers have discovered that the right kind of music, played under the right circumstances, can help increase attention span, improve physical coordination, reduce tensions, boost self-esteem, aid learning and memory, and provide some mental, emotional, and physical relief from disease.[53] Hospitals around the world are beginning to use therapeutic music to improve patients' emotional and mental outlooks and, where possible, speed recovery.

At the same time, there's no doubt that for some people music — no matter how uplifting — interferes with concentration and makes intellectual tasks more difficult. There is also some indication that listening to music for more than twenty minutes at a stretch can fatigue the senses and contribute to anxiety.[54]

Here are several guidelines on music and health:

1 When you need to concentrate on a difficult mental task, skip music. It may interfere.

2 Keep volume low — do not have music blasting through speakers or headphones.

3 Select music based on your emotional/mental needs. It can quickly change your mood. If you're tense and nervous, begin with fast-paced music and change gradually to serene, calming music. If you're depressed or lethargic, start with slow, mellow music and work into light, happy melodies.

4 In general, don't listen to the same music for more than twenty minutes at a stretch.

RESOURCES

▶ Better and Better, Inc. (P.O. Box 1948, Sedona, AZ 86336). A non-profit foundation sponsoring projects to improve health and well-being. Offers music audiotapes, albums, and CDs.

▶ *Bibliography of Noise Publications* (U.S. EPA, National Technical Information Service, Department of Commerce, 5285 Port Royal Road, Springfield, VA 22161).

▶ Institute for Consciousness and Music (P.O. Box 173, Port Townsend, WA 98368). Tapes, newsletter. Widely used therapeutic music for hospitals.

▶ National Association for Music Therapy (1133 15th St., N.W., Washington, DC 20005). Publishes a professional journal and makes referrals to music therapists and programs.

▶ SHHH (Self Help for Hard of Hearing People, Inc., 4848 Battery Lane, Suite 100, Bethesda, MD 20814). National self-help group. Free information.

▶ *Sound Health: The Music and Sounds That Make Us Whole* by Steven Halpern, Ph.D., and Louis Savary, Ph.D. (Harper and Row, 1985).

▶ Source Learning Systems (P.O. Box W, Stanford, CA 94309; 415-328-7171). Free catalog of audiotapes and videotapes.

Your Other Senses

"Because we are used to thinking in terms of the five primary senses," say neuroscientists Miriam and Otto Ehrenberg, "we tend to remain unaware that our sensory potential is much greater. Our total number of senses is still unknown, but current estimates are that they come closer to twenty than five [and are known to include your senses of verticality and balance, receptors for heat, cold, pressure, position, stimulation change, blood sugar, mouth dryness, and so on]. . . . Your perceptions will remain limited if you take for granted that what you see tells you the whole story. . . . It can lead you astray. Many so-called extrasensory perceptions are really sensory experiences that most of us have programmed ourselves not to have because they do not fit in with our preconceptions. Once you stop predefining what the world is like, you will be able to perceive more of it."[55]

38 Other Rejuvenation Priorities

Dental Wellness

Dental disease is preventable, yet it remains a common condition in America. Nearly 95 percent of all United States citizens suffer from tooth decay (dental caries) or gum disease.[56] Many of us take our dental health for granted, assuming that simply brushing and flossing our teeth the way we've done it for decades is the whole dental hygiene picture. It isn't.

More than half of all Americans past the age of sixty-five are toothless. Beyond the age of thirty-five, pyorrhea (gum disease or periodontal disease) causes the loss of most teeth — and much of that loss is unnecessary. Tooth decay and pyorrhea are both bacterial plaque disorders.

Plaque is the name given to the colorless, sticky film composed of colonies of bacteria that attach to the teeth. Even the healthiest mouth contains some three hundred different identified species of bacteria. Plaque that grows above the gum line is aerobic, needing oxygen to survive. Below the gum line, the bacteria are anaerobic; that is, they don't require oxygen to thrive.

Plaque is formed in several stages. The first occurs when a film, derived primarily from saliva, develops on the tooth surface. The bacteria go to work on sugars and soluble food residues in the mouth. One of the by-products of this bacterial activity is a substance called glucan, a thick gel-like substance that sticks to the tooth surface, accelerating the overall buildup of plaque. Glucan can be broken down rapidly by bacteria to form acids. Plaque holds these acids against the tooth surface.

This plaque must be removed every day by brushing and flossing. Studies indicate that regular, dosage-controlled fluoride use helps build a more decay-resistant tooth surface.

In the early stages, periodontal disease is called gingivitis and affects only the gums. It should be prevented before reaching this point but can usually be reversed if caught in the early stages. Like tooth decay, periodontal disease starts with plaque — this time along the gum line. The plaque often becomes mineralized by calcium salts from saliva, forming hard deposits of calculus, or tartar. Over time, these deposits change in color from light yellow to brown.

The calculus irritates the gums every time you chew, swallow, or brush your teeth. Impacted food residue can add to the abrasion effect, causing inflammation and bleeding. This blood is a good source of nutrients for the bacteria, which thrive and contribute to further gum destruction. Over time, the gum separates from the teeth, forming a gingival crevice, which then gradually deepens. Continued formation of plaque and calculus drive the bacterial infection down into the gingival crevice, causing more serious problems, including bone loss, pain, and finally loss of teeth themselves.

Stress and Cavities

Negative stress apparently makes saliva more hospitable to harmful bacteria. In nine studies, a dental research team at Temple University found that as stress increases, overall saliva production diminishes.[57] Saliva is one of the body's natural defenses against decay and periodontal disease. When you're under sustained stress, your saliva has higher levels of bacteria and is more acidic, which is bad for tooth enamel and gums. The saliva is also lower in phosphorus and calcium, two key minerals that rebuild tooth enamel.

Another stress response, jaw clenching, can lead to headaches and other pain syndromes. Grinding of the teeth (bruxism) can loosen teeth, leading to the creation of gum pockets and causing infections.

Selecting Your Toothbrush

A properly used manual toothbrush is the basic tool in controlling plaque. The brush you choose depends to a large extent on the brushing technique you use. Your dentist will help you select the proper size and shape of brush that fits your mouth and is easy to use. The bristles should be soft and have rounded ends. Overzealous toothbrushing with stiff bristles can damage tooth enamel and gums. The brush should be small enough to reach every tooth surface in your mouth. Nylon filaments are better than natural boar bristles, which can more easily trap bacteria in their hollow cores.

Never share toothbrushes with another person, and plan to replace your toothbrush every six weeks or so. A worn-out toothbrush cannot clean your teeth effectively. Researchers at the University of Oklahoma School of Dentistry report that twenty patients plagued with periodontal and other mouth and throat infections improved when they changed toothbrushes every two weeks.[58]

Dr. Richard T. Glass, chairman of the oral pathology department at the University of Oklahoma Colleges of Dentistry and Medicine, suspects that colds, mouth sores, and some rarer infectious conditions keep returning because pathogenic microorganisms flourish on the bristles of your aging toothbrush. On the average, Dr. Glass and his colleagues found that it takes one to four weeks for heavy germ buildup on the bristles.

The researchers offer these suggestions: Rinse your brush thoroughly after each use; replace it routinely at least once a month; replace it when a respiratory infection seems to be starting; replace it again when you begin to feel better; and replace it every two weeks or so on a regular basis if you have gingival or periodontal disease.

Techniques for Brushing and Flossing

The American Dental Association recommends this brushing method: (1) Place the head of the brush beside the teeth, with the bristle tips at a 45-degree angle to the gums. (2) Move the brush with a gentle, vibrating circular motion, brushing the outer, inner, and chewing surfaces of *all* the teeth along with a small area of the gums. (3) Tilt the brush vertically to clean the inside surfaces of the front teeth, making several up and down strokes with the tip of the brush. (4) Brush your tongue to remove bacteria and freshen breath. Some periodontists also recommend gently brushing the inside of your cheeks.

To floss, break off about 18 inches of lightly waxed or unwaxed floss and wind the ends around your middle fingers. Guide it between the teeth with your thumb and forefingers. Gently take the floss down to the gum line until you feel the first resistance, keeping the pressure against the sides of the teeth, not the gums. Scrape all sides of the tooth, moving away from the gum line. Note: Don't snap the floss. Vigorous flossing cuts into gum tissue and creates tiny fissures called "flossing clefts" that may not heal, according to dental researchers at the University of Iowa.[59] Another concern, says Dr. Benny Hawkins, director of the Iowa study, is that bacteria may enter the bloodstream through the small open cuts caused by overzealous flossing.

The American Academy of Periodontology (AAP) offers a booklet on brushing and flossing called "Effective Oral Hygiene," available from AAP (Room 924, 211 East Chicago Ave., Chicago, IL 60611).

Effective brushing helps prevent periodontal disease as well as tooth decay. Studies show that "over a long period of time with the proper technique of toothbrushing plus flossing, people can keep gingivitis practically nonexistent," says Dr. Richard C. Wunderlich, assistant professor at the University of Michigan School of Dentistry. "In [a recent] study, we instructed our test subjects to use a soft brush, direct the bristles at an angle to the edge of the gums, and move the brush in a circular motion."[60]

To periodically check the effectiveness of your brushing and flossing techniques, you can use a "disclosing tablet," a dye tablet that temporarily stains plaque so you can see areas you've missed and adjust your technique accordingly.

As noted in Chapter 22, worldwide studies show that fluoride can be a safe and effective part of dental hygiene if dosages are carefully monitored. The use of fluoride as a tooth decay preventive is endorsed by leading health organizations.

Mouthwash: Don't Use It

Americans spend more than $400 million a year on mouthwash. Because of its alcohol content and the way it's used, researchers suggest that chronic mouthwash use may contribute to the development of malignant oral cancers.[61] It has been known for many years that chronic use of alcohol and tobacco increases the risk of developing cancer of the mouth,[62] but in the past decade new research has linked mouthwash to cancer of the mouth and throat in both nonsmoking and smoking persons.[63]

The problem with mouthwash appears to be the alcohol content, which ranges from 15 to 29 percent (30 to 58 proof) in the leading five mouthwashes in America.[64] While not usually swallowed, mouthwashes are held in the mouth for a longer period of time than alcoholic beverages. This may be the primary problem.

Further studies are necessary and are under way, but there appears to be a cause-and-effect relationship. Solution? Use good basic dental hygiene and skip the mouthwash, unless recommended by your dentist.

Sexual Wellness

Perhaps no other aspect of life commands more attention or is as confusing and laden with myths as our sexuality. We are created as living beings and therefore as sexual beings. Our sexuality is designed to draw on and nurture the full sphere of our sensory existence. Yet in modern society, it has become far too easy to trivialize and depersonalize sex to the level of anatomical organ relationships.

Full sexual wellness depends to a great extent on overall health and fitness. And, in turn, our sexual well-being — or lack of it — affects all dimensions of our lives. An increasing number of authorities suggest that an intimate sexual relationship with a loved one can be as fulfilling at age seventy-five and beyond as at twenty-five.

Separating Stress and Sex: Relaxing for Romance

Lack of time and energy is a major reason for a fall-off in sexual relations, according to a landmark study entitled "American Couples" by sociologists Philip Blumstein and Pepper Schwartz.

"Severe stress not only overloads the mind, it may also shortcircuit sex physically by upsetting the delicate neural choreography of the parasympathetic and sympathetic nervous systems," says psychologist Carol Wade, author of the textbook *Human Sexuality* (Harcourt Brace Jovanovich). "Timing is everything. During the early stages of sexual arousal, the parasympathetic system predominates. It relaxes artery walls in the pelvic area, so they dilate and blood flows in faster than it flows out. In men, increased blood volume produces an erection; in women, vaginal lubrication and swelling of the vulva, clitoris and vaginal walls. This genital engorgement also contributes to the subjective feelings of arousal. . . . Then, as excitement mounts, the sympathetic system takes over."[65]

"Strong emotions," adds Wade, "including those linked to physical or psychological stress, can upset the critical balance, switching on the sympathetic system prematurely." During stressful situations, the human body is designed by nature to put reproductive functions on hold.

It is important to schedule time for yourself to relax and disengage from the day's stress load. If you arrive home from work and immediately dive into domestic chores, you go from one type of stress to another, says psychologist Bernie Zilbergeld of Oakland, California. He suggests a transition period — a regular daily time for couples to release work tensions and simply be together — to chat, stroll, hug, hold hands, perhaps sip a single glass of wine. "A few minutes of peace and quiet can be worth four hours of foreplay," adds Zilbergeld.[66]

Single people set aside time for dates. It's advisable for married couples to do the same, blocking out special times to be together. Of course, there is no need for this to preclude the pleasures of spontaneity. When you are especially busy and stressed, be careful not to let yourself feel that sexual overtures from a loved one are an intrusion that wastes your precious time. Warm, intimate moments can save you time overall by boosting your sense of vitality and well-being so that you perform your job even more effectively during work hours.

Many sexual difficulties arise from four basic causes: lack of communication (both the failure to communicate and the lack of a shared vocabulary about sex), feelings of vulnerability, lack of practice, and "cultural scripting," the myths about how men and women are supposed to feel and act sexually.

"Part of the problem," says sex therapist Lonnie Barbach, "is that sex is intensely personal. We all feel so vulnerable about it."[67]

"Some people can have a satisfying love life without talking about it, but that's very rare, especially in long-term relationships," adds Linda Perlin Alperstein, assistant clinical professor in the department of psychiatry at the University of California San Francisco Medical Center. "The ability to make love is not innate. Most of us have to experiment and learn throughout our lives. But there's a myth that sex is 'natural,' that if people are *really* in love, they shouldn't have to negotiate."[68]

"The idea that a lover should understand intuitively what pleases us is particularly destructive," says Michael Castleman, editor of *Medical Self-Care* magazine and author of *Sexual Solutions*. "It sets up a classic 'damned if you do damned if you don't' situation. If you ask what kinds of caress your lover enjoys, that proves you don't already 'know'; therefore you've failed. But if you don't discuss your lovemaking, you can't possibly know all the fine points of what your partner enjoys; therefore you won't be able to give the pleasure you otherwise might, and again, you've failed."[69]

When you begin a discussion with your loved one on sex, says Alperstein, who teaches workshops called "Speaking Up While Lying Down: Assertive Communication in Sexually Intimate Relationships," acknowledge your fears: "This is difficult for me to say because I really love you and don't want to threaten our relationship, but . . . "[70]

Be as specific as possible: Don't say, "I want more affection." Say: "I want you to hold me and kiss me when I come home from work. I want to cuddle on the sofa when we watch TV together. And I want to be held for a little while each night before we go to sleep without that being interpreted as a sexual invitation."

"It's often helpful," adds Castleman, "to divide your desires into three categories: Needs, wants, and wishes. . . . [This] helps your partner understand your priorities. . . . Your *needs* are your absolute bottomline items. If you don't get your needs met, the relationship cannot work for you. Your *wants* are things you genuinely desire, but wants have less dire 'what if' consequences. If you don't get all your wants, you may feel frustrated, and the relationship may suffer somewhat, but it would still work for you. Finally, your *wishes* are your fantasies. Your wishes would add spice and zing to your love life, but you could live without them relatively easily."

In *Sexual Solutions,* Castleman presents an effective communication technique called the Wish List Game. Over a week or two, you and your lover write down absolutely everything you wish the other would do for you sexually, from more cuddling, hugs, and kisses, to affectionate notes, to taking more responsibility for birth control, to specific intimate caresses. Next, rank your wishes in order from "easiest to ask for" to "the most difficult." Then, once or twice a month, you each reveal the "easiest" items on your lists and eventually work your way down to the more difficult requests. One ground rule: When making a request, you each agree to listen carefully and honor the requests as much as possible; at the same time, the listener always has the right to say no if he or she is uncomfortable with a request.

"The Wish List Game stimulates intimate discussions in several ways," says Castleman. "When a sexual relationship has problems, there's a tendency to lapse into hopelessness, which precludes good communication. Yet, most people's wish lists contain no more than half a dozen items. This can be very reassuring. Suddenly you realize that in your wildest dreams only five or six items stand between you and the best sexual relationship you can imagine. Things start looking up.

"For most people, the sexual wishes that are 'easy' to request are also easy to grant. Typically, they have to do with expressions of affection out of bed: hugs, kisses, and light caresses around the house. The combination of asking for affection and getting it can have surprisingly positive impact on the relationship as a whole. Even in relationships that seem near the breaking point, trust and intimacy begin to deepen. You see that you *can* make positive changes in your relationship. You develop increased confidence in your ability — and your lover's ability — to confront your problems and deal with them successfully.

"The Wish List Game also helps couples *practice* negotiation. By the time you've worked your way down to your more difficult requests, you have several months of experience with intimate conversation. Some wishes may be difficult to request or impossible to grant, but couples who follow through on The Wish List Game gain valuable insights into their lovers and relationships even when they don't get all their wishes. They feel less stuck. This exercise helps transform intimate negotiation from an all-or-nothing heavy talk into an ongoing process. And when things seem tough, simply consult your lists to see how many requests your lover has granted [and] how far you've come."

If men learned to make love the way most women say they prefer, many men's and women's sex problems would disappear. This may sound hard to believe, but it is precisely what many sex therapists are saying.

"When women are asked to critique the men in their love lives," reports Castleman, "their chief complaints are that men make love too quickly, too mechanically, and with too much attention focused on the genitals. Women say men are often so preoccupied . . . with the mechanics of intercourse that they often ignore what most women say really [excites] them — leisurely, playful, whole-body sensuality. Every square inch of the body is capable of sensual arousal through gentle, massage-style caresses. The body is a sensual wonderland. Most women say they like to explore all of it, and have difficulty understanding why so many men concentrate on a few small corners."[71]

"When men are asked to critique women's lovemaking, their chief complaints are that women are too passive and unresponsive. An important reason for many women's lack of enthusiasm is men's rushed lovemaking. Women tend to become aroused more slowly than men. . . . The male lovestyle is largely the result of playground and locker room sex miseducation . . . and the style of the men's magazines. . . .

"To facilitate whole-body sensuality, try not to separate your love-making into 'foreplay' and 'the main event.' There is no such thing as 'foreplay.' There is only 'loveplay.' . . . Extended sensual loveplay means more variety, more playfulness, and more time for both lovers to become fully aroused. . . . A touchy subject like sex feels less threatening when lovers are sensually in touch."[72]

For people who feel especially uncomfortable talking about sex, Linda Perlin Alperstein and other sex therapists recommend a touch exercise called "The Body Tour."[73] Wearing as little or as much as you like, you guide your partner's hands with your own on a special tour of every square inch of your body, showing him or her exactly how you like to be touched. Then you switch and your lover guides you. "Touch," says Alperstein, "can be difficult to discuss with words. What does it mean if I tell you I like 'light' or 'medium' touch? That can mean different things to different people. It's much easier to demonstrate. You let your fingers do the talking. Of course, you can talk while conducting a Body Tour, but simple 'oohs' and 'ahhs' can be just as communicative as words. . . . If you feel ill at ease naming certain parts of the body, the Body Tour allows you to show your partner how you like to be touched there without saying anything."

RESOURCES

In a field filled with myths and contradictory advice, the following resources are noteworthy:

▶ *For Each Other: Sharing Sexual Intimacies* by Lonnie Barbach, Ph.D. (New American Library, 1982). A sensitive book designed to help couples deepen intimacy and trust.

▶ *How to Make Love All the Time* by Barbara De Angelis, Ph.D. (Rawson Associates, 1987). Strategies for overcoming sexual boredom and making loving relationships work.

▶ *The Intimate Male: Candid Discussions About Women, Sex, and Relationships* by Linda Levine, M.S.W., and Lonnie Barbach, Ph.D. (Doubleday, 1983). A collection of candid interviews with 120 men about their sexual preferences. Valuable for encouraging couples to share their sexual feelings with each other.

▶ *Sexual Solutions: An Informative Guide* by Michael Castleman (Touchstone/Simon and Schuster; available from Self-Care Associates, 55 Sutter St., No. 645, San Francisco, CA 94104; revised edition forthcoming). A top-rated self-help book written for men and for the women who want to understand them and better communicate about sex. Solid advice in a wide range of sexual areas.

▶ *Shared Intimacies: Women's Sexual Experiences* by Lonnie Barbach, Ph.D., and Linda Levine, M.S.W. (Bantam, 1983). A compilation of candid interviews with 120 women about their sexual likes and dislikes. A good stimulus to open, clear communication.

▶ *Super Marital Sex: Loving for Life* by Paul Pearsall, Ph.D. (Doubleday, 1987). A practical book containing self-tests, marriage tests, sex assignments, and questionnaires — all designed to encourage discussion and better understanding between partners — by the director of education at the Kinsey Institute for Research in Sex, Gender, and Reproduction.

Professional Sex Therapy Advice

Couples seeking sex therapy should be very cautious in selecting a professional because of the large number of poorly trained individuals calling themselves therapists. For help in finding a qualified sexual therapist near you, write to the American Association of Sex Educators, Counselors, and Therapists (Suite 304, 5010 Wisconsin Ave., N.W., Washington, DC 20016).

AIDS

Acquired immune deficiency syndrome (AIDS) is pandemic in America at the time of this writing. The number of people being infected each year continues to grow at an alarming rate. New facts are needed for safe sexual relationships. The United States Surgeon General believes we must educate even very young children so that they know the behaviors to avoid to protect themselves from exposure to the AIDS virus. By all means, order a copy of *The Surgeon General's Report on AIDS* and related government publications (single copies are free from AIDS, P.O. Box 14252, Washington, DC 20044).

39 Living Environments Design: Introduction

SCIENCE IS UNCOVERING hazards in our environment far more quickly than most of us are learning to cope with them. Pollution threatens the stability — and future — of our natural world. The earth's forests are shrinking, deserts expanding, and soils eroding, all at record rates. Thousands of plant and animal species are disappearing every year. The ozone layer is thinning, and the temperature of the earth is rising.

Overall, it's a most perplexing issue. Do we each need to subscribe to dozens of scientific journals, stop traveling in air-polluting vehicles, and organize protests every time we hear about a new toxic chemical? Or is it time to forget all the warnings, ignore the nagging knot in our stomachs, and just enjoy life while we still can?

It turns out that there *are* things the ordinary person can do. We are not powerless. Solutions to some environmental dangers — such as smoking, overexposure to the sun's harmful rays, and exposure to vapors from unnecessary toxic chemicals in our homes and businesses — are within the control of each of us as individuals. Other problems — such as industrial pollution of the air and water and disposal of nuclear wastes — need to be addressed with strong political measures.

Living environments, the places where we spend our time — to live, learn, work, travel, and vacation — support our well-being or erode it. By taking advantage of current scientific insights, we can pinpoint serious environmental problems and transform our surroundings into more nurturing, health-enhancing spaces. And we don't have to sacrifice our hard-earned comforts. We can still lead good, fulfilling lives without destroying the planet in the process.

Much of the outrage about environmental abuses of the 1960s and 1970s has given way to lukewarm disdain or shoulder-shrugging acceptance. It's one thing to think that we can ultimately survive only if we save the earth first — there is little philosophical disagreement about that — but it's quite another thing to picture yourself doing much of the saving from day to day. In essence, millions of us have been beaten down to cleaning our own corners. And the numbing pace of life in the information age encourages complacency.

But if you look closely at new environmental research, a lot of it coming from European science centers, you will see that there is much we can each do to unpollute our daily lives. At the same time, these simple measures cast a small but significant vote for a sustainable future. This subject of ecological wellness deserves far more space than can be devoted here. But living environments are another inner thread of the golden circle of *Health & Fitness Excellence,* and the next few chapters highlight recent discoveries and new options.

Human Health and the Living Earth

When looking at environmental problems, we can easily forget that our global population is increasing at a monumental rate — and this population increase compounds the challenges we face. "We are taking over larger and larger areas of the Earth," write Dr. Mike Samuels and Hal Zina Bennett in *Well Body, Well Earth,* "covering the surface with new highways, buildings, and factories, clearing billions of acres of what was once wilderness area and cultivating crops needed to feed our growing masses.

"As this growth continues, our global responsibility also grows, and to ensure the quality of life our planet has provided us, scrupulous care must be taken to maintain the Earth's homeostatic mechanisms, those mysterious processes that regulate the Earth's health. . . . It is all too easy to hear only the tolling of the death knell. If we respond to the challenge by merely defending old ways of life, we are, indeed, doomed. But if in the challenge we find the inspiration to create a new and healthier way of life, we can look forward to a better future."[74]

We each have a birthright debt to the planet that has made us possible. And, even more than that, we each have a responsibility to the billions of people yet unborn, each of whom has the right to live in a world at least as beautiful as ours. We cannot blindly assume that human intelligence and technological advancements will enable us to undo ever-deepening environmental damage in the decades and centuries ahead.

Nature's intricate, ancient balance is so complex that it remains far beyond our ability to comprehend, let alone restore if we keep destroying it.

We *can,* however, apply our considerable collective intelligence to bringing humanity into the new century in a prosperous, sustainable way, treading as lightly and respectfully as we can upon the earth. This is both more complicated *and* more achievable than we thought even a few short years ago. Political rhetoric certainly isn't enough. And scare tactics seem to backfire, making millions of people close their ears and minds to the issues. And the answer isn't a few more industrial pollution controls or another fashion wave of Save the Trees T-shirts.

To solve pollution problems, we first need to make some tough-minded, day-to-day personal choices — in what we learn, in what we buy, in how we voice our concerns, and in who we vote into and out of political office. In earlier chapters, we discussed pure water and organic food production. The next few chapters address other areas of importance. Learn all you can, make decisions, schedule specific actions, and support worthwhile organizations (see "Resources" in the next chapter). Once again, be careful not to become fanatical. We cannot solve problems by polluting our own minds with anxious thoughts — about the environment or anything else.

40 Outdoor Pollution Control and Radiation Protection

Outdoor Pollution Control

Outdoor contamination has occurred for centuries. In the past twenty-five years, however, human beings have added toxic pollutants to the environment at a staggering rate.

Airborne pollutants present a serious threat to environmental stability and human health — toxins from accidents, acid rain, and daily emissions of chemicals from motor vehicles and industrial and home sources. The magnitude of the problem makes this a key area about which to stay informed — and that means scheduling some reading time. There are many possible corporate, community, regional, national, and international solutions. Among hundreds of published works on the subject, these are at the top of my list:

▶ *Blueprint for a Green Planet: Your Practical Guide to Restoring the World's Environment* by John Seymour and Herbert Giradet (Prentice Hall, 1987). A book filled with concrete prescriptions for individual and community action to halt and reverse environmental damage. Excellent.

▶ *Well Body, Well Earth: The Sierra Club Environmental Health Sourcebook* by Mike Samuels, M.D., and Hal Zina Bennett (Sierra Club Books, 1983). This well-documented sourcebook presents a detailed, practical program for coping with environmental hazards.

▶ *Gaia: An Atlas of Planet Management,* edited by Norman Myers (Anchor/Doubleday, 1984). This is far from an ordinary atlas; it organizes available environmental data, statistical predictions, and a maze of opinions and solutions into a coherent plan. Each of seven sections — Land, Ocean, Elements, Evolution, Humankind, Civilization, and Management — is considered from three perspectives: potential resources, crises, and management alternatives. Full-color illustrations capture the essence of each topic and make sense of critical issues.

▶ *The Health Detective's Handbook: A Guide to the Investigation of Environmental Health Hazards by Nonprofessionals* edited by Marvin S. Legator, Barbara L. Harper, and Michael J. Scott (Johns Hopkins University Press, 1985). In clear, concise language, this book explains how citizens and community leaders can do their own detective work to find out if potentially toxic chemicals in their midst — in contaminated drinking water, from nearby factories, hazardous waste sites, and workplace exposures — are harming the health and productivity of community members. Shows how to get the attention of appropriate health officials to launch fast corrective action.

▶ *State of the World* by Lester R. Brown (Worldwatch Institute, 1776 Massachusetts Ave., N.W., Washington, DC 20036). Annual report on progress toward a sustainable society. Important reading.

New International Awareness

The world's leading scientific institutions have recently launched a global effort to learn more about what changes in the habitability of the earth are likely in the coming decades.[75] Called the International Geosphere-Biosphere Program: A Study of Global Change, the group is headquartered in Stockholm, Sweden. The sponsoring organization is the International Council of Scientific Unions, with membership that includes scientific academies in more than seventy countries and organizations in all fields of physical and biological science.

The project prospectus states: "Our uses of energy and practices of intensive farming and technology have altered the reflectivity of the earth, the composition of soil and waters, the chemistry of the air, the areas of forests, the diversity of plant and animal species and the balance of the global ecosystem.

"Immediate problems such as acid rain, the increase in deserts, soil degradation and the buildup of atmospheric gases that threaten the climate, all involve interactive processes that transcend the bounds of single disciplines." The plan calls for establishment of observation sites on earth, at sea, and in space. Chemical, physical, and biological measurements will be used to identify long-term changes as early as possible. This is vitally needed.

The U.S. National Aeronautics and Space Administration (NASA) has created an Earth Sciences Committee, with plans to sponsor a Global Geosciences Initiative. Pointing out that every change in a specific environmental area "can propogate through the entire earth system," the committee is launching a new integrated discipline called earth system science.

These national and international efforts deserve our support. Worsening large-scale outdoor pollution problems can be reversed only with a unified effort. Two key federal agencies handle environmental pollution questions: the Centers for Disease Control's Center for Environmental Health in Atlanta (404-488-4380) and the Public Information Center, U.S. Environmental Protection Agency (Washington, DC 20460).

Here is a list of some leading societies and organizations concerned with protecting and improving the environment. All welcome support and participation from new members.

▶ American Farmland Trust (1717 Massachusetts Ave., N.W., Washington, DC 20036).
▶ Citizen's Clearinghouse for Hazardous Wastes (P.O. Box 926, Arlington, VA 22216).
▶ The Cornucopia Project (33 E. Minor St., Emmaus, PA 18049).
▶ The Cousteau Society (930 W. 21st, Norfolk, VA 23517).
▶ Defenders of Wildlife (1244 19th St., N.W., Washington, DC 20036).
▶ Environmental Action Foundation (1525 New Hampshire Ave., N.W., Washington, DC 20036).
▶ Environmental Defense Fund (444 Park Ave. So., New York, NY 10016).
▶ Farm Animal Reform Movement (P.O. Box 70213, Washington, DC 20088).
▶ Greenpeace U.S.A. (2007 R St., N.W., Washington, DC 20009).
▶ Institute for Local Self-Reliance (1717 18th St., N.W., Washington, DC 20009).
▶ National Audubon Society (950 Third Ave., New York, NY 10022).
▶ Natural Resources Defense Council (122 E. 42nd St., New York, NY 10168).
▶ The Nature Conservancy (1800 N. Kent St., Suite 800, Arlington, VA 22209).
▶ Oceanic Society (Stamford Marine Center, Magee Ave., Stamford, CT 06902).
▶ Sierra Club (730 Polk St., San Francisco, CA 94109).
▶ Worldwatch Institute (1776 Massachusetts Ave., N.W., Washington, DC 20036).
▶ World Wildlife Fund — U.S. (1600 Connecticut Ave., N.W., Washington, DC 20009).

Radiation Protection

Radiation is a central pollution issue. It affects every citizen on earth, and exposure is increasing. Radiation — vibrating electromagnetic energy traveling invisibly at high speeds — is divided into two basic types:

High-frequency, ionizing (atomic) radiation, including x-rays, gamma rays, alpha and beta particles, and neutrons

Low-frequency, non-ionizing radiation, including visible light, electric power-line emissions, televisions, computer video display terminals (VDTs), ultrasound, microwaves, radio waves, radar, and even electric blankets

Ionizing Radiation

Ionizing radiation causes cancer and genetic mutation. This high-energy radiation displaces electrons from the molecules in the body, converting them into electrically charged ions. Ionized molecules can biologically mutate cellular structures, including genetic chromosomes, a process that leads to cancer.

"Radiation absorbed dose," or rad, is a measure of energy absorbed per pound of body weight. Rems equal rads multiplied by the mutagenic potential (the ability to biologically damage cellular genetic material) of each specific kind of radiation.

The effects of ionizing radiation are cumulative — they keep adding up throughout a person's lifetime. Government standards for maximum levels of annual exposure have been repeatedly lowered as experts have learned more about the harmful effects of even small levels of radiation.

Ionizing radiation comes from four primary sources:

1 Natural sources radiation, also known as background radiation, comes from elements in the earth (see radon discussion in the next chapter) that have existed since the beginning of history.

2 Medical sources radiation, such as that from x-rays, radiation treatment, and radioactive pharmaceuticals.

3 Consumer products radiation comes from a wide range of artificial products such as television sets, luminous dials on clocks, watches, and other instruments, smoke detectors, ceramics, and cement and other building products made from earth.

4 Nuclear weaponry and fuel radiation comes from nuclear industries and from mining, milling, fuel fabrication, transportation of fuels and wastes, reactor operation, fuel reprocessing, waste disposal, and fallout from nuclear testing, accidents, and weapons.

What You Can Do

Determine, and minimize, your exposure to radon gas (see Chapter 41).

Eliminate unnecessary x-rays. One of the fastest ways you can reduce unnecessary ionizing radiation is to limit your exposure to x-rays and other radioactive materials used by the medical, dental, and chiropractic professions. Here are several recommendations:[76]

Avoid so-called precautionary x-rays, that is, x-rays prescribed for routine medical, dental, or chiropractic checkups. Women of child-bearing age should avoid x-ray examinations except during the ten days following each monthly menstrual period, thereby helping to minimize the risk of irradiation during ovulation and the potential fertilization period. Except for medical emergencies, women should avoid x-ray examinations during pregnancy.

Young children are especially susceptible to radiation damage and should not be x-rayed unless you are convinced there is solid medical evidence that the potential benefits outweigh the risks. Whenever a physician, dentist, or chiropractor recommends high-radiation x-rays for you or a member of your family, insist on learning the comparative risk of x-rays versus the risk of possible health problems if you avoid the x-rays.

Do not submit to x-rays ordered by a doctor for protection against malpractice suits. Be frank. Insist on x-rays for good medical reasons only. Remember that you have the legal right to have x-rays taken by one physician transferred to another physician, thereby avoiding unnecessary duplicate x-rays.

During those times when you *must* get x-rays, be certain the radiologist or dentist uses a lead shield to protect your lower abdomen and all other vital areas. Refuse treatment from chiropractors who recommend full-body x-rays. Whenever possible, select a health professional who uses the newest, most up-to-date equipment and fast films with low exposure levels, automatic photo exposure controls, image intensifiers, pulsed fluoroscopy, and precise monitoring of the radioactive output of every x-ray machine.

Avoid unnecessary radioactive consumer products. Many consumer products contain radioactive materials. Choose alternatives that don't radiate. Remember, radiation damage is cumulative. The more places you can avoid it, the better. Radioactive consumer products not only irradiate the factory workers who make them and the people who buy and use them, but they also pose an increasing risk to future generations since the radioactive elements are extremely long-lived and are accumulating at millions of disposal sites around the country. As long as radiated consumer products are produced, dump site contamination and associated risks will continue to grow.

Radioactive consumer products include the following:

"Luminous," glow-in-the-dark dials on wristwatches and clocks, automobile instrument panels, and switchplates.

Smoke detectors with radioactive cells (choose models with photoelectric cells instead).

Eyeglasses, with lenses made of glass, have reportedly been found to emit radiation since highly refined glass contains thorium and uranium in the glass itself — as much as 30 percent by weight.[77] Select plastic eyeglass lenses instead. Some dental porcelains used in fillings and false teeth also emit radiation.

Natural gas, used as a cooking or heating fuel, emits radioactive radon gas. To minimize radiation exposure, ventilate areas well and provide a reliable source of continuing fresh air.

Minimize risks from the nuclear industries. Nuclear industries include nuclear power plants and nuclear weapons manufacturing facilities. Many people must decide whether to live and work in, near, or downwind from these industrial areas. Political measures are the only certain way to minimize nuclear risks and better ensure global peace.

Non-Ionizing Radiation: Microwave

A growing number of authorities say that there are health dangers from exposure to another type of radiation: non-ionizing. This invisible form of energy is emitted by computer video display terminals (VDTs), microwave communication equipment, microwave ovens, television and radio transmitters, radar, electric wiring and power lines, electric blankets, and other devices. While much of the data have not yet been quantified, prudent people are taking notice of new scientific reports on non-ionizing radiation, of which there are two basic types: microwave and electromagnetic. (Electromagnetic radiation is discussed in the next section.)

Microwaves are close to the low end of the radiation energy spectrum. Although they exist in nature, the predominant sources are human-produced artificial devices. Microwaves are absorbed by the body and start molecules vibrating, in contrast to ionizing radiation, which knocks particles off atoms. While microwaves may not sound like much to be concerned about, scientists have discovered that the vibrational stresses they produce can cause significant, unhealthy alterations to cell structures and functions.[78] Mitosis (cell reproduction or regeneration) and cell membrane permeability can reportedly be disrupted.

Researchers at New York University School of Medicine discovered an increase in cataracts among people working in industries where microwaves were used.[79] That prompted the United States to cut acceptable exposure levels in half. Now preliminary research at Johns Hopkins's Wilmer Eye Institute suggests that microwaves can cause another kind of visual damage at low levels — they kill key cells that line the cornea of the eye, blurring vision.[80] (Note: The danger zone for this visual damage is at higher doses than the current emission levels of household microwave ovens and cellular telephones, however.) Dr. Alan Frey, a biophysicist, recently discovered that humans actually "hear" microwaves, not through the ears but through vibration of brain centers.[81] Microwaves can reportedly change the permeability of the blood-brain barrier, a special filter designed to prevent harmful chemicals from entering the brain from the bloodstream.[82] The implications of this discovery are as yet unknown.

There is also some serious concern about microwaves — in particular, video display terminals (VDTs) — causing or contributing to miscarriages or birth defects.[83] But a recent University of Michigan study of four thousand pregnant women concluded that those who work at a VDT less than 20 hours per week do not increase their risk of miscarriage.[84]

There is still no consensus of opinion on how much microwave radiation humans can withstand without health damage.

What You Can Do   Learn more about microwave exposure levels where you live and work. Seek independent scientific opinions, since those offered by industry may be misleading or deliberately inaccurate. Community problems, such as radiation dangers from large radar facilities near work sites or residential areas, should be approached on a political action basis.

If you choose to cook with a microwave oven, use a recent model since emission levels are much lower with current design improvements. Be very aware of safety procedures. Representatives from the FDA's Center for Devices and Radiological Health recommend that people never operate an oven with a warped door or damaged seals or when an object is trapped in the door.[85] Be scrupulous about keeping the seals clean. Never stand in front of the oven while it is on. If you have any reason to suspect radiation leakage from your oven, do not test it with an inexpensive home testing device. Contact your local appliance service center along with state consumer protection officials or health department representatives.

If your job requires frequent VDT time at work, or if you use a home computer regularly, the following practices are recommended:

1 Test your computer and other devices for radiation emission levels. A sensitive home test kit is available from Radiation Safety Corporation (140 University Ave., Palo Alto, CA 94301).
2 If you are pregnant, limit VDT work to less than 20 hours a week or consider requesting assignment to a non-VDT job.
3 Take 15-minute rest breaks at least once every 2 hours, and whenever possible restrict VDT use to 50 percent or less of the working day.
4 Have an eye examination before starting to use a VDT and have annual exams thereafter.

5 Reduce VDT screen glare by keeping general room lighting soft, illuminate source material with a small separate lamp, and use window blinds when necessary.

6 Remain up to date on the results and recommendations of new scientific studies in this area (see Resource list of recommended periodicals at the end of this book).

Non-Ionizing Radiation: Electromagnetic Fields

Electromagnetic radiation, the lowest-wave energy in the radiation spectrum (called ELF for extremely low frequency), is produced by high-tension, high-voltage electric power lines; electric railways, subways, and buses; electric wires and telephone lines in businesses and homes (wires shielded in metal conduit have significantly reduced electromagnetic emissions); and household items such as electric blankets.

Electromagnetic radiation doesn't produce the kind of severe damage associated with ionizing radiation, in which electrons can be knocked out of their orbit in living tissue, or the reported damage linked to microwaves, in which vibrations disrupt molecules. But new evidence suggests that artificially generated electromagnetic radiation may cause more subtle damage by interfering with delicate electromagnetic force fields that are involved with cellular communication in the body.[86] Activities that are crucial in cell membrane structure and neural (nerve) development also appear to be affected.[87] Studies have shown that electromagnetic radiation can change the permeability of cell membranes and alter the flow of calcium into tissues perhaps because electromagnetic fields influence the alignment of molecules forming cell membrane structure.[88]

While exposure to electromagnetic fields — such as those from electric power lines — may not cause cells to become cancerous, there is evidence that it stimulates human colon cancer cells to grow faster, proliferate, and survive longer, according to research at San Antonio's Cancer Therapy and Research Center and the University of Texas Health Science Center.[89] Animal studies show that living in an artificial electromagnetic field may reduce immune system white-cell activity and lower resistance to disease.[90] Disproportionately high mortality from leukemia has been reported among workers whose occupations exposed them to strong magnetic fields.[91]

Researchers have also reported changes in body rhythms (which may interfere with normal sleep patterns),[92] changes in pain reactions, and slowing of learning responses in both humans and animals when they were exposed to electromagnetic fields.[93]

Epidemiological studies have reported an association between residential exposure to magnetic fields — from home electrical wiring configurations or electrical wires near the home — and the incidence of cancer in children[94] and adults.[95] A recent follow-up study confirmed a positive association between electromagnetic field exposure and increased cancer risk.[96]

A recent major research project by the State of New York Department of Health on the biological effects of electromagnetic fields offered this conclusion: "The variety of effects of magnetic fields have not been previously appreciated. Several areas of potential concern for public health have been identified, but more research must be done before final conclusions can be drawn. Of particular concern is the demonstration of a possible association of residential magnetic fields with incidence of certain childhood cancers. Further study of this possible association and mechanisms to explain it is important. The variety of behavioral and nervous system effects may not constitute a major hazard because most appear to be reversible, but they may impact temporarily on human function. Further research should also be done in this area."[97]

What You Can Do   If you work in or around concentrated electromagnetic fields, you may want to explore methods for shielding the sources of radiation or limiting the duration of your exposure. Don't rely on industry-generated studies, which all too often present a slanted viewpoint about safety. Become aware of the results of new and ongoing health studies in this field (see Resource list of recommended periodicals at the end of this book).

41 Indoor Pollution Control

WE CAN EACH TAKE steps to create home and work spaces that are more healthful, comfortable, quiet, and inviting. We can throw out the clutter, get rid of toxic chemicals, brighten the color scheme, increase fresh air ventilation, turn down noise, and surround ourselves with pictures and other decorations that remind us of the best, happiest aspects of life. Part of this living environments plan involves dealing with indoor pollutants, the focus of this chapter.

Surprisingly, many of the worst air pollutants aren't outside — they're in our homes and automobiles. That's the finding of a five-year research project by the Environmental Protection Agency (EPA).[98] The seven-city project found toxic pollutant levels as much as five times greater inside homes as outdoors, even for people living near chemical plants. In fact, in some homes the level of pollutants was *100 times higher* than that outdoors.[99] A growing number of studies in Europe and America have compared indoor and outdoor pollution and have reached similar conclusions to those of the EPA.[100]

The National Academy of Sciences recently estimated that indoor air pollution may add nearly $100 billion to national health care costs every year.[101] The worst offenders include tobacco smoke, household cleaning products, poorly maintained gas heaters and other carbon monoxide sources, asbestos, insecticides, radon gas, paints, mothballs, solid air fresheners, dry-cleaned clothes, and even hot chlorinated water in showers, dishwashers, and washing machines. And, in most cases, the "tighter," more energy-efficient the dwelling, hotel, school, or office building, the greater the pollution problem.

Determining the exact extent of health damage from indoor contaminants will require many years of further study. But the levels of indoor air pollutants recently measured already "suggest significant risks" to health, warns Paul J. Lioy of Rutgers University Medical School.[102] It appears that people who expose themselves even to low-level repeated contact with common household and office chemicals may gradually develop subtle brain and nerve impairments.

Major Indoor Pollutants

Some of the major indoor pollutants include the following:

Asbestos

This carcinogen is found in fibers used for many years to fireproof and insulate furnace ducts, oven linings, floor and ceiling tiles, siding, and shingles. The cancer-causing danger results from inhaling the microscopic asbestos fibers. Some asbestos products — but not all — are now banned by the federal government. The National Consumer Product Safety Commission (CPSC) and Environmental Protection Agency have published a guide for identifying and handling asbestos, a job only for professionals. For a copy of "Asbestos in the Home," a booklet published by the EPA and CPSC, write Superintendent of Documents (U.S. Government Printing Office, Washington, DC 20402; hotline for information: 800-835-6700).

Carbon Monoxide

Improperly adjusted, poorly sealed, or inadequately vented heaters using carbon-containing fuels — natural gas, oil, propane, kerosene, and so on — can produce clouds of invisible carbon monoxide (CO) gas that quickly reach health hazard levels.[103] Stoves and heaters that burn charcoal and wood can also give off CO. According to estimates by the National Center for Health Statistics, 2 percent of Americans — nearly 5 million people — are regularly exposed to indoor CO levels that exceed the EPA's standard.[104]

Smokers and people in the immediate vicinity of smokers are at even greater risk, since burning tobacco can produce blood CO levels equal to or higher than EPA levels, where harm to the nervous system can set in. The American Lung Association offers a booklet called "Air Pollution in Your Home." Carbon monoxide detectors — some as small as a key chain — are now available in pharmacies. They use small ceramic disks that change color when exposed to 50 parts per million or more, the highest CO concentration allowed by law.[105] Although the new units are

valuable because they can warn of dangerously high levels of CO exposure, they do not detect chronic low-level concentrations, which may be
a long-term health risk.

Chlordane

Chlordane — a carcinogenic insecticide that persists for at least twenty
years once it's sprayed in homes, schools, and offices for termite protection — has been used in more than 30 million American homes.[106] The
EPA is currently studying this poison to determine the exact extent of
contamination and to determine what, if anything, can be done about it.
A ban on future use has been proposed.

**Chloroform from
Chlorinated Water**

Many toxic organic compounds are easily absorbed through the skin. In
some cases skin absorption of pollutants may be an even greater exposure
risk than consumption of contaminated water, according to a report in
the *American Journal of Public Health*.[107] For example, an adult taking a
15-minute shower or bath may be exposed to twice the level of contaminants he or she would have consumed through drinking 2 quarts of tap
water. And the risks are even higher for children. These projections may
be conservative and do not take into account a wide range of factors
known to increase skin absorption — wetness of the skin, higher water
temperatures (like whirlpools, hot showers and baths, heated swimming
pools, and hot tubs), breaks in the skin (cuts, abrasions, rashes, sunburn),
or the use of soap.[108]

Since most Americans use chlorinated water, the problem is of special concern. A recent Environmental Protection Agency report identified
chloroform as a major indoor pollutant. It is emitted from, among other
sources, hot running shower and bath water. This carcinogen is a by-
product of chlorinated water. The hotter the showers you take and the
longer you stay in them, the more pollutants you will breathe — including toxic chloroform gas.[109] To minimize risks, take brief showers or a
short bath — the body absorbs only about half the toxic chemicals in a
bath compared with a shower of the same time length.

One water filter designed to remove chlorine from hot running
water is called the Niagra Shower Filter (Niagra Enterprises, 5699 Ka-
nan, Agoura, CA 91301). This granular carbon device fits right on the
shower head.

Formaldehyde

This preservative chemical, used in embalming fluids, is found in small
amounts in hundreds of consumer products in America, ranging from
cosmetics, perfumes, and soaps to permanent-pressed fabrics, upholster-
ies, resin-treated drapes, carpets, dry-cleaning fluids, and paper towels.[110]
Building materials such as laminated wood paneling, plywood, particle
board, and urethane foam insulation give off — "out-gas" — formaldehyde.

Formaldehyde is a strong irritant to the respiratory, sensory, and nervous systems and may cause brain damage. Surprisingly, studies by the National Space Technology Laboratory reveal that certain house-plants — notably spider plants (*Chlorophtum comosum*) — may significantly reduce formaldehyde levels inside closed spaces.[111] Consumers desiring more information on formaldehyde should call the Consumer Product Safety Commission toll-free (800-638-2772). For a copy of "Formaldehyde: Everything You Wanted to Know But Were Afraid to Ask," send a stamped, self-addressed envelope to Consumer Federation of America (1424 16th St., N.W., Washington, DC 20036).

Household Cleaners and Disinfectants

Cresol and phenol are two of the corrosive poisonous chemicals found in many products used for disinfecting, sanitizing, and deodorizing homes, farms, schools, and businesses. These chemicals can harm the body by penetrating the skin and entering the lungs, where they damage nerve tissues.[112] Cleaning supplies are among the most hazardous products in many homes and because of this are labeled DANGER, POISON, WARNING, or CAUTION and regulated by the Consumer Product Safety Commission under the federal Hazardous Substances Act. But the government focuses only on immediate dangers, not on long-term health effects from limited contact with the skin or lungs. And loopholes in labeling laws make it nearly impossible for consumers to know exactly what is in most commercial cleaning products.

"The easiest way to begin your transformation to a nontoxic home," suggests Debra Lynn Dadd in *The Nontoxic Home,* "is by replacing cleaning products — ammonia, oven cleaners, furniture polish, scouring powder, disinfectant, glass cleaner — all the heavy-duty chemicals we use to maintain our homes. The replacement products are simple and inexpensive — in fact, most cleaning jobs can be done quite well using natural materials you probably already have in your kitchen. These substances are odorless or have natural fragrances and work *every bit as well* as the chemicals you are accustomed to cleaning with."[113]

"Nontoxic cleaning requires very few special ingredients," adds Dadd. "I do *all* my cleaning with a squirt bottle of 50/50 vinegar and water, liquid soap, and a can of nonchlorine scouring powder, available at most supermarkets and hardware stores. It couldn't be simpler." To learn a complete series of least-toxic chemical options — for drain cleaners, all-purpose cleaners, oven cleaners, furniture and floor polish, mold and mildew cleaners, germ-fighting disinfectants, rug and carpet shampoos, and air fresheners, see *The Nontoxic Home* (J. P. Tarcher, 1986).

Organic Solvents

Federal scientists in Oak Ridge, Tennessee, recently conducted a survey and found between 20 and 150 solvents and other volatile organic compounds in every house.[114] They are used in cleaners, adhesives, finishes, paints, art supplies, spot removers, furniture-stripping solutions, and some cosmetic and hair care products. Organic solvents are known to depress brain function and create other debilitating behavioral changes.[115] Further studies are badly needed to determine exact danger levels and toxic effects from combinations of various chemicals.

In the meantime, if it's absolutely necessary to use these chemicals, do so with protective gloves and mask in a well-ventilated space, preferably outdoors. Inside areas must be ventilated from the ground up with an exhaust fan since solvent fumes are heavier than air and accumulate near floor level. Sources of alternative products that reportedly produce no toxic fumes when applied or dry are LIVOS Plant Chemistry (614 Agua Fria St., Santa Fe, NM 87501) and AMF Enterprises, Inc. (1140 Stacy Ct., Riverside, CA 92507).

Radon

Over half of a typical American's exposure to ionizing radiation may come from radon. By current estimates, this naturally occurring radioactive gas causes up to 10 percent of all lung cancer deaths and a total of 20,000 to 30,000 cancer deaths each year, according to the Environmental Protection Agency.[116] The colorless, odorless gas is emitted from natural underground uranium deposits in soil and bedrock into at least 10 percent of all American homes — more than 1 million — at a rate considered too high for safety, according to the National Council on Radiation Protection and Measurements, a nonprofit scientific group in Bethesda, Maryland. Measurements in some homes have reportedly been as high as 300 times the allowable limit in uranium mines.[117] Radon is not just a problem in mining towns or isolated areas of the country. It's everywhere. Above-limit levels have been measured in public and private drinking water supplies in New England and several other areas of the country. In addition, the EPA estimates that about one-fourth of all U.S. homes have water that is radon-contaminated.[118] The EPA hotline for information is 800-334-8571, ext. 713.

EPA booklets are available at public libraries and local health offices. They include "A Citizen's Guide to Radon" (OPA-86-004), which describes what radon is and how to test for it, and "Radon Reduction Methods: A Homeowner's Guide" (OPA-86-005), which explains how to decrease radon pollution if it exists. Also refer to *Radon: A Homeowner's Guide to Detection and Control* by Bernard L. Cohen (Consumer Reports Books, 540 Barnum Ave., Bridgeport, CT 06608; 1987). Radon gas concentrations can be reduced by fans and heat exchangers, although some dwellings require more elaborate measures, such as installation of a perforated pipe system beneath the building to vent radon away.

Note: Special Concern for Children

"Children are particularly vulnerable to the health effects of household toxics," writes Debra Lynn Dadd in *The Nontoxic Home*. "For example, simply because of children's size and physiology, they are exposed to more indoor pollutants than adults standing nearby in the same room! Children inhale more air per body weight than adults, their respiratory rates are faster than those of adults, and, since pollutants are generally heavier than air, they are at greater concentrations at the height of a child's nose than they are at the height of an adult's nose."[119]

Do You Work in a "Sick" Building?

Many of us feel sick for awhile when the buildings where we live and work are remodeled. "Sick buildings" are a growing concern across America and Europe. "Occupants of a building, usually [a] large [building], but sometimes modest in size, may complain of a set of symptoms which have collectively been named the 'sick-building syndrome,'" says Jan A. J. Stolwijk of the department of epidemiology and public health at Yale University School of Medicine.[120] At other times it has been referred to as the "tight" or "stuffy" building syndrome.[121]

By some estimates, up to half of the work force in Europe and North America may be affected by sick-building syndrome. As energy-conscious construction sets the theme for new buildings worldwide, there has been a corresponding increase in indoor pollution. Poor ventilation systems that lock in stale air; poorly maintained air filters, humidifiers, and cooling towers that spread airborne infections; and hundreds of new manmade materials that "out-gas" toxic fumes are all part of the problem.

Other concerns include poor lighting, seating, noise control, chemicals, and video display terminals — all addressed in previous or subsequent chapters. What can you do right now? First, adopt a *Health & Fitness Excellence* work style: Take frequent short breaks that get you outside in fresher air, eat regular small meals and light snacks, take a basic broad-spectrum vitamin-mineral supplement (see Chapter 28), drink plenty of extra water between meals, and begin action steps to correct specific pollution problems. For job-related safety information, contact your local or regional office of the Occupational Safety and Health Act (OSHA), or the OSHA National Office (U.S. Department of Labor, 200 Constitution Ave., N.W., Washington, DC 20210).

For answers to home, business, and institutional pollution questions, contact the CPSC (800-638-2772) or your state health department or regional office of the EPA. Basic resource books include *The Nontoxic Home* by Debra Lynn Dadd (J. P. Tarcher, 1986); *Office Work Can Be Hazardous to Your Health* by Jeanne Stellman, Ph.D., and Mary Sue Henifin, M.P.H. (Pantheon, 1983); and *Indoor Air Quality and Human Health* by Isaac Turiel (Stanford University Press, Stanford, CA 94305; 1985).

Dangers Related to Smoking

Smoking is health-destructive, not just for smokers themselves but for everyone who comes in close proximity to them while they are smoking. "The right of a smoker to smoke stops at the point where his or her smoking increases the disease risk in those occupying the same environment," says the United States Surgeon General.[122] In addition, most of us pay higher taxes and wrestle with exorbitant insurance premiums resulting in part from accidents, diseases, and early deaths attributable to the smoking habits of some policyholders.

From a health perspective, data on the harms of cigarette smoke continue to mount. The National Research Council and National Academy of Sciences have published research reports documenting many of the ways that "passive smoking" (also called "slipstream smoking," "environmental tobacco smoke," and "involuntary smoking") is linked to health risks, particularly among the children and spouses of smokers. For a free copy of the Surgeon General's report, "The Health Consequences of Involuntary Smoking," write to Office of Smoking and Health (Room 1010, 5600 Fishers Lane, Rockville, MD 20857).

According to the American Cancer Society:[123]

Workers who smoke have an absentee rate 30 to 40 percent higher and a 5 percent greater chance of hospitalization than their nonsmoking colleagues.

Thousands of nonsmokers die each year from lung cancer caused by secondhand or passive smoke.

The cost to the economy each year from smoking is estimated at $38–$95 billion by the U.S. Congress Office of Technology Assessment.

Each smoker costs his or her employer more than $4,000 a year, according to figures compiled by William L. Weis, assistant professor at the Albers Graduate School of Business, Seattle, Washington. In addition, a recent study of nearly 4,000 Massachusetts drivers indicated that smokers had 50 percent more car accidents and got 46 percent more traffic tickets than nonsmokers.[124]

For health-concerned smokers who wish to quit, the best nonjudgmental guide to date is *The Smoker's Book of Health: The No-Nag, No-Guilt, Do-It-Your-Own-Way Guide to Quitting* by Tom Ferguson, M.D. (Ballantine, 1989). Updated monographs, audiotapes, and related products are available from Self-Care Productions (3805 Stevenson Ave., Austin, TX 78703; 512-453-0484).

For action-oriented information on nonsmokers' rights and the movement toward smoke-free workplaces, see *The Smoke-Free Workplace* (Prometheus Books, 700 E. Amherst St., Buffalo, NY 14125), which lists addresses of about seventy-five nonsmokers' rights groups in the United States and Canada; *Smoke in the Workplace: An Action Manual for Non-Smokers* (Non-Smokers' Rights Association, Suite 308, 344 Bloor St., W., Toronto, Ontario, Canada, M5S 1W9); Action on Smoking and Health (2013 H Street, N.W., Washington, DC 20006); Americans for Non-Smokers' Rights (P.O. Box 668, Berkeley, CA 94701); and Health at Work (Group Health Cooperative, 1625 Terry Ave., Seattle, WA 98101).

42 Personal Safety and Medical Resources

IT'S EASY TO TAKE the subjects of this chapter for granted. But we can't afford to abdicate our personal responsibility for family safety and ready access to medical resources and emergency care — integral factors in health and psychological well-being.

Personal Safety

Personal safety goes far beyond government law enforcement, the judiciary, national defense policy, and the United Nations. It also transcends insurance policies, which provide us with monetary compensation in case of fire, accidental injury, vandalism, or death.

Science has confirmed what common sense told us for centuries: we each need a sense of *inner* security, of control, in our lives.[125]

Anticipating emergencies and minimizing safety risks doesn't mean that you're a pessimist; it means you are living a smart, alert life, prepared for the worst and planning for the best. The subject of personal and family safety and security goes far beyond the space available here. However, one particular issue merits special attention.

Driving Safety: The Easiest Way to Live Longer

Don't get caught in a typical shortsighted situation in which you exercise regularly and do your best to eat a good diet but fail to buckle your seatbelt. By one estimate, 75 percent of Americans still don't buckle their seatbelts when traveling in a motor vehicle.[126] That's missing the boat — it's far more likely that you'll die in an auto accident than from pesticide poisoning. Driving safety is a preventive health habit that none of us can afford to overlook.

Safety Belts and Harnesses

The National Highway Safety Administration estimates that 17,000 lives could be saved every year if all of us buckled our seatbelts.[127] What's the risk without them? Death, certainly. One prevailing myth is that seatbelts aren't really necessary at speeds of 30 miles per hour and less. Fact: In a head-on collision at 30 miles an hour, an unbelted driver or passenger is hurled into the dashboard and windshield with a force equal to diving head first into a concrete sidewalk from three stories up in the air. The body has exactly one-hundredth of a second to stop! Fact: Automobile fatalities have occurred in parking lots at speeds as low as 12 miles an hour when seatbelts weren't worn.[128]

A landmark research project at the University of Colorado Medical School studied 256 crashes in which one front-seat occupant was wearing a safety belt while a companion in the other front seat was not. The results indicated that the unbelted occupant was *five times* more likely to die and three times more likely to be injured as the person wearing the safety belt. These results are especially noteworthy since they compared matched pairs in which the accident severity, car size, crash speed, and road conditions were identical for both occupants.[129]

Two recent reports in the *Journal of Trauma* issued these warnings:[130] To cut the risks of internal injury in case of an accident, sit up straight in the car seat and wear the seatbelt low across the pelvis, not the abdomen.

Another concern is the slack in shoulder harnesses in American-made cars.[131] Most U.S. car makers use safety straps that relock at a new length whenever pulled, the way a window shade does. This design isn't allowed in Europe because it's considered dangerous. Excess harness slack can be very unsafe: "Safety experts agree that anything more than an inch or two of additional slack can have profound consequences for safety," says Robert Dewey of the Center for Auto Safety. More than that inch or two of slack can allow the head to hit the steering wheel or dashboard in the event of a sudden stop or crash.

Don't tuck the shoulder strap under your arm or across your neck when you drive. Even though this common habit keeps the strap from irritating the breastbone, neck, or chest or rubbing against jewelry, it's dangerous. A recent study found that it dramatically increases your chances of major injury or death in case of an accident, causing you to be thrown against the windshield or dashboard or ejected from the car.[132] It's essential for short people to have the shoulder portion of the three-point safety strap lowered to prevent choking. Your car dealer can easily provide this service.

Finally, wear safety belts in the rear seat. New automobiles are being equipped with lap-shoulder straps for back seat passengers, but wearing a properly adjusted lap-only belt is still better than wearing none at all.[133]

Another factor enters the picture: money. The National Highway Safety Adminstration estimates that America pays $40 billion a year in motor vehicle crash costs, much of it incurred because of a lack of safety belt use.[134]

Headrest Adjustments

Be certain that your headrest is properly adjusted each time you sit down in a car. A recent report in the British medical journal *Lancet* indicated that if your car doesn't have headrests or if they aren't adjusted properly to fit your height, you are risking potentially fatal injury similar to that which occurs to victims of a hanging. This study reported that about 75 percent of patients admitted to the hospital with "hangman injury" — resulting from sudden-impact accidents in which the head is whipped backward and there's no head support from a high seat back or properly adjusted headrest — were involved in auto accidents while wearing safety belts but had no headrests.[135]

Child Restraints

Automobile accidents are the leading cause of death and serious injury for children over six months of age.[136] Use a high-quality children's safety restraint that meets or exceeds all National Safety Council standards *every time your child is in a motor vehicle*. Follow the recommendations of your family physician or pediatrician for the safest designs that match the size and age of your child. Children who have outgrown infant or toddler safety seats — usually after age four — pose a special challenge. Lap-shoulder straps tend to cross their necks or faces. The answer, says the National Safety Council, is to put children from 40 to 65 pounds (four to nine years old) in a restraining seat called a booster chair. Different designs work for lap-only belts and lap-shoulder straps. For details, send for the free booklet "Child Safety Seats for Your Automobile" (U.S. Government Printing Office, Washington, DC 20402).

Emotional Stability on the Road

It's not enough to simply adjust your headrest, wear your safety harness properly, and obey the speed limit. Emotional stability is a crucial part of safe driving. In a recent survey, one of every five drivers killed in auto crashes had experienced some major emotional upset within a 6-hour period preceding the fatal accident.[137] Get in the habit of checking your driving fitness before you turn the key, and if you are upset and *must* drive, use an instant calming sequence (see Chapter 7) to regain a measure of balance and then drive defensively.

The person who uses his or her car as an instrument of aggression is probably aggressive in other areas of life, reports a recent University of Illinois study.[138] Research shows there really *is* such a thing as an accident-prone personality, according to Dr. Ming T. Tsuang, professor of psychiatry at the Harvard Medical School.[139] These hot-tempered traffic hazards have certain defects: a hair-trigger temper, emotional immaturity, and difficulty accepting authority. In many cases, these individuals are unaware that their personality puts other people in jeopardy.

Nighttime Driving Safety

Do you realize the increased risks you face during nighttime driving, even in good weather and road conditions? Human night vision is far inferior to daylight vision. In fact, by some estimates, you can see only one-seventh as well at night.

Before starting off on a nighttime drive, first be certain your headlights, turn signals, and windshield are clean. Next, never exceed the speed limit. And go slower whenever conditions warrant. To maximize safety, don't flash your bright lights at an oncoming car with its bright lights on. If the driver is elderly, driving a strange car, on drugs, or drunk, you may inadvertently cause an accident.

To learn more, send for "How to Drive After Dark," a brochure available from the National Safety Council (444 N. Michigan Ave., Chicago, IL 60611).

Medical Resources

Preventing illness and disease is one goal of *Health & Fitness Excellence*. But nearly all of us have occasional accidents, injuries, and symptoms that require medical attention.

The American College of Emergency Physicians lists seven warning signs of potential medical emergencies:

1 Pain or pressure in your upper chest or abdomen
2 Vomiting, when it is severe or continuous
3 Fainting
4 Dizziness, a sudden feeling of weakness, or a severe change in vision
5 Shortness of breath or trouble breathing
6 Severe pain anywhere in your body
7 Homicidal or suicidal feelings

Health-conscious people can learn to be intelligent medical consumers — to make good, basic decisions about when to seek medical advice or care and how best to handle emergency situations for themselves and their families. Excellent resources include the following:

▶ *The People's Book of Medical Tests* by David S. Sobel, M.D., and Tom Ferguson, M.D. (Summit, 1985). "A complete guide to more than 200 diagnostic and home medical tests that answers questions about each test: Do I need it? What will it cost? How should I prepare? How long does it take? How is it given? Does it hurt? What is the risk? What will it tell me?"

▶ *Take Care of Yourself: A Consumer's Guide to Medical Care* by Donald M. Vickery, M.D., and James F. Fries, M.D., revised edition (Addison-Wesley, 1985). Dr. Fries, professor at the Stanford University School of Medicine, and Dr. Vickery, founder of the Center for Corporate Health Promotion in Reston, Virginia, emphasize prompt decision making for more than seventy common emergency situations. Using unique algorithms (mathematical equation charts), readers can answer short questions to quickly decide whether to seek immediate emergency help, make an appointment for routine medical care, or treat themselves at home. Filled with practical tips for each problem and corresponding home treatments when indicated. Has sections on choosing a doctor and tips on saving money in medical care.

▶ *Take This Book to the Hospital with You* by Charles B. Inlander and Ed Weiner (People's Medical Society, 14 E. Minor St., Emmaus, PA 18049). Subtitled "a consumer's guide to surviving your hospital stay," this publication is designed to help everyone who faces emergency or elective hospital stays. Information is included on limiting hidden costs, keeping accurate records, avoiding doctor-caused (iatrogenic) and in-hospital (nosocomial) infections, and maximizing safety. Includes a list of medical terminology, checklists for evaluating a hospital's features, and key questions to ask in various situations.

▶ *Taking Care of Your Child* by Robert H. Pantell, M.D., James F. Fries, M.D., and Donald Vickery, M.D. (Addison-Wesley, 1984). Provides clear diagrams and decision-making flowcharts to enable parents to deal appropriately with most childhood health problems at home. Lists home treatments and includes a useful section on family medical records.

Emergency Life Support Skills

Millions of Americans have advanced cardiovascular diseases and other ailments. In ideal circumstances, these conditions can be prevented for future generations. But right now, heart attacks occur frequently throughout the modern world. What specifically are your capabilities if someone nearby suddenly starts choking, has a heart attack, or experiences some other emergency situation?

New CPR

Cardiopulmonary resuscitation (CPR) may save 40 percent of heart attack victims who are stricken outside the hospital. The American Heart Association and American Red Cross recently updated their guidelines for CPR to make the procedures easier and more effective. The Heimlich maneuver — to clear blocked airways for all choking victims except infants and pregnant women — is also taught. Both organizations emphasize the importance of teaching CPR to family members, friends, neighbors, and co-workers of people at high risk for heart attack, as well as parents of babies. Contact your local chapter of the American Heart Association or American Red Cross for details.

Step 7

UNLIMITED MIND AND LIFE UNITY

43 Unlimited Mind: Introduction

What lies behind us and what lies before us are small matters compared to what lies within us.

— *RALPH WALDO EMERSON*

MYTH: Most of us use only about 10 percent of our brain power.

FACT: Neuroscientists now estimate that we only use about *one-hundredth of one percent* of our potential brain power! And the brain can steadily deteriorate, becoming flabby like unused muscles. Another discovery: senility is *not* a normal part of aging. With the right mental exercises and environment, the size, number, and function of many types of brain cells can be increased at any age.

MYTH: We find solutions to emotional distress by zeroing in on it, by thinking and talking about our shortcomings and problems, and getting all our negative feelings "out in the open."

FACT: Most of us have been led to believe this — but in most cases, it's simply not true. Thinking and talking about difficulties and inadequacies is precisely what keeps these problems alive and growing. Learn fast, simple ways to switch negative moods into positive ones. (*See Chapter 44.*)

MYTH: Stress is bad — but it just changes some hormones, tightens up muscles, and makes people tired. It doesn't really affect the brain.

FACT: Negative stress lowers intelligence test scores and can cripple your ability to think, learn, and remember. Worse, heavy loads of unresolved stress can destroy brain cells. Now you can learn ways to prevent this from happening. (*See Chapter 45.*)

MYTH: Some of us are born with good mental concentration, others with minds that wander. It's the same with creativity — you either have it or you don't.

FACT: Mental concentration and creativity aren't inherited, they're *learned*. These and other mental skills can be developed at any age. (*See Chapter 48.*)

MYTH: "Positive thinking" is simply a matter of filling your mind with "good" thoughts and blocking out the "bad."

FACT: Surprising new research reveals that much so-called positive thinking is really negative. Whether or not we consciously notice the many thoughts that flash through our minds, we *feel* their effect because thoughts create or influence emotions. You can learn two key elements in positive thinking and five steps for forming mental images that help you relax, boost immune power, and achieve your goals. Discover how to tap into your vast mental potentials and let go of whatever self-defeating thoughts and attitudes are holding you back. (*See Chapter 44.*)

Your Unlimited Mind. This powerful phrase is turning out to be far from fantasy. Recent studies show that the brain/mind is profoundly more capable and complex than had been previously imagined. Neuroscientists — specialists in neurophysiology, neurosurgery, neuropsychology, neuropharmacology, psychology, physics, education, and mathematics — are at the crest of a global wave of research on the brain, mind, and nervous system. What most of us consider normal intelligence is just a faint shadow of our mammoth mental potential.

This section of *Health & Fitness Excellence* focuses on unlocking your unlimited mind by transcending restrictive or destructive thoughts and attitudes and offering new options to expand your brain power.

Your Untapped Mental Potentials

Let's begin with some startling estimates about your untapped mental potentials. The human brain is a three-pound universe; a state-of-the-art computer with the same number of information "bits" would be one hundred stories tall and cover the entire state of Texas.[1] Researchers now estimate that, over a lifetime, most of us use as little as *one-ten-thousandth* of our brain potential.[2]

The *brain* is the physical site and fluctuating physical-chemical state where the body's nervous system activities originate, are moderated, or are controlled. To some scientists, this is all there is; no mind, only the brain. Other experts have thrown their formidable scientific weight behind the idea that the mind is far more than the brain organ. The *mind* is an interpretative state, influenced by emergent properties of the brain, and represents the totality of all that makes us human, or as *Webster's* dictionary defines it, "the element or complex of elements in an individual that feels, perceives, thinks, wills, and especially reasons; the organized conscious and unconscious adaptive mental activity of an organism."

The capabilities of the human brain to create, learn, and store are virtually unlimited. "Throughout our lives we only use a fraction of our thinking ability," wrote the prominent Russian scholar Ivan Yefremov. "We could, without any difficulty whatever, learn 40 languages, memorize a set of encyclopedias from A to Z, and complete the required courses of dozens of colleges."[3]

Your brain processes information using special cells called neurons. There are about 100 billion in your brain, each making between 5,000 and 50,000 connections with surrounding nerve cells. Even using the most conservative estimates, there are 100 trillion neuron junctions in your brain.[4] And a growing number of scientists insist that these numbers are much too small.

By some estimates, there are 2 to the 100 *trillionth* power connections among the brain's nerve cells. According to Dr. Carl Sagan of Cornell University, this means that *there are more possible mental states in each human being's brain than there are atoms in the known universe.*[5]

The Magic of the Synapse

One of the ways your billions of nerve cells communicate is using chemical messengers called neurotransmitters. When a neurotransmitter molecule seeps across a microscopic gap, called a synapse, between nerve cells, it locks on to a specially shaped and coded receptor on the receiving cell. This is how our brains transmit the signals that process information, keep us alive, transform thoughts into emotions and emotions into thoughts, and allow us a great degree of control in shaping our physical destinies.

Neurons, the most glorified of nerve cells, are complex things. Each neuron is busy most of the time. As each one receives a message at its receptor sites, it must instantly — in a fraction of a thousandth of a second — assess its own state, listen to what other neurons are saying to it, and decide whether to stop the stimuli there or send a particular message impulse to another nerve cell and, if so, to which one. In a hundredth of a second, an individual neuron may adjudicate hundreds of messages from other neurons as to what each of them advises it to do. The impulse can be stopped, delayed, increased, reduced, or transmitted exactly as it arrives. Even more amazing, this phenomenon takes place at speeds of 200 miles an hour and more. If the brain were merely electrical, then human beings might be deterministic machines similar to robotic computers. But it isn't and we are not.

The more scientists learn, the more awe-inspiring are the functions and capabilities of the human brain and nervous system. For example, it has recently been discovered that nerve cells not only produce chemicals that are sent to adjoining nerve receptor sites but also produce and transmit chemicals that affect nerves at far distant locations in the body. Moreover, rather than being one-way signals, nerve communication is conducted *in two directions* like a telephone conversation.[6]

The Neuroplastic Brain

As myths have been cast aside, we have learned that brain function is remarkably changeable and that we possess nearly unfathomable capacities for healing, learning, achieving, and remembering. This quality is called neuroplasticity.[7]

"The brain is not a machine in which every element has a genetically assigned role; it is not a digital computer in which all the decisions have been made," says neuroscientist Michael Merzenich, of the University of California at San Francisco. "Anatomy lays down a crude topographic map of the body on the surface of the cortex [the upper brain's outer covering where the cerebral hemispheres are located], which is fixed and immutable in early life. But the *fine-grained* map is not fixed. Experience sketches in all the details, altering the map continually throughout life."[8]

Another long-unchallenged scientific truth was that while other cells of the body could reproduce or regenerate themselves after injury, damaged brain cells could never repair or regain full function. But in recent years, medical journals have reported remarkable recoveries by people with severe brain injuries.[9] It now seems that, under the right conditions, nerve cells are capable of regeneration and growth throughout our lives.

The Brain, like Muscles, Can Become "Flabby"

It has long been assumed that once we reach maturity, brain growth ceases, signaling the beginning of a steady, unavoidable loss of nerve cells as we grow older. Finally, or so the tradition goes, we end up elderly and stuck in some inevitable web of senility, confusion, fatigue, and boredom. But scientists are discovering that, in most cases, there is just no need for this mental collapse.

Here's why. Without the right activities and stimulation, we know that the brain can steadily deteriorate, becoming "flabby" in certain vital areas as do unused muscles. But scientists at Yale University School of Medicine, the National Institute on Aging, and other research centers have discovered that with the right series of mental exercises, active intellectual interests, and an enriched, complex, challenging environment, your mind can keep developing toward its full potential and may be as sharp — or sharper — at age ninety as at age twenty.[10]

Brain Cell Loss Not Inevitable

Faulty scientific research is responsible for the myth that all of us lose a large number of brain cells as we age. The brains studied were inactive, degenerate brains, and consequently many cells had died. Except in rare cases, this loss appears unnecessary. In long-term human studies, researchers have found that people who are healthy and mentally active can actually improve on intelligence tests at sixty years of age and beyond.[11] The key words are *healthy* and *active*.

We can protect and nourish our brain cells. How? In part with a wise diet, good posture, regular physical exercises, stress management, social support, and other aspects of *Health & Fitness Excellence*. Beyond that, with a mental development program, introduced in the upcoming chapters.

New Knowledge, New Explanations

Many models have been developed to describe the brain/mind. As subatomic physicists break down the brain into ever-finer particles, some scientists still struggle with a computer-like, "hard-wired" model of the brain. At the same time, there is growing support for a model based on synergy — the concept in which large collections of neurons or the whole brain generate emergent properties that are greater than the mere mathematical sum of the individual neurological pieces.

"The deep error in the machine, switchboard, and computer metaphors is that nothing is happening until you *do* something," says Dr. Arnold Mandell, biological psychiatrist at the University of California at San Diego.[12] His brain model is a place where millions of things happen at once in a fluid, probabilistic universe within the cranium.

"Up until recently," says Dr. Candace Pert, "I've visualized the brain in Newtonian terms. I've pictured the neurochemicals and their receptors as hard, little locks, keys, and balls, like the drawings in textbooks. . . . But now I see the brain in terms of quantum mechanics — as a vibrating energy field. . . . I've stopped seeing the brain as the end of the line. The brain is just a receiver, an amplifier, a little wet minireceiver for collective reality. We make maps, but we should never confuse the map with the territory."[13]

The holonomic brain theory has been developed by Dr. Karl H. Pribram, National Institutes of Health professor of neuroscience, professor of Psychology and Psychiatry at Stanford University, and director of Stanford's Neuropsychology Laboratory. Using new scientific data and the laws of physiology, physics, and mathematics (including processes such as the Fourier and Gabor transforms and Hilldebrant space), Dr. Pribram has described the existence of a "spectral domain" where the brain/mind functions instantaneously — without time-space limitations.[14] This holographic model of the brain suggests that it is capable of storing nearly infinite amounts of information in virtually no space at all. Every part of the brain contains the image of the whole, and holographic codes automatically — instantaneously — take care of imaging from different distances and angles, enabling us to simultaneously compare size, shape, color, texture, luminosity, distance, and many other sensory criteria. There's no doubt: our potentials are dazzling.

The Brain Develops in Response to How You Use It

The path to lifelong mental development is becoming clear: We must learn to welcome change, acquire the flexibility to appreciate challenges, ambiguity, and unpredictable experiences, and continue to seek out and assimilate new information and skills. By choosing this kind of psychological road map, we can expand our wellness and wisdom as we grow older in years.

RESOURCES

▶ *Maps of the Mind: Charts and Concepts of the Mind and Its Labyrinths* by Charles Hampden-Turner (Macmillan, 1982). Sixty different maps of the mind are summarized and organized under nine headings, each compared and cross-referenced. A whole-picture view of theoretical perspectives on the mind. An interesting, accessible book.

▶ *The Three-Pound Universe: Revolutionary Discoveries About the Brain* by Judith Hooper and Dick Teresi (Macmillan, 1986). An intriguing look at the field of modern neuroscience and its diversity of people and visions.

▶ A listing of periodicals that discuss discoveries in brain/mind science is included in the Resource list at the end of this book.

44 Positive Thinking, Good Moods, and Guided Imagery

What we nurture in ourselves will grow: that is nature's eternal law.
— *GOETHE*

You become what you think about most of the time.
— *EARL NIGHTINGALE,*
THE STRANGEST SECRET

Do you control your thoughts, words, emotions, and mental images? Or do they control you? Are you the beneficiary or the victim of their power? Most of us are regularly assaulted by our own minds, and have years of practice hearing and using negative comments. Far too many of us have learned to specialize in ignoring what's right and pinpointing everything that's wrong. We get stuck seeing specks of dust on the window of the world.

Over the years, "positive thinking" books and seminars have suggested innumerable slogans and phrases that, if repeated often enough, purportedly catapult us to bliss and happiness. But positive mental and emotional states rarely ever come from reciting pep talk jingles. Mind-mood success requires a lasting shift in awareness and actions.

Thoughts are brief electrical flashes in the brain. Although they happen so fast we often don't "hear" them, we *feel* their effect because our thoughts create or influence our perceptions, emotions, and behaviors.[15]

In fact, there is evidence suggesting that *every one of your thoughts affects every cell in your body*.[16]

Why is thinking so powerful? Because the brain is extremely precise in its interpretation of, and response to, incoming messages. That's why so much "positive thinking" ends up being negative.

The more we focus on preventing and inadvertently magnifying what we *don't* want — anxiety, body fat, interpersonal conflicts, fear of speaking, fatigue, or memory loss, to give just a few examples — the more likely the dreaded results will occur. And a sense of emotional upset often results from looking at an unpleasant situation in a narrow, painful way without including other, more objective assessments.

Separate Realities

As unique individuals, each of us sees reality differently — it is what *appears* to be happening within us and around us at this moment. Our thoughts help formulate that reality. We each give acceptance and life to our thoughts. Accordingly, our perceptions, feelings, and behaviors are our own. They are not thrust on us by an outside force (other people, our job, or a particular situation). Only when we can learn to step outside our limited, habitual patterns of thinking can we view circumstances and other viewpoints with objectivity and without judgment. When we reach that point, conflicts diminish, productivity surges, and there's room for greater happiness to fill our lives.

The Mood-Thought Connection

When our moods are positive, we feel optimistic, motivated, productive, and creative. Regardless of external events and stress pressures, when our consciousness or mood is high we have a general sense of well-being and hope for the future. We are more helpful and generous toward others and experience improved cognitive processes such as judgment, problem solving, decision making, and creativity.[17] We have a higher psychological vantage point from which to view the challenges and conflicts that enter our lives.

In contrast, negative feelings and emotions are a sharp signal that we are dropping into a lower psychological state of functioning, reverting into patterns of negative thinking. We start attacking ourselves with our thoughts and lose our conscious ability to make commonsense decisions. We feel insecure and emotionally fragile and become poorer in various intellectual capacities.

Most of us have been led to believe that we can find solutions to our emotional distress if we think or talk about it enough. But that is rarely true. Thinking or talking about our difficulties and inadequacies — dwelling on them in our mind and conversations — is precisely what keeps most problems alive and growing.

Self-suggestion, or self-talk, magnifies the dilemma. We live with this inner mind chatter all day, every day. It's a natural human tendency and, unfortunately, most of us have learned to emphasize self-defeating messages. We often have trouble being as compassionate or rational with ourselves as we would be with a friend or loved one. Perhaps this is because critical parents, teachers, bosses, and peers have inadvertently led us to believe many negative things about ourselves. Nonetheless, these thoughts sink our moods.

When work stress starts to pile up, for example, it's easy to feel overloaded and anxious. Just as soon as our thoughts become negative, our mood drops. We begin to feel stuck, things start looking bleak, our work becomes more of a struggle. Our thoughts then become twisted, distorted. To break out of this pattern, we first need to look at some of the common ways we use our minds to attack ourselves and others.

Cognitive Distortions

Distorted thoughts are automatic, specific, discrete messages. They have the power to tie us in emotional knots. Our daily conversations and mental dialogues are filled with these bombshells but, amazingly, most of us are unaware of them. We end up living on an emotional roller coaster that is running out of control. To take charge of our mind and mood, we need to identify distorted thinking patterns and replace them with clear, positive alternatives.

Traditional cognitive psychotherapy has established a solid research foundation for this approach to psychological health.[18] No matter how irrational they are, distorted, automatic thoughts are almost always believed, and they often appear in incomplete sentences — several key words or a visual image flash. When we are emotionally distressed, anxious, or under pressure, cognitive distortions flourish.

The good news is that, with practice, automatic, twisted thoughts can be straighted out. Once you have read this section and are aware of problem thinking habits, deal with them using the solution strategies presented later in this chapter. To help sharpen your awareness and thought-correcting actions, consider these sixteen examples of typical distorted thinking patterns (listed alphabetically):

1 *Being right.* You need to always prove that your statements and actions are right. You are quick to launch into defensive rationalizations whenever your "rightness" seems in question.

2 *Blaming.* Your problems are either *never* your fault (other people and situations cause whatever goes wrong) or *always* your own fault.

3 *Change illusion.* Your happiness and success depend on other people changing their bad habits — "bad" from your perspective of reality — and you believe they will make these changes if you keep pressuring them enough.

4 *Control illusion.* You either feel externally controlled — and therefore victimized — by other people and circumstances or internally controlled — which leaves you feeling that you cause everyone else's unhappiness.

5 *Disqualifying the positive.* You reject positive experiences on the grounds that they somehow "don't count" when compared with the endless list of problems in your life.

6 *Either/or thinking.* There is no middle ground — things are either good or they're bad. Either you perform perfectly or you're a total failure.

7 *Emotional reasoning.* You automatically assume that your feelings are facts and therefore must reflect the way things really are. If you *feel* incompetent and unattractive, then you must *be* incompetent and unattractive.

8 *Fairness illusion.* You think you know exactly what's fair in all situations but feel victimized when other people often don't agree with you.

9 *Filtering.* You find negative details in any situation and dwell on them so exclusively — ignoring the positive — that no matter how bright an experience may initially be, it soon looks bleak.

10 *Jumping to conclusions.* You quickly leap to negative interpretations of statements and situations even though you usually lack the facts to support your conclusion.

> *Mind reading.* Without checking to find out the truth, you assume that you know precisely why other people are thinking, feeling, and acting the way they are.

> *Fortune telling.* You anticipate that a future event will turn out badly and act as if this is a predetermined fact.

11 *Labeling and mislabeling.* This is an extreme version of overgeneralization. When you make an error or become irritated with others, you emotionally assign a label to yourself ("I'm a loser"; "I'm an idiot"), another person ("He's a quitter"; "She's a cheater"), or situation.

12 *Magnification (catastrophizing) and minimization.* You exaggerate risks, anticipating disaster; you overplay your mistakes or the importance of someone else's achievements; or you erroneously shrink your positive attributes or another person's imperfections until they appear insignificant.

13 *Overgeneralization.* You make a sweeping assumption based on only a shred of evidence — a single negative event becomes a never-ending pattern of defeat.

14 *Personalization.* You see yourself as the cause of some negative occurrence for which you were not primarily responsible. You think that everything other people say or do is a reaction to you. You keep comparing yourself to others, wondering who's smarter, more successful, better looking, and so on.

15 *"Shoulds."* You try to motivate yourself and others with guilt, using statements filled with "shoulds" and "shouldn'ts," "musts," and "oughts." When you or others break your rules you feel anger, resentment, and frustration.

16 *Ultimate reward illusion.* You talk and act as if monumental daily sacrifices and self-denial are what will ultimately bring you great rewards. You feel resentful when the rewards don't seem to come.

Self-directed cognitive distortions are closely related to explanatory style — the way we describe experiences to ourselves and others.[19] According to researchers, if you explain bad things that happen to you in terms that are internal ("It's all my fault"), stable ("It's going to last forever"), and global ("It's going to spoil everything I do"), you are at increased risk for depression, poor performance, and illness.

Distorted thinking is contagious — the habit spreads. "If you consistently respond to events pessimistically," says psychologist Martin E. P. Seligman, "that negative style can actually *amplify* your feelings of helplessness and spread to other areas of your life."[20] The best advice? Begin paying closer attention to the way you explain unpleasant situations and outcomes to yourself and others. Catch negative, stressful thoughts and begin replacing them with constructive, positive ones. It comes down to building new habits of mind.

Ways to Elevate Your Mood

We each have the natural ability to disengage ourselves from pointless, negative thinking. The fastest, surest way to do that is to raise our mood. Although we all experience mood fluctuations, some of us — many of us — get stuck in low moods. New research shows that that's usually unnecessary. In fact, when we learn to notice shifts in our feelings we can use that awareness as a cue to keep us oriented in a positive direction. How? By quickly adjusting our thinking and raising our mood.

To begin with, there is little point in trying to suppress negative thoughts. Researchers have confirmed that struggling to block thoughts often backfires — leading to obsession about the thoughts we try to suppress.

Psychologists have identified some fast, simple ways to elevate mood.[21] (These techniques can be included in each rejuvenation-in-motion routine during the day, as explained in Chapter 10.) First, fully *acknowledge* your current circumstances so that you can move forward. Disengage your mind from a lock grip on stressful thoughts. Shift your thinking *away* from problems and emotional storms. Think about what you want, not what you don't want.

Second, choose not to take negative thoughts seriously if you happen to be in a lower mood. To make it easier to notice the twists and turns of negative thinking, some experts advise writing down your thoughts and feelings on a piece of paper and next to each enumerating a rational response. Some people find that talking aloud to themselves, instead of engaging in a silent dialogue, quickly helps to give them a better sense of perspective whenever they're in a down mood.

Third, take action — balance your posture, breathe deeply, think in a new direction, get up and move around, exercise, talk to someone new about something new. Taking action steps, no matter how small, tends to raise moods.[22]

Your choice of food for snacks and meals also influences your state of mind and mood. This connection is discussed in Chapter 27.

Another mood-raising tool is mental imagery.

Imagery: The Power of Pictures in the Mind

Beginning in the 1950s, researchers and clinicians in Europe, the United States, Asia, and the Soviet Union began systematically exploring the role of mental imagery in health, education, and human performance. There is now an extensive body of knowledge affirming the power of pictures in the mind.[23]

Thoughts. Images. What's the difference? "*Thoughts* are basically [short-lived] electrical events in the brain, like electric sparks, they *come* quickly and they *go* quickly — dozens in each moment," says Dr. Emmett E. Miller, author of *Power Vision: Mastering Life Through Mental Image Rehearsal.* "Look back at the thousands of thoughts you've already had today. . . . They can easily distract you. But if you [guide and] hold your thoughts to a single *focus* for a while, something quite interesting and important occurs . . . a *mental image* begins to form. . . . This image is represented in the brain by a pattern of chemicals . . . hormone-like substances secreted by the nervous system. . . . The quality of this chemical state influences how we *feel*. Thus, each image stimulates the creation of a particular chemical state, which in turn produces emotions and behaviors consistent with that image. Our emotions, in turn, have a direct effect on our muscular system . . . on how we stand, speak and approach our [lives and] work."[24]

Thoughts and mental images can now be measured by computer, using tests such as positron emission tomography (PET scans) — "windows to the brain" that permit us to see precise mental actions in thousandths of a second, mapping blood flow in the cerebral hemispheres as thoughts, images, and feelings change our cells.

Researchers have found that nearly all of us in the Western world fall far short of our potential in forming mental images. "Imaging abilities are vastly underdeveloped in most of us," says Harvard University psychologist Stephen Kosslyn, who has directed several recent studies. "With training and a bit of practice, people can improve immensely in their capacity to use images."[25]

Dr. Kosslyn recommends finding the separate parts of a mental picture, fitting them together properly, then scanning the image, moving it around, zooming in on one aspect of the image, moving it farther away, panning it to capture a better view of the whole picture, and more. With practice, we can each develop our ability to create intense images, richly woven sensory tapestries filled with sounds, lights, colors, touches, textures, temperatures, movements, emotions, and so on.

Before we discuss positive imagery techniques, let's identify two widespread problem areas or stumbling blocks.

Watch Out for Negative-on-Negative Thinking

Argue for your limitations, and sure enough, they're yours.
— *RICHARD BACH,* ILLUSIONS

Bleak negative-on-negative statements are easy to spot. They are often a judgmental put-down of yourself, someone else, current circumstances, or the world in general, followed by a prediction of failure or suffering.

The problem, of course, is that negative suggestion works. It is a self-fulfilling prophecy, bringing about in reality the inadequacy, worthlessness, and other victimizing traits that are imagined. We are masters at making ourselves miserable.

People are amazed to learn how many negative and judgmental statements they tend to make in a day. Most of us have years of practice with put-downs. As mentioned in Chapter 6, the national average of parent-to-child criticisms is 12 to 1 — a dozen criticisms for every single compliment or positive comment. And in the average secondary school classroom, the ratio of criticisms to compliments from teacher to student is 18 to 1.[26] Stanford University researchers have found that in business situations the negative-to-positive ratios range from 4 to 1 to 8 to 1.[27]

We can each learn to favor constructive attributions and control negative thoughts in a positive way. In addition to the strategies already mentioned in this chapter, you can (1) prepare yourself to use negative thoughts as a trigger for positive responses, acting immediately to do something productive instead of destructive, and (2) identify the source of negative thoughts and then remove the origins. For example, negative thoughts caused by tension or anxiety tend to get bigger if you use mental warfare, but they can be controlled through stress management techniques or relieved by physical exercise.

Negative-on-Positives: Saboteurs of Self-Talk

It is important to notice — and correct — the mixed-up statements that slip by most of us in everyday self-talk and conversation. Here, one part of the image or comment is positive, another negative. The net result is often negative.

For example, even if you mentally picture yourself in a positive way, how do you describe your choices and actions? Are you avoiding a problem (negative focus) or building a constructive outcome (positive focus)? This subtle difference in mental direction can create a major difference in results. Are you making choices or taking actions to keep from becoming flabbier or fatter, making repeated mistakes, feeling aches and pains, becoming more tired or anxious, or losing your memory (in each of these cases you are focusing on a negative or destructive image)? Or choosing or acting in specific ways to tone muscles and burn excess fat, improve your concentration and coordination, take charge of stress, move with greater ease and comfort, increase energy and confidence, or boost your thinking abilities (all positive or constructive images)?

Positive-on-Positive Thinking: A Solution

Pictures in the mind generally have two predominant emphases: the subject and the event. *Both* must be positive to avoid self-sabotage:

1 Is the subject of your attention (the specific person, group, place, feeling, action, or circumstance) positive and enhancing?
2 Does something good happen (the actual statement about the subject of your thought) once your concentration is focused there?

The first part of the picture. How do you envision yourself and others throughout the day? Take several minutes right now to relax and examine some of your statements in slow motion. In a typical image or statement, when you say or think *I*, do you automatically sense your best self? Or do you see a composite self-image that you don't like very much?

Slow down your mind so you can look at a number of your mental pictures more closely. As you review them, do you notice any patterns in your thoughts and images of yourself, other people, places, and circumstances? Is there a predominant negative or positive slant? As mentioned earlier, many of us have an unconscious tendency to amplify — and hold on to — the distrustful, anxious, angry, hurtful parts of our experiences.

Sit quietly now, relaxing, and roll your mental videotape in slow motion. Here comes the subject of your thought. Imagine: yourself, a parent, child, sibling, loved one, former loved one, associate, former associate, friend, or other subject. What is the view of this person in your mind? Your imagery choice will quickly affect your mood.

With some practice, you can teach your mind to choose the most vivid, positive, competent view of yourself (and most other subjects) every time you think or say the name or pronoun. Whenever possible, choose meaningful, nurturing images — and give them a little extra magnitude. Remember, you're not required to permanently banish bad memories — you are just deciding to stop dragging up the negative again and again.

The same principles apply to events and situations. Go out of your way to think of the best, most productive, or most constructive elements of each. Instead of seeing *problems*, which tend to get bigger each time they're shown in technicolor, learn to draw out the bright spots and embrace *opportunities* and *solutions*, however "minor" they may seem.

All right, you may be thinking, but what about those people and circumstances for which you have no positive memories at all? In these cases, imagery experts often suggest "rewriting the script" of the past to create a temporary positive thought or feeling. As discussed in Chapter 6, you can imagine the past hurt, mistake, or situation as if the outcome had been positive. This helps you let go of emotional baggage and find some growing room right now.

What about inanimate objects — like your home, car, office, desk, computer, checkbook, and so on? Have you had this feeling before: Returning from an out-of-town trip, the closer you get to home or the office the more anxious you become? Subconscious negative responses can be associated with a variety of places and things in our lives. If you have experienced heated arguments in a particular room of your home or office, for example, you may associate those tensions with your image of that spot, in spite of the fact that you may have also had hundreds of good, nurturing moments there.

When you think of your home right now, do you picture a confluence of the great times you've enjoyed there? Or a parade of problems — broken things to fix, stressful memories, the mortgage, or some other burden of responsibility? If you don't control images like these, they can flood the mind and hit you with waves of anxiety.

The bottom line is that images are a choice. Whenever possible, why not choose the warmest, brightest memories of places and things in your life — your home, for example, as a "safe haven," gathering place for special occasions, site of quiet, fulfilling moments? Roll these positive memories into one "homing thought." Whenever you'd like to take a quick break from pressure you can think "home" and feel especially good.

The second part of the picture. Now look at the predicate — what's happening to the subject in each image or sentence. Do you tend to catastrophize or empower? Anticipate failure or success? Remind yourself of what's right or pinpoint what's wrong? Find ways to solve dilemmas or wallow deeper in conflict? Our assessments and predictions make a dramatic difference in our lives.

Choose accurate, empowering descriptions. Surround yourself with people who are committed to doing the same. Start a mental campaign to cut out doom and gloom — the distorted backward thinking that locks us in stress closets. As discussed in Chapter 9, experts recommend honest, specific statements that focus on the positive. We need to think and speak in ways that prompt our best feelings, perceptions, and actions.

Five Steps to Successful Positive Imagery

Mental imagery skills are expanded through practice. In the beginning, mental training often works best using audiotapes. Without a tape, you need to give yourself specific suggestions as well as carry them out. Sometimes this is too complicated for fast results.

You can either create your own written scripts and listen to a friend's voice or your own voice reading them on a recorded tape or memorize the instructions "in a relaxed fashion, then close your eyes and let yourself drift through [the message]."[28] As an alternative, consider purchasing pre-recorded tapes (see "Resources" at the end of the chapter). In every case, the voice (including your own internal voice) should be calm, interested, and pleasing.

Powerful, positive mental images can be formed using five key steps:

1. Establish a Relaxed, Receptive State

The most effective guided imagery training is preceded by deep relaxation, which helps free the brain from unnecessary chatter and distraction.

Breathing helps you relax quickly and deeply, changing the body's center of gravity, increasing the feeling of inner calm, and enhancing your ability to focus. With regular practice, you can link sensory signals (words, thoughts, sounds, touch, fragrances, or other stimuli "anchors") with deep relaxation. You can then use these cues to quickly enter a re-laxed state.

2. Recall a Successful Past Experience

"To take charge of your life and create your own positive future, it is absolutely essential that your images be based on a foundation of high-quality, successful experiences from your past," says imagery expert Dr. Emmett E. Miller.[29] To tackle something new or a task you have never been able to do, you can invent a positive image by watching or reading about others performing the feat successfully, or relating some similar ex-perience from your past. For example, athletic confidence in one sport can often be transferred to another. Images of speaking eloquently to a close friend can be used to help prepare for your first public speaking appearance. And so on.

"We all have within us the key to feeling stronger, more confident, more resourceful, and more successful," observe psychologists Bernie Zilbergeld and Arnold A. Lazarus. "By recalling and focusing on times when you were successful, you recreate the feelings of confidence, power, and accomplishment that are associated with these successes, and that helps to ensure good feelings and positive results in the present and fu-ture. Recollection of past achievements is one of the most powerful kinds of imagery available to anyone. . . . All of us have been successful and effective at something, but it's amazing how quickly we forget or mini-mize these experiences."[30]

You can assemble a collection of past success images to call upon whenever you need a boost of confidence or strength. This sets a positive emotional tone for the next step in the mental training sequence.

3. Imagine a Positive Outcome

Imagining a desired outcome — also called goal imagery or result imag-ery — helps you focus on what you really want. This unlocks your cre-ativity, gives you a precise direction, and helps you organize the steps necessary to achieve that result. If you regularly, vividly imagine achiev-ing your goal — your vision of the future — you will begin to think about yourself in a brighter light, improving your self-image or per-ception.

For best results, make certain the image is an achievable one, some-thing you truly believe can happen, something motivating, satisfying, ful-filling that serves your higher values and purposes. Use all of your senses and describe the image in the present tense as if it were happening right now.

If you are recording your own audiotape, be certain to give enough detail to get yourself deeply involved with the next step — process imag-ery — and be certain to include frequent positive reinforcements: "You're doing fine," "That's great," "Wonderful," "That's it," "Very good," and so on.

4. Imagine the Process to Achieve Your Positive Outcome

This part of the guided imagery experience, called outcome imagery, clearly identifies the challenges you face in achieving your goal and creates a specific action plan of thoughts, behaviors, and resources that will help it become a reality. Precisely what skills, feelings, attitudes, words, performance adjustments, shifts in awareness, and so on are essential to the results you desire? Be clear and supportive. Remember to focus on the precise ways to solve each challenge or problem rather than dwelling on the problem itself.

5. Anchor Success

Form an "anchor." Anchors are multisensory cues that can be associated with successful outcomes and make it faster and easier to achieve subsequent positive results. For more about creating your own anchors, see Chapter 46.

Slow Things Down and Practice, Practice

It is unrealistic to assume that you can change your thinking simply by agreeing to. It takes regular practice — you may be unraveling *years* of experience making unpositive choices. To change thinking patterns and imagery habits, work on them several times a day, devoting a few minutes to sitting quietly, relaxing your body, becoming meditative or mindful, and practicing positive-on-positive imagery. As noted in Chapter 10, one of the easiest ways to do this is to include mental training techniques each time you go through a 30-second rejuvenation-in-motion routine.

"Imagine Your Blessings"

Here's a success secret you can begin using right now: "Don't just count your blessings, *imagine* them," suggests Anees A. Sheikh, chairman of the department of psychology at Marquette University and a leading expert on mental imagery.[31] First, write down descriptions of ten specific blessings in your life. Over the next month, add two or three new blessings to this list each week. At least once a day, sit quietly for a few minutes and relax. Then imagine each blessing on your list for a minimum of 10 seconds — see it, hear it, touch it . . . use *all* your senses.

Dr. Sheikh reports that in many cases this simple exercise can transform an individual's whole view of life. Instead of struggling or being overwhelmed with the bad events that happen every day, you'll feel your awareness shift toward good things, to the positive occurrences all around you that, until now, may have rarely been noticed.

The Golden Circle

A number of psychologists and motivational speakers suggest that all we really need to master stress and be in great mental health is the right self-talk. That's a myth. By itself, positive thinking just isn't enough.

Moreover, it's all but impossible to think truly positive thoughts (you can recite empty mental jingles perhaps, but not thoughts with meaning) when stress hits and you have halted your breathing, frowned, collapsed your posture, tensed your muscles, and opened the floodgates to negative emotions — all about as fast as you can blink your eyes.

In addition to honing your awareness and practicing ways to elevate your mind and mood, mental health and well-being depend on the golden circle of *Health & Fitness Excellence*. All areas of this program — nutrition, exercise, stress management, balanced posture, and the others — merge to form an inner environment where constructive thoughts and images are easier to create, believe, and express.

RESOURCES

Mental development warrants considerable attention by everyone interested in *Health & Fitness Excellence*. In addition to the periodicals included in the Resource list at the end of this book, the following resources are especially noteworthy:

▶ American Imagery Institute (P.O. Box 13453, Milwaukee, WI 53213). This institute, directed by Dr. Anees Sheikh, offers publications in a wide range of mental imagery areas.
▶ *How to Stubbornly Refuse to Make Yourself Miserable About Anything — Yes, Anything!* by Albert Ellis, Ph.D. (Lyle Stuart, 1988). Clear, no-nonsense advice from a leading psychologist.
▶ Insight Publishing (P.O. Box 2070, Mill Valley, CA 94942; 415-388-8225) offers a collection of guided mental imagery tapes by Martin L. Rossman, M.D., author of *Healing Yourself: A Step-by-Step Program for Better Health Through Imagery* (Walker, 1987).
▶ Institute for Rational-Emotive Therapy (45 East 65th St., New York, NY 10021; 212-535-0822). Founded by psychotherapist Albert Ellis, Ph.D., the institute offers a catalog of publications, research monographs, and audiotapes.
▶ *Mind Power: Getting What You Want Through Mental Training* by Bernie Zilbergeld, Ph.D., and Arnold A. Lazarus, Ph.D. (Little, Brown, 1987). A practical, step-by-step guide. Accompanying audiotapes are available from MindPower Distribution Services (2847 Shattuck Ave., Berkeley, CA 94705).
▶ *Power Vision: Mastering Life Through Mental Image Rehearsal* by Emmett E. Miller, M.D. (Nightingale-Conant Corp., 1987). Audiotape

album and manual by a leading stress management authority. A complete series of Dr. Miller's audiotape programs are available from Source Cassette Learning Systems (P.O. Box W, Stanford, CA 94309; 415-328-7171).

▶ *Rapid Relief from Emotional Distress* by Gary Emery, Ph.D., and James Campbell, Ph.D. (Fawcett, 1986). A book about rapid cognitive therapy by two experts in the field. Audiotapes are available from L.A. Center for Cognitive Therapy (630 S. Wilton Pl., Los Angeles, CA 90005; 213-387-4737).

▶ *Sanity, Insanity, and Common Sense* by Rick Suarez, Ph.D., Roger C. Mills, Ph.D., and Darlene Stewart, M.S. (Fawcett, 1987). A groundbreaking book on nco-cognitive psychology. A practical program on understanding true sources of our perceptions, feelings, thoughts, and behaviors. Audiotapes are available from the Advanced Human Studies Institute (P.O. Box 140223, Coral Gables, FL 33114).

▶ *Seven Steps to Peak Performance* by Richard M. Suinn, Ph.D. (Hans Huber, 12–14 Bruce Park Ave., Toronto, Ontario, Canada M4P 2S3; 1987). A training manual for "visual motor behavior rehearsal" for athletes.

▶ *Software for the Mind* by Emmett E. Miller, M.D. (Celestial Arts, 1987). A practical book filled with examples and exercises for selective awareness and guided imagery.

▶ Whole Person Associates, Inc. (P.O. Box 3151, Duluth, MN 55803; 218-728-6807). Offers a popular collection of imagery and relaxation audiotapes by psychologist Donald Tubesing, Ph.D.

45 Concentration, Neuronutrition, and Protecting Your Brain from Negative Stress

Concentration

Mindfulness is the ability to focus your complete attention on the world around you and within you exactly as it is this moment — slowing your pace and releasing tensions while increasing your energy, objective intelligence, and productivity. It is a mental health trait we desperately need in our helter-skelter society.

Yet there are growing indications that our modern culture is drifting farther and farther away from mindfulness, that an escalating sensory invasion is taking its toll. A recent Stanford University study, for example, estimated that a majority of people may now be spending an average of 58 minutes of every hour dealing with the past or anticipating the future, and *only about 2 minutes* focused on the present.[32]

"Mindfulness requires a change in attitude," explains Joan Borysenko, director of the Mind/Body Clinic at Harvard Medical School. "It means being open to an awareness of the moment as it is and to what the moment could hold. It is a relaxed state of attentiveness to both the inner world of thoughts and feelings and the outer world of actions and perceptions. . . . The joy is not in finishing an activity — the joy is in doing it. . . . You can train yourself to be mindful by cultivating awareness of where your mind is and then making a choice about where you want it to be."[33]

"Mindfulness frees us of forgetfulness and dispersion and makes it possible to live fully each minute of life," says Zen master Thich Nhat Hanh, who was nominated for a Nobel Peace Prize by Dr. Martin Luther King, Jr. "You might well ask: Then how are we to practice mindfulness? My answer is: keep your attention focused on the work, be alert and ready to handle ably and intelligently any situation that may arise — this is mindfulness."[34]

"I would like to offer one short poem," adds Hahn, "you can recite from time to time, while breathing and smiling.

Breathing in, I calm body and mind.
Breathing out, I smile.
Dwelling in the present moment
I know this is the only moment.[35]

One time-tested way to increase mindfulness is to practice meditation (see Chapter 4 for some basic guidelines). Another important mental strength is concentration.

Concentration is defined as bringing one's faculties and efforts into focus on a single task or thought. Many people assume that it's possible to pay attention to several events simultaneously — for example, reading a book while listening to a news report on the radio or writing detailed notes while you listen to a public speaker or instructor in school. What actually happens is that your attention must shift back and forth between the two stimuli, causing your attention to oscillate and creating fatigue. When you add other distractions — sights, sounds, scents, uncomfortable seating, and so forth — the stress soars. This promotes mental tension.

By strengthening your concentration, you can cut down on random, energy-wasting shifts in attention. With heightened concentration, you increase your power to choose *where* and *when* you focus your mind — on what you wish to feel, see, hear, think, and do; on foreground or background, inside or outside, good or bad. Research suggests that it's even possible to slow or reverse some common aging symptoms by sharpening your senses (Chapters 35–37) and concentration.[36]

Concentration can also often be improved with the right food. As discussed in Chapter 27, nutrients in your meals and snacks affect the production and balance of brain neurotransmitter chemicals that influence mental focus and mood. The right personal food choices may help you gain greater control over your powers of concentration, although this is only one part of the picture. Varied exercises, such as the following, for your hearing, sight, touch, and thinking are also important in strengthening your attention-focusing abilities.

Hearing: By listening to two radios, each on a different news channel with the volumes set equally, you can practice "tuning in" one station and "tuning out" the other. Alternate your focus from one station to the other every 20 seconds or so for up to two minutes several days a week. Progressively reduce the volume as your hearing acuity improves.

Sight: Place a single object on a table. Study it meticulously for about one minute and then close your eyes. Visualize it in your mind for about 15 seconds and then open your eyes and compare your exact image with reality. Over a period of weeks, expand the exercise: increasing the number of objects visualized at one time, varying the colors, lighting, positioning, and distance from you as you reduce the allotted time.

Touch: Sit or lie down quietly, with your eyes closed, and take several moments to become maximally aware of a specific feeling — tension, temperature, touch, and so on — in a selected area of your body. After 15–30 seconds, switch your attention to another part of your body. Spend several minutes at least once a week developing this aspect of concentration. You can also create sensory "tests" by collecting a variety of small objects and pieces of material of different shapes, sizes, and textures and placing them in separate envelopes. After shuffling the envelopes with your eyes closed, open each envelope one at a time as you describe the object by touch.

Thinking: Your powers of mind can be developed in countless ways. The biggest problem is lassoing your mental faculties often enough and long enough to focus them in precise new ways. This chapter and the following three chapters provide examples of mental development exercises.

Here's a simple strategy: In the midst of important daily tasks, notice whenever your mind begins to wander or concentration starts to wane. As soon as you catch this happening, actively, assertively refocus your attention. "It's one thing to *look* and another to actively *see*," says performance psychologist Richard M. Suinn of Colorado State University. "If you find yourself looking but not seeing, then ask yourself questions [about what you are seeing] to direct your attention."[37]

Neuronutrition

Are we nourishing our brain's full potential or merely its survival? That's a question being investigated by neuroscientists around the world. "Neuronutrition" goes beyond what most people call "a good diet." The full-spectrum *Health & Fitness Excellence* approach — with stress strategies, exercise, nutrition, balanced posture, and the other golden circle elements — puts you squarely on the path to peak brain function. Let's take a look at several key points.

Oxygen

Optimal brain function depends on maximizing your body's ability to take in and process high levels of oxygen. How is this accomplished? Diaphragmatic breathing patterns and regular aerobic exercise are essential. At both young and older ages, individuals with top physical fitness display higher levels of fluid intelligence, the ability to actively, creatively use their minds.[38] In addition, the disease-free heart can pump oxygen-carrying blood to brain cells as well at age eighty as at age twenty.[39]

Regular, balanced exercise programs help sharpen mental capabilities, including memory, sensory acuity, reaction speed, learning abilities, practical intelligence, and emotional control.[40] Insufficient oxygen supply to cerebral nerve cells reportedly leads to a decline of certain neurotransmitters and diminished brain function.[41]

Pure Water

This is another forgotten nutrient for mental health. The gradual loss of water during the day contributes to fatigue and muscular discomfort.[42] Water also plays a critical role in keeping the brain adequately hydrated, say sports medicine authorities Dr. Bob Goldman and Robert M. Hackman. "Even a slightly dehydrated body can produce a small but critical shrinkage of the brain, thereby impairing neuromuscular coordination, concentration, and thinking."[43] Dehydration stresses are particularly high in modern office buildings and during air travel. Follow the fluid intake guidelines presented in the nutrition and exercise sections of *Health & Fitness Excellence*.

Avoid Neurotoxic Chemicals

Few of the contaminants in America's food supply have been adequately tested for neurotoxicity. And some poisons — including pesticides, fungicides, and molds — show potential for adversely affecting the nervous system. See Chapter 23 for details and a step-by-step action plan.

Widely Varied Diet

Eating a widely varied diet of fresh, wholesome foods taken at frequent small meals and light snacks helps ensure peak nutrient availability for the brain. Don't forget those often overlooked "nutritional factors" such as relaxation and good circulation, which help determine whether the nutrients ever reach the cells in your brain.

Mind-Mood-Food Connection

Once you have organized a healthful diet, specific choices among various good foods can influence your brain power. What, when, how much, and in what order you eat certain foods appear to affect the production and concentration of brain neurotransmitters, which in turn influence mental alertness, concentration, attitude, mood, and performance.[44]

Chapter 27 reviewed compelling new evidence that low-fat snacks that include a small amount of protein-rich food (such as fish, shellfish, skinless chicken or turkey breast, soy tofu, skim milk, low-fat or nonfat cottage cheese or yogurt, lentils, dried peas or beans) can promote faster thinking, increased attention to detail, and quicker reaction speed. Low-fat, low-protein snacks that are high in complex carbohydrates (such as pasta/fruit salad, whole-grain bread, bagel, muffin, pita chips, or crackers with fruit preserve) can often help produce a calm, focused state of mind and relaxed emotions.

Nutritional Supplements	Recent studies suggest that even slight deficiencies of certain vitamins and minerals may contribute to mental deficits, even among people in otherwise excellent health. Researchers in one study published in the *Journal of the American Medical Association* found "an association between poor performance on cognitive tests and low intake and serum levels of riboflavin, folate, vitamin B_{12}, and ascorbate [vitamin C]."[45] Consider taking a broad-spectrum multivitamin-mineral supplement on a regular basis (see Chapter 28).
The Rest of the Picture	There is solid evidence that posture, muscular tension levels, the precise way we each deal with daily stresses, the type and frequency of our work breaks, sensory stimulation, communication patterns (including self-talk and verbal/written dialogues), the quality of our nightly sleep, our focus of mind and mood, and a variety of other *Health & Fitness Excellence* factors each influence changes in blood and oxygen flow to the brain.

Protecting Your Brain from Negative Stress

Negative stresses — pressure-filled situations in which you feel helpless, hopeless, or hassled to the point where there's no relief in sight — can destroy brain cells. Lower levels of distress cause mental difficulties, too.

This damage or loss of function takes place in many ways. For example, when fear or anxiety makes your muscles tense or your posture collapses even slightly, blood flow to the brain is restricted. This can interfere with cerebral access to oxygen and nutrients.[46] A recent Georgetown University study of four thousand schoolchildren concluded that high stress reduced IQ scores by a full 13 percent.[47]

Negative stress is also implicated in premature aging of the adult brain.[48] Scientists performing research under grants from the National Institute on Aging have discovered that stress-related hormone levels in the blood correlate with the degree of age-related function loss in the brain tissues.[49] Neuroscientists studying this phenomenon believe it may lead to a weakening of the hippocampus's ability to "turn off" the stress reactivity system and, through a feedback loop with the brain's emotional control center — the limbic system — the hippocampus gradually destroys itself.[50]

Physical and emotional tensions also have profound effects on our thought and memory processes. Many memory deficiencies connected with "aging" appear to be reversible, according to Stanford University psychiatrist Dr. Jerome Yesavage.[51] Dr. Yesavage and colleague Danielle Lapp started an ongoing memory research project at Stanford in 1978, centered on the hypothesis that the anxiety created by forgetfulness literally hurts the memory, among both young and old people. They discovered that many people can restore their memory by simply learning relaxation techniques. "Anxiety clutters the channels of memory," says Lapp. "Relaxation opens these channels."

46 Anchors and Patterning Excellence

Anchors

You can learn to instantly elicit surges of your best energy and reduce or eliminate many common anxiety reactions using a technique called *anchoring*.[52] Anchors call forth positive physical-emotional-mental states by linking sensory cues to images of competence. This technique can be used to enhance your mental abilities and ease in handling stressful situations.

Anchoring happens throughout our lives — in both good and bad ways — since we live in a stimulus-response world. Anchors hook on to a bodily sense and prompt us to change our thoughts, feelings, or actions whenever a particular sensory signal is given.

Examples: Think of the instant wave of memories when you hear a special song, even many years after you last heard it; or the strong feelings you immediately get from vividly recalling any of your "great moments" or "worst moments" in sports, speaking, art, music, dating, parenting, working, traveling, a hobby — *any* peak experience.

Traumatic or painful events condition us to anticipate trauma whenever certain similar stimuli are present. Advertising jingles, symbols, and pictures are targeted our way to sensitize us to automatically think or feel about a particular product or service in a special way. What about a police car with lights flashing and siren sounding? It brings an immediate "anchored" response to most people — perhaps a flash of anxiety if you're concerned with the speed at which you are driving or a sense of reassurance if you live in a crime-ridden neighborhood.

Anchors can be good or bad, strengthening or weakening, empowering or victimizing. The important fact is that they're everywhere. We can chose to take greater charge of our own lives by forming positive anchors or make no effort at all and let our environment and the people around us do the conditioning.

Experts say the most effective anchors are multisensory; that is, they involve several senses (touch, sound, sight, gesture, smell, or taste) unified into a single nervous system cue that recaptures the sensation of being your best.

Anchors are not a panacea, however. They are only one of many factors contributing to best fitness and performance. But they can help you in a wide range of personal and work situations, big and small. For example, it is ideal to add an anchor to the instant calming sequence presented in Chapter 7. No matter what pressures you face — serious personal crises and "it's-all-on-the-line" performance challenges or quiet, nagging self-doubts, guilt about the past, or worries about the future — anchors are a fast, powerful way to help conquer them.

Forming an Anchor

To create an anchor, first sit in a comfortable, quiet place and take some time to relax deeply. Then, vividly imagine yourself thinking, feeling, looking, sounding, and performing with excellence in a specific past circumstance — real-life experiences are best, but imaginary moments are also effective. Keep the mental picture moving in slow motion. "Summon an image of yourself at your best, a time when you were able to respond effortlessly no matter how demanding or intricate the challenge," advises a recent scientific report. "Recall your finest moment in every detail, using every sense . . . etch it into your consciousness so that you can summon it in an instant when facing a crisis."[53]

Develop every aspect of the mental image: Were you indoors or out? In sunlight or shade, clear air, rain, or snow? What was the temperature? Did you notice air currents? What were you wearing and how did it feel on your skin? What could you see in all directions from the surface (hard, soft, cold, warm) where you sat, stood, or lay? What did it smell like there? Forest or floral scents in the air? How did the muscles in your body feel? Were you breathing fast or slow? What were all the sounds around you and off in the distance? And so forth.

At the peak moment of the imagined experience, make a unique sensory signal. For example, choose a touch (such as your thumb against the second knuckle of your index finger with a specific amount of pressure), a mental picture (of yourself in a fluid state of confidence and control, performing at your best), and a sound (a silent, personally meaningful word or phrase — "calm," "confident," "clear mind," "joyful," "creative," "I *can* handle this," or any other choice). This combined sensory signal becomes your anchor.

Wait half an hour or so and repeat the process. Later that day, test your anchor. Re-create the quiet, relaxed scene. Then, as you imagine the first sign of a stressful situation in which you'd like to recapture your sense of the "best moment" state, initiate your anchor by "firing" the sensory signals — in this example we used touch, mental picture, and a cue word. When the anchor works, you will feel a quick surge of energy, inner peace, and confidence. With practice, you can make the anchor stronger.

If your anchor doesn't seem to be effective at first, you probably haven't used a vivid enough image. Rehearse it several more times. Go back through the process of forming the anchor, increasing the richness and brilliance of the scene. How *exactly* did your best moment look, feel, sound, smell? Sense the lighting, colors, shapes, temperatures, textures, movements, tastes, physical sensations, and feelings. Be certain your sensory cues are unique — try modifying your touch or gesture to see how that works.

Examples of Anchoring

We've all had moments of excellence. Those are the experiences to anchor, and add new ones as they arise. Here's an example. If you want to improve your ability to speak before certain individuals or groups of people to advance in your job, you may wish to form an anchor to help you. Sit quietly, relaxing thoroughly. With sensory brilliance, recall a time when you were speaking confidently to another person or a small group, a time when you were excited, communicating clearly and from the heart. Use this image to form your anchor.

But, you may be wondering, how do you form an anchor for situations where it seems you have no related experience? Authorities confirm that you can create anchors by creatively *imagining* a new personal strength and then anchoring that image.

Begin using positive anchors whenever you are faced with a difficult situation. You'll be surprised at how helpful anchors can be in boosting your resourcefulness and responsiveness.

Here's one example. Anchors can make a dramatic difference in relationships. Much traditional psychotherapy focuses on negative attitudes and actions in relationships. The idea is to bring the problems to the surface to better confront them. But each time the hurtful, anxiety-producing actions and events are replayed, the negative anchors associated with them get strengthened. In our communications with loved ones, bringing up negative patterns again and again can add to the relationship's destruction rather than resolution.

Well-known marriage and family therapist Virginia Satir emphasizes positive anchors.[54] Her success record is remarkable. Rather than having a married couple replay a negative situation, Satir first has her clients sit close together and look at each other in the way they did when first falling in love, and then she asks them to begin speaking to each other in that way too.

Throughout her counseling sessions, she creates positive anchors with her voice and touch and has the couple do the same for each other. From this positive state, the two people can better resolve their problems by communicating clearly and not hurting each other's feelings. They can establish — and anchor — such a degree of sensitive caring that they can call on this new pattern to help resolve future problems as well. A growing number of psychophysiologists and psychologists are using and expanding on Satir's anchoring techniques.

Become Aware, Then Practice, Practice

Forming effective anchors takes concentrated effort. Begin to recognize the stimuli that trigger negative anchors in your life. Find ways to reduce their influence and then substitute positive anchors in their place.

Patterning Excellence

Every one of us longs to nurture our hidden talents — those exemplary human qualities we each possess and see occasionally mirrored in exceptional people we meet during our lives. Yet for many reasons, that longing goes unfulfilled. Imagined limitations block our paths.

Competence and excellence, say scientists, can in many cases be transferred from one person to another using a simple set of instructions. In observational (vicarious) learning, or "guided mastery modeling," we help acquire or reinforce a behavioral pattern simply by watching another person. By observing and interacting with peak performers — people who are committed, inspirational, and powerfully active — and patterning their behaviors, we can thereby help change our own lives.

Behaviors and performance can be enhanced through modeling because it "programs neuromuscular traces into the body," says Richard M. Suinn, performance psychologist and chairman of the department of psychology at Colorado State University. "Each time the [individual] rehearses a movement in imagery, the body replicates the experience, possibly storing the results in muscle memory or the right brain hemisphere."[55]

The concept of patterning competence is supported by recent psychological research at the University of London,[56] in health behavior studies,[57] in sports performance research,[58] and in other reports applicable to many dimensions of education, business, and personal life.[59] It is important to realize, of course, that this is but one of many factors in improving behavior and performance.[60]

Take a moment to think about who you have been modeling and what habits you have accepted unconsciously by patterning. Take a close look at the individuals you associate with, the television shows you watch, the ways you spend your time. Carefully observe those whose behavior(s) you wish to emulate — in any physical, emotional, mental, or social way.

"If you want to become more creative as an individual, start spending more time around creative people," advises James L. Adams, chairman of the Values, Technology, Science, and Society Department at Stanford University.[61] Wherever possible, arrange to spend more time with the people you'd like to be more like — those who fit your own definitions for being successful, aware, joyful, health-conscious, well-organized, athletic, artistic, or possessing whatever other qualities you want to draw forth in yourself.

At the same time, reduce the time you spend with people whose behavior distresses, or at least doesn't nurture, you. And cut back on nonproductive television viewing and mind-numbing background music in your home, office, and car. In place of these distractions — which can end up pushing you out of touch with your goals and dreams — devote some quality time to studying new subjects and people who inspire you; use personal contacts, books, audiotapes, and videotapes to learn more about them.

Here are several basic steps to pattern a selected behavior in another person, your "model."

1. Choose your desired outcome, stating it specifically and positively in terms of what you want, instead of what you don't want. Put your goal — thinking ability, attitude, feeling, or skill — in context: *precisely* what you want, where you want it, when you want it, and with whom you want it.

2. Select the person to model, someone who exemplifies your desired outcome. Learn clear, warm-hearted communication skills from a clear, warm-hearted communicator; inner joy and calmness from someone who is joyful and calm; creative art from a creative artist; exemplary sports skills from an exemplary athlete; and so on.

If you stand on the ski slope watching beginning skiers fall down or stand in the lodge laughing at the video collection of the worst spills of the year, without realizing it you're most likely learning to fall down, not ski. That's one reason why Sybervision Systems, Inc. of Newark, California, chose Jean Claude Killy as its video model for downhill skiing, and why it continues to select world-class athletes for each of its sports videotape programs and business leaders to exemplify business success skills.

You certainly don't need to spend time chasing down top-ranked experts in everything. But you *can* make the best available choices in the friends, neighbors, and associates you model, the seminars you elect to take, the books you choose to read, and the movies and videos you spend time watching. That's the key.

3. Elicit all the pertinent information you can — by observation and if possible by asking the model to describe and perhaps give you a step-

by-step demonstration of the behavior you want to reproduce. Get as much detail as possible. Find out everything you can about thought processes, emotions, and physical actions that precede, are part of, and follow the behavior you wish to pattern.

4. Turn this knowledge into action. First relax; then practice slowly, emphasizing perfection. Learning something new takes practice — in some cases lots of it. One determining factor is the clarity of your mental image. "In the early stages of practicing a skilled movement, we begin by contracting many more muscles than we really need," explains Emilio Bizzi, neurophysiologist at MIT. "Gradually, however, through practice, unnecessary movements are eliminated."[62]

Even if you can't find a good model, you can learn new behavior sequences by *imagining* people performing the desired behavior successfully. This is called "covert modeling."[63] Another technique, known as visual motor behavior rehearsal (VMBR), was developed by performance psychologist Richard M. Suinn of Colorado State University. VMBR begins with a slow, well-organized sequence of steps. It is "a total sensory experience which replicates visual, tactile, proprioceptive, emotional, autonomic, and auditory sensations."[64]

VMBR can be used to enhance specific techniques or actions, correct errors, prepare for important events, and increase confidence. When compared in controlled studies to imagery (mental practice) only, and relaxation only, and/or placebo training, VMBR has proved superior.

The basic steps are (1) selecting the scene (in this case the modeled behavior); (2) "centered breathing" and progressive relaxation; (3) vividly visualizing the scene and performance of the behavior you have chosen to emulate, being fully aware of positive bodily sensations such as fluidness, ease, and confidence; and (4) anchoring the results.[65]

Whichever technique you choose, begin by practicing slowly, striving to re-create the perfect movements or behavior qualities you have chosen to pattern. This way your brain has plenty of time to receive and precisely process sensory input. This feedback, says Dr. Bizzi, is essentially a measure of how far the actual movement is from the brain's original intent. If on the other hand, like so many Americans, you practice absentmindedly or haphazardly with lots of uncoordination and errors, your brain and nervous system get bogged down with bad habits. As a result, it's easy to become frustrated and abandon the effort altogether.

RESOURCES

Books

▶ *The Emprint Method: A Guide to Reproducing Competence* by Leslie Cameron-Bandler, David Gordon, and Michael Lebeau (FuturePace, Inc., P.O. Box 1173, San Rafael, CA 94915; 1985).

▶ *Peak Performance: Mental Training Techniques of the World's Greatest Athletes* by Charles A. Garfield, Ph.D. (Warner Books, 1984).

▶ *Peak Performers: The New Heroes of American Business* by Charles A. Garfield, Ph.D. (Morrow, 1986).

▶ *Seven Steps to Peak Performance* by Richard M. Suinn, Ph.D. (Hans Huber Publishing, P.O. Box 51, Lewiston, NY 14092; 1986). Excellent manual for athletes.

▶ *Software for the Mind* by Emmett E. Miller, M.D. (Celestial Arts, 1987). Practical book with ideas for turning negative mental-emotional conditioning into positive.

Achievement-Oriented Audiotape and Videotape Programs

▶ Advanced Excellence Systems (P.O. Box 1085, Bemidji, MN 56601; 218-854-7300).

▶ Blanchard Training and Development, Inc. (125 State Pl., Escondido, CA 92025; 619-489-5005).

▶ Nightingale-Conant Corporation (7300 N. Lehigh Ave., Chicago, IL 60648; 800-323-5552).

▶ Performance Sciences, Inc. (3921 E. Bayshore Rd., Suite 201, Palo Alto, CA 94303; 415-960-0700).

▶ Source Cassette Learning Systems (P.O. Box W, Stanford, CA 94309; 415-328-7171).

▶ Sybervision Systems, Inc. (Fountain Square, 6066 Civic Terrace Ave., Newark, CA 94560; 800-255-9666).

▶ Whole Person Associates, Inc. (P.O. Box 3151, Duluth, MN 55803; 218-728-6807).

47 Mind-Emotions-Immunity: Science Discovers Your Inner Healer

New knowledge about the brain is transforming our understanding of why we get sick and what to do about it.

— *BLAIR JUSTICE, PH.D.,*
WHO GETS SICK?

Scientists have begun to confirm what many people have suspected for centuries: our thoughts and emotions influence our immune system's ability to protect us from disease. "The relations between emotion and immunity may prove to be another strong argument for a return towards whole-person medicine," says a recent editorial in the *Lancet,* one of Great Britain's leading medical journals, reflecting a growing consensus in some medical circles.[66]

Beliefs, moods, mental attitudes, explanatory style, hardiness, and self-talk habits all play a role — scientists have yet to calculate precisely how large a role — in determining how susceptible you are to certain illnesses, how quickly you recover, and — in serious diseases — perhaps your very survival.

While there is still much we don't know about the relationship of brain, mind, emotions, body, environment, and society, scientists are making the connections clearer. New research areas have opened up, attracting social psychologists, psychiatrists, experimental psychologists, immunologists, neuroendocrinologists, neuroanatomists, oncologists, biologists, epidemiologists, pharmacologists, and many other professionals.

One of the new specialty areas is neuroimmunomodulation, which attempts to determine the manner and degree to which the brain and immune system interact. Another discipline, psychoneuroimmunology (PNI), examines interactions among stress, change, brain reactions, immune function, psychological interpretation of events, and the relationship of thoughts to wellness.

While the results are not yet conclusive, compelling studies now link the mind, emotions, and immunity.[67] Research suggests the following:

▶ The immune system is affected by mismanaged minor daily hassles and tends to weaken following severe psychological stress.

▶ Pessimism, negative personal beliefs, disillusion, despair, and a sense of helplessness in day-to-day life can weaken the immune system.

▶ Tumors grow more rapidly in animals exposed to uncontrolled stress than in those exposed to pressures they can control.

▶ The onset and course of viral infections may be linked with stress-reduced immune processes.

▶ Feelings, expressed or not, can be associated with immune system function and the course of disease.

These studies confirming popular folk wisdom would be pretty discouraging except that we have also learned we can do something about it. In more and more cases, evidence confirms that we can voluntarily improve our immune function by improving our emotional and mental health.

"An explosion of knowledge in the neurosciences has uncovered dozens of chemical messengers that the brain uses for its far-ranging influence in the body and communication between cells," says Blair Justice, professor at the University of Texas Health Sciences Center and author of *Who Gets Sick? Thinking and Health*. "Among these potent compounds are stress hormones and fast-acting neurotransmitters that vary in magnitude or kind depending — at least, in part — on our attitudes, moods and ways of reacting to problems. . . . Throughout the body, the systems most important to our health — the brain, the glands and the immune system — connect up and communicate . . . by way of 'informational substances,' chemical messenger molecules that are exquisitely sensitive to our thoughts and reactions."[68, 69] Studies report that we can even control single cells with our thoughts.[70]

"We are entering a new level in the scientific understanding of mechanisms by which faith, belief, and imagination can actually unlock the mysteries of healing," observes Joan Borysenko, cofounder of the Mind/Body Clinic at Boston's Beth Israel Hospital and author of *Minding the Body, Mending the Mind*. "What we see . . . is a rich and intricate two-way communication system linking the mind, the immune system, and potentially all other systems, a pathway through which our emotions — our hopes and fears — can affect the body's ability to defend itself."[71]

Germs Alone Aren't Enough

Contrary to popular belief, in most cases we don't "catch" illnesses. Viruses and bacteria usually need other contributing factors — such as weakened immune response, low moods, and inadequate coping — to produce illness. Disease is bio-psycho-social, which means that an individual's body, mind, and environment together determine whether he or she gets sick.[72]

According to Justice, "Disease is not so much the effect of noxious, external forces — the 'bugs,' both literal and figurative in our lives — as it is the faulty efforts of our minds and bodies to deal with them.[73] Most of the 'bugs,' the literal kind, already reside in our bodies. When our responses to problems in life are excessive or deficient, the central nervous system and hormones act on our immune defenses in such a way that the microbes aid and abet disease. The balance is upset between us and our resident pathogens."[74]

And it's not just the big hassles that hurt our disease resistance, it's the little daily ups and downs too.[75] New studies suggest that "minor, daily mood fluctuations are associated with immune functioning."[76]

Hopefulness and Hardiness: Two Factors That Really Matter

Our mental outlook affects the stress burden we feel.[77] Research indicates that individuals who handle life's stress pressures in an immature way tend to become ill much more often than those who handle stress positively. According to Harvard University psychiatrist George E. Vaillant, the degree to which we are able to master stress and remain in touch with our innermost feelings and thoughts may turn out to be as strong a predictor of heart disease as smoking cigarettes.[78]

Our psychological reactions are related to how much stress we perceive ourselves to be under and how much control, if any, we feel we have over the circumstances in our life. The attitude of helplessness that typifies pessimists is associated with weakening of the immune system's protection against infections and tumors.[79]

Demoralized, joylessly striving people who are cynical about life appear to be even more susceptible to heart disease than those with classic type A behavior, according to a recent study published in the *New England Journal of Medicine*.[80] The researchers found that it may be clusters of negative thoughts and emotions that can push the immune function out of balance, causing it to underact or overact.

The early, simplistic medical view of the body as an automaton is being discarded by a growing number of scientists around the world. One outspoken supporter of the mind-emotions-immune system connection is Candace B. Pert, chief of brain biochemistry at the Clinical Neuro-science Branch of the National Institute of Mental Health. Pert, her colleagues, and other top researchers have been studying neuropeptides, small protein-like chemicals made by cells in the brain.[81] The endorphins, one type of neuropeptide, are joy-related neurochemicals that have been frequently discussed in recent years.

Neuropeptides, which Pert describes as the biochemical units of mood and emotional tone, exist in high concentrations in the brain's main control center for emotions: the limbic system. "I believe that *neuropeptides* [which are secreted by the brain, the immune system, and nerve cells in various other organs and tissues of the body] and their receptors are a key to understanding how mind and body are interconnected and how emotions can be manifested throughout the body," says Pert. "These emotion-affecting chemicals actually appear to control the routing and migration of monocytes [special cells], which are so pivotal in the immune system. . . . The more I look, the more I'm convinced that emotions are running the show."[82]

"Thoughts, beliefs, imaginations are not ephemeral abstractions but electrochemical events with physiological consequences," adds Justice. Researchers have forged the link between mind, emotions, and health. A sense of helplessness, hostility, distrust, cynicism, or despair can depress the immune response and increase the risk of illness and death. In contrast, a sense of control, openness to change, and an attitude of involvement can increase resistance to disease.[83]

RESOURCES

To learn more about discoveries in the mind-emotions-immunity field, see the periodicals given in the Resource list at the end of this book and the following publications:

▶ *Healing Yourself: A Step-by-Step Program for Better Health through Imagery* by Martin L. Rossman, M.D. (Walker, 1987). A clear, pragmatic manual for guided mental imagery in the healing process.

▶ *In Self-Defense: The Human Immune System — The New Frontier in Medicine* by Steven B. Mizel and Peter Jaret (Harcourt Brace Jovanovich, 1985). An intriguing descriptive journey into the human immune system.

▶ *Minding the Body, Mending the Mind* by Joan Borysenko, Ph.D. (Addison-Wesley, 1987). A very practical book by the director of the Mind/Body Clinic at Boston's Beth Israel Hospital. Recommendations on changing attitudes and ways of living, eliciting a relaxation response through meditation, breathing, and related exercises.

▶ *Who Gets Sick? How Thoughts, Moods and Beliefs Affect Your Health* by Blair Justice, Ph.D. (J. P. Tarcher, 1988). This highly readable encyclopedic book on thinking and health was written by an award-winning medical writer and professor at the University of Texas Health Sciences Center. It focuses more on clear, useful information than on advice. Justice has divided the book into five sections: Germs and Stress, Neurotransmitters, Coping, Vulnerability, and Self-Repair.

If your personal physician or psychologist is presently unreceptive to the concepts in this chapter, the following reference books — in addition to the publications listed above — may go far in increasing his or her awareness of recent scientific discoveries.

▶ *Mind and Immunity: Behavioral Immunology,* edited by Steven E. Locke, M.D., and Mady Hornig-Rohan (Institute for the Advancement of Health, 16 E. 53rd St., New York, NY 10022; 212-832-8282; 1983). An annotated bibliography of 1,453 scientific and medical studies from 1976 to 1982.

▶ *Psychological and Behavioral Treatments for Disorders Associated with the Immune System,* edited by Steven E. Locke, M.D. (Institute for the Advancement of Health, 1986). Annotated bibliography of 1,479 recent scientific and medical studies has been edited by Dr. Locke, faculty member at Harvard University Medical School.

▶ *Psychological and Behavioral Treatments for Disorders of the Heart and Blood Vessels,* edited by Mady Hornig-Rohan and Steven E. Locke, M.D. (Institute for the Advancement of Health; 1985). Annotated bibliography of 916 recent scientific and medical studies.

48 Developing Your Brain/Mind at Any Age

Man's mind, once stretched by a new idea, never goes back to its original dimensions.

— *OLIVER WENDELL HOLMES*

No magic pill unlocks the further reaches of brain power. Only a wide array of mental challenges will enable each of us to break down the barriers to our mind's optimal function. Exercises to develop the brain benefit the nervous system, of course, but they also enhance the health, fitness, and longevity of your entire body and can pay great dividends in terms of performance and accomplishments in life.

Beyond IQ

We are smarter than we think, say the experts. The human brain has levels of thought that go far beyond intelligence quotient (IQ). What's more, your mental powers can steadily increase with age.

Intelligence may be broadly defined as the capacity to learn. *Learning* is the acquisition of new knowledge — personal, interpersonal, environmental, societal, and more. *Memory* is the retention of knowledge. And *thinking* is the operating skill with which intelligence and knowledge act on experience for a purpose, applied to life's experiences and challenges.

Until recently, most intelligence experts thought that brain/mind development stopped in late adolescence and that adults reached their peak intelligence by about age twenty. That theory is now being challenged.

IQ tests have been used as standard mental measurements since the early 1900s. Based largely on studies of children, the results of those tests have been widely applied to adults. At best, IQ has an incomplete relationship to intelligence. At worst, it has little correlation at all. Neuroscientists have discovered a number of new stages of intellectual growth that continue throughout our lives.

Among those leading the fight to abolish the IQ test, or at least put it in proper perspective, are psychologists Howard Gardner of Harvard University and Robert Sternberg of Yale University. In his book *Frames of Mind: The Theory of Multiple Intelligences,* Gardner defines an intelligence as "the ability to solve problems, or create products, that are valued within one or more cultural settings." He introduces eight distinct criteria for measuring intelligence and proposes seven human competences that fulfill those criteria. Three of the seven are intellectual in the traditional view — linguistic, spatial, and logical-mathematical. The others — bodily-kinesthetic, musical, self-knowledge, and social adroitness — take into account the variety of ways people excel using their mind.

In *Beyond IQ: A Triarchic Theory of Human Intelligence,* Sternberg emphasizes the *practical intelligence* that's sorely missing from traditional IQ theories and schoolroom skills. He suggests three distinct dimensions of intelligence: internal problem-solving ability, practical day-to-day skills that reflect "common sense," and the ability to creatively face new challenges and assimilate the experiences.

These new theories of intelligence underscore the lifelong need to activate the brain and senses in a wide variety of ways to keep our minds developing and flourishing. "A brain cell needs to be stimulated," says Marian Diamond, neurophysiologist at the University of California at Berkeley. "If you cut off that stimulation, you lose the dimensions of that cell. . . . You lift weights to get more efficient muscles, and you challenge the brain to get more efficient brain cells."[84]

Age Is No Barrier

Learning actually changes the qualities of nerve cell endings and increases the strength of nerve impulse transmission.[85] Scientists project that a major part of the neurological deficits attributed to "aging" are really the result of a lack of stimulation of the nerves involved with learning. Becoming a lifelong learner has never looked so important.

Aging business executives whose work required sharp concentration and diversified intellectual focus showed little or no weakening of their brain and nervous system when compared in a recent study with production workers of the same age.[86]

The human brain is much more capable of longevity than was once thought. Even in our later years, from the time we reach sixty into our nineties, brain cells can keep creating new growth connections, reports Paul Coleman of the University of Rochester.[87] In long-term studies of humans, it has been shown that people who continue to actively develop their intellectual abilities can keep improving on intelligence tests beyond their sixtieth birthday[88] and probably well into their nineties.[89]

There can be an actual increase in the dendrites — key parts of nerve cells — in the cortex of the aged brain, report neuroscientists at the University of California at Berkeley.[90] Changes have also been measured in the synapses, the gaps between nerve cells where information is exchanged and the nerve cell is either fired into action or blocked from reacting. Specific learning activities not only resulted in adding or subtracting synapses but in altering the strength of such contacts. After studying three thousand people over a period of years, Pennsylvania State University researchers reported that people who lead active, challenging lives show little or no deterioration in word recognition and usage, the ability to solve problems, and the ability to adjust to unfamiliar situations, even when they're in their sixties or seventies.[91]

The central message is clear: *You must regularly challenge all aspects of your brain to expand its performance and slow or prevent its aging.* Here are some important additions to the recommendations for learning, performance, sensory-enhancement, and memory skills presented in earlier chapters of *Health & Fitness Excellence*.

Mind-Body Integration

When most people think of building mind power, they think of mental exercises. But you can also strengthen your mind by developing your body. The more sensitively aware the surface of your body is and the more fit your muscles, the larger the "map" in your brain. Recent discoveries suggest that this map can be expanded in many directions and at virtually any age. For example, you can augment the area of the brain assigned to your fingers simply by increasing and varying the use of your fingers.[92]

A deterioration of the cerebellum area of the brain is now associated with many common aspects of aging — slowness of movement, poor pacing, loss of coordination and balance.[93] How do you prevent this decline? In part, by strengthening existing movement patterns and adding new ones.

To increase your overall coordination, choose a variety of regular physical exercises and sensory enhancement techniques. Beyond that, any safe activity that challenges your balance and coordination can be beneficial. Playing the piano, hand-eye coordination drills, stacking coins, using tweezers to pick up small objects, playing jacks, completing puzzles requiring you to trace through dot-to-dot, connect-the-numbers, mazes, and so on, are among the exercises recommended by neuroscientists for improving hand dexterity and hand-eye coordination.[94]

Activities like these help develop *fluid intelligence*.[95] Also known as performance intelligence, fluid intelligence is essentially nonverbal and involves the timing and integration of muscular movements and sensory acuity in situations where reaction speed and quick judgment are important. In contrast, *crystallized intelligence* — also called verbal intelligence — depends on well-established habits of judgment and experience to solve problems. Sudden, unexpected changes cannot be handled by this aspect of the mind.

To a great extent, fluid intelligence depends on physical fitness and nervous system proficiency, which require that we pursue challenging mental and physical activities throughout our lives. At both young and older ages, more fit individuals consistently display higher levels of fluid intelligence.[96]

Creativity and Problem-Solving Skills

To endure life's parade of challenges and particularly to thrive in it, we must be able to create and change. "Not only do we seek more creativity and change for winning and for stimulation, but our environment also changes over time and, if we do not accommodate, the strain becomes intolerable," writes Stanford University professor James L. Adams in *The Care and Feeding of Ideas*.[97]

Creativity is shrouded in myth. For millions of us, it's as mysterious as sex appeal or charisma. But there's no need for it to be puzzling. Creativity is the ability, the learned skill, to form something new — a thought, emotion, perception, or behavior. Creativity is related to variety, which researchers say is the spice of memory. In fact, much age-related memory loss can reportedly be prevented if people seek a great diversity of fun-filled, challenging activities.[98]

Creativity is more than simply generating new ideas. "Over the years I've become increasingly frustrated with the belief that more ideas alone mean better results," says Adams. "If you're serious about encouraging creativity in yourself or others and if you want to deal with change effectively, then implementing ideas is at least as important as generating ideas. You need to understand the entire process — from concept to reality."[99]

Your Inner Creative Resource

The creative process begins when you face a problem or need and moves in a variety of ways through a series of stages, say Stanford University professors Michael Ray and Rochelle Myers, "consisting of information-gathering, digestion of the material, incubation or forgetting the problem, sudden inspiration (when the conditions are idiosyncratically right), and, finally, implementation."[100]

In *Creativity and Business,* Ray and Myers point out that creativity consists of intuition (a direct knowing without conscious reasoning), will (the part of you that can take responsibility), joy (which you receive from creativity in spite of all the hard work it entails), and strength (which you need to break through the wall of fear and criticism that might otherwise stop you).

Virtually every aspect of *Health & Fitness Excellence* contributes to the physical, emotional, and mental harmony that leads to creative insights. One recent study, for example, confirmed that regular bouts of aerobic exercise spark brainstorms of creative thinking. The researchers concluded that exercise is "not frills, but should be central to our learning and educational processes."[101]

According to Professor Adams, key principles of increased creativity include the following.[102]

1 When solving problems remain aware that the information you have in your mind is not complete and not identical to that of those around you.

2 Be aware that your brain would like to follow a traditional pattern — to simplify your life by applying solutions that have successfully worked before. Be grateful for that, but suspicious that the creativity you are looking for may not occur automatically.

3 The brain is efficient in business-as-usual situations. It is able to make use of past experience and apply it quickly and unconsciously. However, it may be less efficient in new situations.

4 Conscious effort is both able and necessary to pursue new directions. Perspiration is, in fact, an excellent investment.

Brainstorming. "The ability to analyze and judge the products of our intuition is of crucial importance," writes Philip Goldberg in *The Intuitive Edge.* "But we tend to do it too quickly and peremptorily, forcing premature closure and killing fragile intuitive ideas before they have a chance to develop and reproduce. . . . To counteract this critical urge, it is a good idea to set aside a judgment-free period for generating solutions to specific problems. *Brainstorming,* created by Alex Osborn in 1948, is a formal method . . . where the collective interaction yields extra power because each person's thoughts spark the others'. The rules are easily enforced, and the principles can be adapted to individual use. There are essentially four rules":[103]

1 There is to be no judgment or criticism of any ideas presented. Evaluation is done in a subsequent session. Otherwise you interfere with the creative flow.

2 Quantity is desirable; the more ideas the better. As the Chinese proverb states, The best way to catch a fish is to have many lines.

3 No idea is too bizarre, too wild, or too irrelevant. The purpose is not to be correct but to fuel the process of generating imaginative alternatives.

4 Combinations, modifications, and improvements on previously mentioned ideas are encouraged.

Once the facts are in, decide yes or no right away. Life comes down to the decisions we make. Big ones and little ones, all day long. Good decisions are clear-sighted and tend to produce positive action. Bad decisions are often made from poor perceptions and result in inappropriate action. The most paralyzing decision of all, however — and one far too many people specialize in making — is no decision.

"The correct decision is always within, waiting to express itself," say Ray and Myers. "Living with yes/no develops a positive attitude about change. At its base, procrastinating about decisions because of fear of making mistakes is really an attempt to avoid change. In contrast, love of change characterizes successful . . . people, even the change that comes from what others might think of as a mistake."[104] Once the facts are in, decide yes or no and move on.

Sidestepping creativity-stifling criticism. When you come up with new ideas, you invite criticism. This criticism ultimately causes many of us to forgo even our fondest dreams and projects. One way to head off critical remarks or deal with them more effectively is to anticipate such responses, says Vincent R. Ruggiero, professor at the State University of New York. This can help us prevent discouragement when we hear them and enable us to improve certain aspects of our ideas before making them public. In his book *The Art of Thinking*, Ruggiero suggests knowing — and perhaps changing — your ideas in advance if they are impractical; too expensive; illegal; immoral; inefficient; unworkable; disruptive of existing procedures; unesthetic; too radical; unappealing to others; or prejudiced against one side of a dispute.[105]

RESOURCES

▶ *Care and Feeding of Ideas: A Guide to Encouraging Creativity* by James L. Adams (Addison-Wesley, 1986). Adams is chairman of the Values, Technology, Science, and Society Department at Stanford University and author of the best-selling book *Conceptual Blockbusting: A Guide to Better Ideas*.

▶ *Creativity in Business* by Michael Ray and Rochelle Myers (Doubleday, 1986). One of my favorite books on creativity, written by two innovative Stanford University business professors.

▶ *Lateral Thinking: Creativity Step by Step* by Edward de Bono (Harper Colophon, 1973). A classic.

49 Life Unity

ONE GOAL THROUGHOUT this book has been to chart a new direction that points toward integration of knowledge about health, fitness, and performance. The word *integrated* means "lacking nothing essential." It symbolizes filling in empty spaces, completing the whole picture. When we step back and look at *Health & Fitness Excellence* and how the seven steps complement each other, it becomes clear that the golden circle awaits a final thread: life unity.

According to *Webster's, unity* is "the quality or state of ONENESS; a totality of related parts; an entity that is a . . . systematic whole." Life unity is more than a quality of thinking, feeling, and doing. It is a quality of *being*. It encompasses elements overlooked in nearly all traditional health programs.

"[In] our current collective approach to health promotion," writes health educator Larry S. Chapman, "we generally feel somewhat embarrassed to mention things like love, joy, peace, sense of purpose, connectedness, reverence for living or achieving one's full potential in the context of most health promotion programs. Should we not strive to broaden our concept of health promotion to include these kinds of issues? After all, what is life worth if there is no love in it? Or joy? Or peace? Or an overriding sense of purpose? Or connectedness to others? Or the goal of being all that we can be? Are we only interested in prolonging life and unclogging arteries? I hope not."[106]

We are living at a turning point in history, a time of unprecedented challenges and opportunities. Our society is whirling with change and complexity. Stress meters read "overload." But it's actually a blessing in disguise, a new kind of energy that we can learn to guide wisely — to keep us growing, flourishing, moving toward our higher potentials.

Here are several final considerations.

Meaningful Living

Strong beliefs and sense of purpose have profound effects on health.[107] The search for meaning in life is as old as humanity. But in recent years this search has turned into a crisis, reflected in the large number of young adults who are "isolated, self-centered, tolerant of everything and committed to nothing." Those are the words of University of Chicago professor Allan Bloom, author of *The Closing of the American Mind*. Bloom and others are convinced that institutes of higher education have become like factories and this has impoverished the intellectual lives of millions of Americans and led to "a loss of deep significance in the choices we make."

"There is philosophic wonderment," says Bloom. "Around us people say, 'I'm getting my act together,' 'I'm just being myself,' 'These are my values.' But there is an enormous sense of emptiness in our talking about what it means to live. We are obviously disconnected, and all this is a script written by Nietzsche."[108] That's philosopher Friedrich Nietzsche, who said, "If we have our own *why* of life, we shall get along with almost any *how*."[109] Is *your* "why of life" clear?

Getting in Closer Touch with Your Inner Direction

There are many ways to clarify the values, mission, and meaning in our lives. I'd like to share one example from my work for several years with elderly people — hundreds of wonderful individuals who were, in their own minds, nearing the end of their lives and suddenly aware of that "enormous sense of emptiness" of which Professor Bloom speaks.

Here's a pearl of wisdom that came to light from their collective experiences: Beginning as early as possible in your adult life, regularly — perhaps once every month or two — enter in a diary your observations under the heading "How I want to be remembered at the end of my life." Then ask yourself whether you are devoting some time every single day to living that kind of life.

It's easy to forget that time passes so quickly. How many people have awakened at age sixty, seventy, or eighty to realize that they haven't stopped once in all those years to clearly match the direction of their lives with the values and purpose deep in their hearts? Act right now to commit some time every week — best of all, every day — to "Activities from the Heart."

Again and again I have heard retirees say, "If only I had paused several times a day to be certain I was taking the best care of myself and supporting the people around me," "If only television hadn't pulled me away from my family and close friends," "If only I had taken that extra time on weekends to help young children the way I wanted to," "If only I had written one postcard every week to a politician, school board member, person in charge of a cause I believed in, or someone who did something worthwhile in my community," and so on. "If only . . . " life could have been — *and can be* — so different, so meaningful.

Love

Love is the pursuit of the whole.

— *PLATO*

Love is a dazzling, intriguing mixture of caring, inner joy, expansiveness, and concern. The experience of love changes thinking, feelings, and lives. Nearly all of us seek love, yet few of us believe we ever truly attain it or learn how to keep it. This a gripping, disturbing point since the quest for love speaks to us all.

While good health habits are important to staying healthy, being loved and giving love are just as important. Scientists are finding that love can bolster our resistance to disease and speed healing.[110] The edict "Love your neighbor as you love yourself" is more than just a moral mandate, it's a physiological and psychological mandate. We *need* to live with compassion, we need to care.[111]

"Love is not primarily a relationship to a specific person; it is an *attitude,* an *orientation of character* which determines the relatedness of a person to the world as a whole, not toward one 'object' of love," writes Erich Fromm. "If I truly love one person I love all persons, I love the world, I love life. If I can say to somebody else, 'I love you,' I must be able to say, 'I love in you everybody, I love through you the world, I love in you also myself.'"

Reflect for a moment: In what specific ways can you become more compassionate, more loving to yourself and others?

Sense of Community

One often overlooked factor in health and well-being is a sense of community.[112] Throughout history, extended families, tribal networks, farming cooperatives, small villages, rural townships, and neighborhood enclaves in metropolitan areas all have served as communities. Earlier, we reviewed ways that social support boosts our sense of control and improves our health. But community goes beyond the social aspects of a close-knit network of family and friends. It also provides a shared vision and strengthens our sense of permanence and continuity, our roots. This attachment to home, place, or religion has been shown to help neutralize stress and promote inner joy and meaningful living.[113]

Until recent years in America, neighborhoods often filled our need for a sense of community. Here the spirit of helpfulness and altruism was nurtured outside the immediate family. But in recent decades our society has become more urban, transient, technological, and wealth-oriented. People have begun to lose contact with their community. Individual freedom and social isolation have grown in direct proportion.

"A close-knit community can act as a protective envelope against the stresses of the environment," says psychologist Dennis T. Jaffe. "Evidence is mounting that overinvolvement with oneself, at the expense of the community, leads to psychological dislocation that results not only in anxiety, but in various psychological ailments as well."[114]

"You may have been raised believing that if everyone concentrated primarily on his or her own self-interest, the community as a whole would prosper," adds Jaffe. "Yet take a look at the world around you. Has commitment to the self created the paradise we've sought? The communities in which we live show that signs of decay, marriage and other forms of personal commitment are dispensable, and few individuals are concerned about the environment as a whole. In general, our sense of collective purpose and meaning is languishing."

A 13-year study of people between the ages of sixty and ninety-four concluded that maintaining a useful and satisfying role in society is one of the most important ways to enhance longevity.[115] French studies of seven hundred people (with documented ages of one hundred or more) typically found these individuals to be enthusastic and interested in public affairs.[116]

One recent study on altruism concluded that an attitude of selflessness made it 2.4 times more likely that an individual would be happy, whereas an attitude of selfishness made it 9.5 times more likely that the person would be unhappy.[117]

Findings like these have led researchers to propose that the need for community is part of our evolutionary heritage. In *The Healing Brain*, Drs. Robert Ornstein and David Sobel present a convincing argument that one of the brain's primary purposes is to guard the body against illness — and part of the formula for this protection is "community." According to Ornstein and Sobel: "It now appears that the brain cannot do its job of protecting the body without contact with other people. It draws vital nourishment from our friends, lovers, relatives, lodge brothers and sisters, even perhaps our co-workers and the members of our weekly bowling team."[118]

It begins with helping others, say Ram Dass and Paul Gormon in *How Can I Help? Stories and Reflections on Service.* "At times, helping happens simply in the way of things. Caring is a reflex. Someone slips, your arm goes out. A car is in the ditch, you join the others and push. It all seems natural and appropriate. You live, you help."[119]

People in all walks of life have overcome pain and gained strength and happiness through service to others in need, reminding us how much we have to give and how serving others can lead to some of the most joyous and satisfying moments of our lives.

"We can, of course, help through all that we *do*," say Dass and Gormon. "But at the deepest level we help through who we *are*. We help by appreciating the connection between service and our own progress on the journey of awakening. We work on ourselves in order to help others. And we help others as a vehicle for working on ourselves."

One inspiring newsletter called *Regeneration* (33 E. Minor St., Emmaus, PA 18098) reports on ways that individuals, families, neighborhoods, and communities across America are working together to regenerate and revitalize their way of life. This periodical highlights ways to create thriving local and regional economies that are both self-generating and self-improving.

For all of us with a global view of community, Windstar Foundation (Box 286, Snowmass, CO 81654) merits our attention. This nonprofit foundation publishes the *Windstar Journal* and provides on-site educational programs in renewable energy and food production technologies, land stewardship and global resource management, conflict resolution, international citizen exchange, and personal and community growth.

Spiritual Wellness

When you awaken or renew your awareness of the spiritual aspect of life, the world around you appears in a new light. The beauty of nature is harder to overlook, love and compassion have room to grow, children's effervescent excitement becomes more of a wonder to behold and less of a mutinous commotion to be silenced, rush-hour traffic jams and airline delays are better tolerated, conflicts are more easily resolved, and the meaning of life peeks up at us over the top of our daily to-do lists and monthly budgets.

Spiritual wellness is vital to *Health & Fitness Excellence*. The body, emotions, mind, and spirit are integral parts of every human being. Although most commonly nurtured through organized religions, spiritual wellness can certainly thrive independent of them. It is both a personal and global concern, reaching from families to communities and from business organizations to entire nations.

In an *American Journal of Health Promotion* article entitled "Spiritual Health: A Component Missing from Health Promotion," Larry S. Chapman suggests a definition for *spiritual health:* "Optimal spiritual health may be considered as the ability to develop our spiritual nature to its fullest potential. This would include our ability to discover and articulate our own basic purpose in life, learn how to experience love, joy, peace and fulfillment and how to help ourselves and others achieve their full potential."[120]

Spirituality encompasses faith, which in its truest sense goes far beyond platitudes. Faith is what your heart tells you is true when your mind can't prove it. It's one of the final extensions of your powers of perception, your higher self.

Many of us benefit greatly from setting aside time every day — even just a minute or two — for spiritual renewal, for our own personal choice of prayer, meditation, contemplation, or reflection.

There are many spiritual paths. Whichever is yours, follow it, exemplify it. I deeply hope that in the years ahead a far greater sense of *spiritual oneness* will be felt around the world; that people of various religions, faiths, and beliefs will transcend their differences. There is a pressing need for world religions to join together in fostering global spirituality, forging an alignment based on spiritual similarities, of which there are so many. This may be the only way to create a unified humanitarian response to the crises of our time.

Global Consciousness, Local Action

As you can well see by now, *Health & Fitness Excellence* isn't a path for fanatics. It's a program about balance, integration, opportunities, and actions. We are about to enter the twenty-first century with a culture in which many of the brightest people have become obsessed with caring for their bodies and minds — at the same time that the world around them is falling apart due to a lack of mutual caring.

Of course, individual good health habits are vital — look around you and you will see people jogging, meditating, lifting weights, growing their own vegetables and fruits, and taking all kinds of other actions to improve their health, enhance their performance, and promote longevity. But while all of this is happening, as valuable as it may be, many of these same individuals are showing little concern for the health and well-being of the planet from which their food derives and of which they are a part.

The ability to create a worldwide commitment to wellness resides within each of us as individuals and can flourish only when we take action to make it a reality.

I have come to realize that the planetary goals I believe in — right human relations, peace, and the end of hunger, homelessness, and despair — can't simply be proclaimed or legislated. Mahatma Gandhi said: "You must *be* the change you wish to see in the world." You must *be* the health, fitness, integrity, compassion, cooperation, performance, and peace that you wish to see in the world. Global changes are the collective reflection of personal inner development.

Conclusion

One scientific message is loud and clear: Human excellence can become far more than a trite accolade. It's time to begin weaving it into the fabric of society, into every aspect of our daily lives. In closing, I would like to share a short message I wrote for my son, Christopher, about my philosophy of *Health & Fitness Excellence:*

The influence that each of us has
   on the hours, days, months, and years ahead
is created each new moment
   — moment by moment by moment —
in our perceptions, thoughts, images, attitudes,
   words, emotions, and actions.
What are *you* choosing to perceive, to think, to imagine, to believe,
   to say, to feel, and to do?

The world of tomorrow
will be better in direct proportion
to the excellence you bring
to each fleeting instant of time.

May you always remain aware
that the greatest contributions you can make
— to yourself, to your loved ones, to your work, to humanity —
begin, are nurtured, and are expressed
   right now, right now, right now . . . .
because *right now* is the only time on earth that is ever truly yours.

If you choose *Health & Fitness Excellence*
then you must choose it again and again.
It isn't a faraway goal or endpoint.
It's a day-by-day, moment-by-moment opportunity.

So what will it be?
"Common" and "normal" — or what's truly possible?
Myths, fads, fragments, and tangents —
or a philosophy and action plan based on the whole picture?

The choice is up to you.

I wish the brightest and best for you, my reader, this moment and always.

Resources

In this rapidly changing world, it's important to stay up to date on scientific developments in health, fitness, performance, cooperation, and achievement. The following periodicals, listed alphabetically within general categories, may prove very valuable in this regard. Write each publication for descriptive information and current subscription rates.

General Health Education, Wellness, and Medical Resources

► *American Health* (P.O. Box 3016, Harlan, IA 51593).
► *American Journal of Health Promotion* (746 Purdy St., Birmingham, MI 48009).
► *The Edell Health Letter* (Dean Edell, M.D., P.O. Box 57812, Boulder, CO 80322).
► *FDA Consumer* (Superintendent of Documents, Government Printing Office, Washington, DC 20402).
► *Harvard Medical School Health Letter* (P.O. Box 10945, Des Moines, IA 50340).
► *Health* (P.O. Box 359030, Palm Coast, FL 32035).
► *Health Values: Achieving High Level Wellness* (Slack, Inc., 6900 Grove Rd., Thorofare, NJ 08086).
► *Healthlines* (University of Michigan Fitness Research Center, 401 Washtenaw, Ann Arbor, MI 48109).
► *Healthy Living* (2727 Fairview Ave., E., Seattle, WA 98102).
► *Hippocrates: Magazine of Health & Medicine* (P.O. Box 52431, Boulder, CO 80321).
► *Medical Self-Care Journal* (349 Healdsburg Ave., Healdsburg, CA 95448).
► *Melpomene: A Journal of Women's Health Research* (2125 E. Hennepin Ave., Minneapolis, MN 55413).
► *Omni Longevity* (P.O. Box 11301, Des Moines, IA 50340).
► *The People's Medical Society Newsletter* (14 E. Minor St., Emmaus, PA 18049).
► *Prevention* (Emmaus, PA 18099).
► *The Public Citizen Health Research Group Health Letter* (2000 P St., N.W., Washington, DC 20036).

▶ *Sun & Skin News* (Skin Cancer Foundation, 475 Park Ave. So., New York, NY 10016).

▶ *University of California, Berkeley, Wellness Letter* (P.O. Box 10922, Des Moines, IA 50340).

▶ *Wellness Management* (National Wellness Association, South Hall, University of Wisconsin at Stevens Point, Stevens Point, WI 54481).

▶ *The Wellness Newsletter* (3451 Central Ave., St. Petersburg, FL 33713).

Nutrition

▶ *Environmental Nutrition* (52 Riverside Dr., New York, NY 10024).

▶ *Nutrition Action Healthletter* (Center for Science in the Public Interest, 1501 16th St., N.W., Washington, DC 20036).

▶ *Tufts University Diet & Nutrition Letter* (475 Park Ave. So., New York, NY 10016).

Also see *American Health, FDA Consumer, Hippocrates, Medical Self-Care, Prevention,* and *University of California, Berkeley, Wellness Letter.*

Exercise and Fitness

▶ *The Aerobics News* (Institute for Aerobics Research, 12330 Preston Rd., Dallas, TX 75230).

▶ *Dance-Exercise Today* (IDEA, 6190 Cornerstone Court East, Suite 204, San Diego, CA 92121).

▶ *Fitness in Business* (Williams and Wilkins, P.O. Box 23291, Baltimore, MD 21203).

▶ *President's Council on Physical Fitness and Sports Newsletter* (450 5th St., N.W., Washington, DC 20001).

▶ *Shape, Men's Fitness,* and *Muscle & Fitness* (all published by Weider, 21100 Erwin St., Woodland Hills, CA 91367).

▶ *Soviet Sports Review* (P.O. Box 2878, Escondido, CA 92025).

▶ *Sports Research Monthly* (8033 Sunset Blvd., Suite 483, Los Angeles, CA 90046).

▶ *Women's Sports & Fitness* (P.O. Box 472, Mt. Morris, IL 61054).

Also see Resources listed in Chapters 16–19 and *American Health, Healthlines, Medical Self-Care, Prevention,* and *University of California, Berkeley, Wellness Letter.*

Stress-Brain-Mind-Emotions

▶ *Advances* (Institute for the Advancement of Health, 16 E. 53rd St., New York, NY 10022).

▶ *Brain/Mind Bulletin* (Box 70457, Pasadena, CA 91107).

▶ *Journal of Applied Imagery: Applications of the Imaging Process in Health,*

Education, Relationships, Communication, Business, Sports, and Related Areas (P.O. Box 13453, Milwaukee, WI 53213).

▶ *Living Well* (Emmett E. Miller, M.D., P.O. Box W, Stanford, CA 94309).
▶ *The Omni Whole Mind Newsletter* (P.O. Box 11208, Des Moines, IA 50347).
▶ *Psychology Today* (P.O. Box 2562, Boulder, CO 80321).

Also see *American Health, Hippocrates, Medical Self-Care, Omni Longevity,* and *Prevention.*

Posture and Massage Therapy

▶ *Massage Magazine* (P.O. Box 1969, Kealakekua, HI 96750).
▶ *Massage Therapy Journal* (American Massage Therapy Association, 1130 W. North Shore Ave., Chicago, IL 60626).
▶ *Somatics* (1516 Grant Ave., No. 220, Novato, CA 94947).

Also see *American Health, Medical Self-Care,* and *Prevention.*

Environment, Global Wellness, and a Sustainable Future

▶ *East West* (P.O. Box 6769, Syracuse, NY 13217).
▶ *Harrowsmith* (The Creamery, Box 1000, Charlotte, VT 05445).
▶ *Mother Earth News* (P.O. Box 3122, Harlan, IA 51593).
▶ *New Age* (342 Western Ave., Brighton, MA 02135).
▶ *Regeneration* (33 E. Minor St., Emmaus, PA 18098).
▶ *Sierra* (Sierra Club, 530 Bush St., San Francisco, CA 94108).
▶ *Whole Earth Review* (P.O. Box 428, Sausalito, CA 94965).
▶ *Windstar Journal* (P.O. Box 503, Snowmass, CO 81654).
▶ *Worldwatch Institute* (1776 Massachusetts Ave., N.W., Washington, DC 20036).

Also see resources in Chapter 39, *FDA Consumer, Harvard Medical School Health Letter, Nutrition Action, Prevention, Public Citizen Health Letter,* and *University of California, Berkeley, Wellness Letter.*

Notes

Chapters 1–2

1. Haynes, R. B., et al. "How to Keep Up With the Medical Literature." *Annals of Internal Medicine* 105 (2)(Aug. 1986): 309–312.
2. Foege, W. H. "Public Health and Preventive Medicine." *Journal of the American Medical Association* 254 (16)(Oct. 25, 1985): 2330–2332; the Carter Center of Emory University. *Closing the Gap: National Health Policy Consultant* (Atlanta, 1985).
3. Goldsmith, M. *The Science Critic* (New York: Methuen, 1986): 12.
4. Weil, A. *Health and Healing* (Boston: Houghton Mifflin, 1986): 48.
5. Green, L. W. "Health Education Models." In Matarazzo, J. D., et al. (Eds.). *Behavioral Health: A Handbook of Health Enhancement and Disease Prevention* (New York: John Wiley, 1984): 181–198.
6. Taylor, C. W. "Promoting Health Strengthening and Wellness Through Environmental Variables." In Matarazzo et al. *Behavioral Health:* 130–148.
7. Christopher, G. M. Lecture at the Center for Health & Fitness Excellence, Bemidji, MN (Jun. 15, 1987).

Step 1: Stress Strategies (Chapters 3–10)

1. Eliot, R. S. *Is It Worth Dying For?* (New York: Bantam, 1984); Rosch, P. "The Health Effects of Job Stress." *Business and Health* 1 (1984): 5–8.
2. Cummings, N., and VandenBos, G. "The Twenty Year Kaiser-Permanente Experience with Psychotherapy and Medical Utilization." *Health Policy Quarterly* 1 (2)(1981); Elite, A. "Stress Management Program." Internal paper, California Department of Mental Health (Jul. 25, 1986); "Stress: Can We Cope?" *Time* (Jun. 6, 1983): 48; Weiss, J. "Stress: The Invisible Killer." *Gallery* (Feb. 1985): 44.
3. Witkin, G. *The Female Stress Syndrome* (New York: Berkley, 1985): 1.
4. Orioli, M. S., Jaffe, D. T., and Scott, C. D. *StressMap* (New York: Newmarket Press, 1987): 11.
5. Selye, H. *Stress Without Distress* (New York: Signet, 1974): 11.
6. Vaillant, G. E. *Adaptation to Life* (Boston: Little, Brown, 1977).
7. Rozanski, A., et al. "Mental Stress and the Induction of Silent Myocardial Ischemia in Patients with Coronary Artery Disease." *New England Journal of Medicine* 318 (16)(Apr. 21, 1988): 1005–1012; Boston University School of Medicine study, reported in *Internal Medicine News* (Jun. 15–30, 1987); Eliot. *Is It Worth Dying For?*; Baker, G. B. H., et al. "Stress, Cortisol, Interferon and Stress Diseases." *Lancet* 1 (8376)(1984): 574; Cooper, K. H. *Controlling Cholesterol* (New York: Bantam, 1988): 266–273, 310; McClelland, D. C., et al. "Stressed Power Motivation, Sympathetic Activation, Immune Function, and Illness." *Journal of Human Stress* 6 (2)(1985): 11–19; Pelletier, K. R., and Herzing, D. "Psychoneuroimmunology: Toward a Mindbody Model — A Critical Review." *Advances* (Journal of the Institute for the Advancement of Health) 5 (1)(1988): 26–56; "Cholesterol Level Is Affected by Stress: Duke University Research." *Environmental Nutrition* 11 (7)(Jul. 1988): 5.
8. Sapolsky, R. "Glucocorticoids and Hippocampal Damage." *Trends in Neurosciences* 10 (1987); U.S. Department of Health and Human Services. *Special Report on Aging.* NIH No. 80-2135 (Aug. 1980); Troell, S. J. "Cerebral Atrophy in Young Torture Victims." *New England Journal of Medicine* 307 (21) (Nov. 18, 1982): 1341.
9. Winter, A., and Winter, R. *Build Your Brain Power* (New York: St. Martin's Press, 1986): 153.
10. "Research on Stress Hormones: Powerful Agents in Health and Disease." *Salk Institute Newsletter* (Summer 1986): 2–3.
11. Pelletier, K. R., and Lutz, R. "Healthy People — Healthy Business: A Critical Review of Stress Management Programs in the Workplace." *American Journal of Health Promotion* 2 (3)(Winter 1988): 5–12.
12. Brodish, A., et al. *Brain Research* 426 (1987): 37–46.
13. Lazarus, R. S. *American Psychologist,* 30 (1975): 553–561; DeLongis, A., et al. "Relationship of Daily Hassles, Uplifts, and Major Life Events to Health Status." *Health Psychology* 1 (1982): 119–136; Kanner, A. D., et al. "Comparison of Two Modes of Stress Measurement: Daily Hassles and Uplifts Versus Major Life Events." *Journal of Behavioral Medicine* 4 (1981): 1–39.
14. Witkin. *Female Stress:* 12.
15. Witkin, G. *The Male Stress Syndrome* (New York: Newmarket Press, 1986): 2–3.

16. Nathan, R. G., Staats, T. E., and Rosch, P. J. *The Doctors' Guide to Instant Stress Relief* (New York: Putnam's, 1987).

17. Eliot, R. S., quoted in "Stress: Can We Cope?" *Time* (Jun. 6, 1983): 48.

18. Friedman, M., and Ulmer, D. *Treating Type A Behavior and Your Heart* (New York: Knopf, 1984).

19. "Type A Behavior Identified in Women and Children." *Brain/Mind Bulletin* 10 (17)(Oct. 21, 1985).

20. Ragland, D. R., and Brand, R. J., "Type A Behavior and Mortality from Coronary Artery Disease." *New England Journal of Medicine* 318 (2)(Jan. 14, 1988): 65–70.

21. Fischman, J. "Type A on Trial." *Psychology Today* (Feb. 1987): 42–50; Barefoot, J. C., et al. *Psychosomatic Medicine* 45 (1)(1985): 59–64.

22. Maddi, S. R., and Kobasa, S. C. *The Hardy Executive: Health Under Stress* (Homewood, IL: Dow Jones–Irwin, 1984).

23. Borysenko, J. *Minding the Body, Mending the Mind* (Reading, MA: Addison-Wesley, 1987): 24.

24. Kraus, H., and Raab, W. *Hypokinetic Disease* (Springfield, IL: Charles C. Thomas, 1962).

25. Pelletier, K. R. "Reading Your Own Stress Signals." *Medical Self-Care* (Summer 1985): 15.

26. Borysenko. *Minding the Body:* 105.

27. Maslow, A. *The Farther Reaches of Human Nature* (New York: Viking, 1972).

28. Stroebel, C. F. *QR: The Quieting Reflex* (New York: Berkley, 1982): 121; Loehr, J. E., and Midgow, J. A. *Take a Deep Breath* (New York: Villard, 1986): 91–100; Hymes, A., et al. *Science of Breath* (Honesdale, PA: Himalayan Institute, 1979): 47.

29. Hahn, T. N. *The Miracle of Mindfulness* (Boston: Beacon Press, 1976).

30. Borysenko. *Minding the Body:* 37–38, 50.

31. *International Journal of Neuroscience* 16 (1982); Carrington, P., et al. "The Use of Meditation-Relaxation Techniques for the Management of Stress in a Working Population." *Journal of Occupational Medicine* 22 (1980): 221–231; Fiebert, M. S., and Mead, T. M. "Meditation and Academic Performance." *Perceptual and Motor Skills* 53 (1981): 447–450; Hoffman, J. W., et al. "Reduced Sympathetic Nervous System Responsivity Associated with the Relaxation Response." *Science* 215 (1982): 190–192; Kutz, I., et al. "Meditation and Psychotherapy." *American Journal of Psychiatry* 142 (1985): 1–8.

32. Benson, H. *The Relaxation Response* (New York: Avon, 1975).

33. Benson, H., with Proctor, W. *Your Maximum Mind* (New York: Times Books, 1987).

34. Crum, T. F. *Windstar Journal* (Fall 1986): 73.

35. Pelletier, K. R., quoted in Ferguson, T. "Dr. Pelletier's Do-It-Yourself Stress Management." *Medical Self-Care* (Sep./Oct. 1986): 54.

36. Miller, E. E. *Self-Imagery: Creating Your Own Good Health* (Berkeley, CA: Celestial Arts, 1978/1986): 75–76.

37. Eliot. *Is It Worth Dying For?*: 225.

38. Everly, G. S. "Time Management: A Behavioral Strategy for Disease Prevention and Health Enhancement." In Matarazzo, J. D., et al. (Eds.). *Behavioral Health: A Handbook of Health Enhancement and Disease Prevention* (New York: John Wiley, 1984): 363–369; Everly, G. S. "Time Urgency and Health-Related Coping Behavior." Unpublished research report, Loyola College, Baltimore (1982).

39. Lakein, A. *How to Get Control of Your Time and Your Life* (New York: Signet, 1973): 15.

40. Ferguson, T. "Getting Organized to Deal with Stress." *Medical Self-Care* (Spring 1982): 22.

41. Miller, E. E. *Power Vision: Mastering Life Through Mental Image Rehearsal* (Chicago: Nightingale-Conant Corp., 1987).

42. Pribram, K. H. Lecture at the Center for Health & Fitness Excellence, Bemidji, MN (Jun. 13–14, 1987).

43. Ferguson. "Getting Organized."

44. Curran, D. *Stress and the Healthy Family* (Minneapolis: Winston Press, 1985): 25.

45. Bliss, E. C. *Doing It Now* (New York: Bantam, 1984): 154–155.

46. Pearsall, P. *Superimmunity: Master Your Emotions and Improve Your Health* (New York: McGraw-Hill, 1987): 301.

47. Douglass, M., and Baker, L. *The New Time Management* (Chicago: Nightingale-Conant Corp., 1983): 25.

48. Ferguson. "Getting Organized."

49. Buscaglia, L. *Bus 9 to Paradise* (New York: Slack, 1986): 229–231.

50. Ferguson. "Getting Organized."

51. Johnson, S. *One Minute for Myself* (New York: Morrow, 1985): 19, 43.

52. Curran. *Stress;* Curran, D. *Traits of the Healthy Family* (Minneapolis: Winston Press, 1983).

53. Peterson, P., and Seligman, M. E. P. "Causal Explanations as a Risk Factor for Depression: Theory and Evidence." *Psychological Review* 91 (3)(1984): 347–374; Seligman, M. E. P. "Helplessness and Explanatory Style: Risk Factor for Depression and Disease." Paper presented at the annual meeting of the Society for Behavioral Medicine, San Francisco (Mar. 1986).

54. Beck, A. T. *Cognitive Therapy and Emotional Disorders* (New York: New American Library, 1979); McKay, M., Davis, M., and Fanning, P. *Thoughts and Feelings: The Art of Cognitive Stress Intervention* (Richmond, CA: New Harbinger Publications, 1981); Burns, D. *Feeling Good: The New Mood Therapy* (New York: Signet, 1981).

55. Segal, J. *Winning Life's Toughest Battles: Roots of Human Resilience* (New York: McGraw-Hill, 1986): 80–81.

56. Dyer, W. *The Sky's the Limit* (New York: Pocket Books, 1980): 21–22.

57. Burns. *Feeling Good:* 187.
58. Burns. *Feeling Good:* 199–200.
59. Viscott, D. *Risking: How to Take Chances and Win* (New York: Pocket Books, 1979): 13.
60. Jeffers, S. *Feel the Fear . . . and Do It Anyway* (San Diego: Harcourt Brace Jovanovich, 1987): 1.
61. Paul, J., and Paul, M. *Do I Have to Give Up Me to Be Loved by You?* (Minneapolis: CompCare, 1983).
62. Branden, N. *Honoring the Self: The Psychology of Confidence and Respect* (New York: Bantam, 1983): 3, 4, 7.
63. Maddi and Kobasa. *Hardy Executive.*
64. Crum, T. F. *The Magic of Conflict* (New York: Simon and Schuster, 1987): 120.
65. Tavris, C. *Anger: The Misunderstood Emotion* (New York: Simon and Schuster, 1982).
66. Julius, M., et al. *American Family Physician* (May 1986).
67. Cummings, E. M., et al. *Developmental Psychology* 21(3)(1985).
68. Weisinger, H. *Dr. Weisinger's How to Give Criticism and Get Results* (New York: William Morrow, 1986); Blanchard, K., and Johnson, S. *The One Minute Manager* (New York: Berkley, 1983).
69. Kohn, A. *No Contest: The Case Against Competition* (Boston: Houghton Mifflin, 1986).
70. Johnson, D. W., et al. "Cooperation in Learning: Ignored but Powerful." *Lyceum* 5 (1982): 22–26; Johnson, D. W., et al. "Effects of Cooperative, Competitive, and Individualistic Goal Structures on Achievement: A Meta-Analysis." *Psychological Bulletin* 89 (1981): 47–62.
71. Kohn. *No Contest:* 24–25.
72. Chapman, A., and Foot, H. *Handbook of Humor and Laughter: Theory, Research and Applications* (New York: John Wiley, 1982); Dillon, K. M., et al. "Positive Emotional States and Enhancement of the Immune System." *International Journal of Psychiatry in Medicine* 15 (1)(1985–1986): 13–18; "Laughing Toward Longevity." *University of California, Berkeley, Wellness Letter* (Jun. 1985): 1; "The Mind Fights Back: Scientists Study How Smiles and Laughter Boost the Immune System." *Washington Post* (Jan. 9, 1985); Brody, J. F. "Increasingly, Laughter as Potential Therapy for Patients Being Taken Seriously." *New York Times* (Apr. 7, 1988).
73. Cousins, N. *Anatomy of an Illness* (New York: Berkley, 1980).
74. Curran. *Traits of a Healthy Family:* 125–132.
75. Rabow, G. "The Cooperative Edge." *Psychology Today* (Jan. 1988): 54–58.
76. House, J. S., et al. "Association of Social Relationships and Activities with Mortality: Prospective Evidence from the Tecumseh Community Health Study." *American Journal of Epidemiology* 116 (1)(1982): 123–140; Berkman, L. F., and Syme, L. O. "Social Networks, Host Resistance, and Mortality: A Nine-Year Follow-up of Alameda County Residents." *American Journal of*

Epidemiology 102 (2)(1979): 186–204; Eisenberg, L. "A Friend, Not an Apple, a Day Will Keep the Doctor Away." *Journal of the American Medical Association* 66 (1979): 551–553; Syme, L. "People Need People." *American Health* (Jul./Aug. 1982): 49–51; Cohen, S., and Wils, T. "Stress, Social Support, and Buffering Hypothesis." *Psychological Bulletin* 98 (1985): 257–310; Caplan, G. "Mastery of Stress: Psychological Aspects." *American Journal of Psychiatry* 138 (1981): 413–420; Lynch, J. J. *The Broken Heart: Medical Consequences of Loneliness* (New York: Basic Books, 1977); Ornstein, R., and Sobel, D. *The Healing Brain* (New York: Simon and Schuster, 1987).
77. Segal. *Winning:* 18.
78. Ferguson, T. "Social Support Systems as Self-Care." *Medical Self-Care* (Winter 1979/1980): 3.
79. Ferguson. "Support."
80. Buscaglia. *Bus 9:* 17, 235.
81. House, J. S., et al. "Association"; Rimland, B. "The Altruism Paradox." *Psychological Reports* 51 (2)(Oct. 1982): 521–522; Palmore, E. B. "Physical, Mental and Social Factors in Predicting Longevity." *Gerontologist* 9 (2)(Summer 1969): 103–108; Palmore, E. B. "Predicting Longevity: A Follow-up Controlling for Age." *Gerontologist* 9 (4)(Winter 1969): 247–250.
82. Ferguson, T. "Self-Help Groups in the Computer Age." *Medical Self-Care* (Sep./Oct. 1987): 73–80.
83. Ford, M. R., et al. "Quieting Response Training: Predictors of Long-Term Outcome." *Biofeedback and Self-Regulation* 8 (3)(1983): 393–408; Ford, M. R., et al. "Quieting Response Training: Long-Term Evaluation of a Clinical Biofeedback Practice." *Biofeedback and Self-Regulation* 8 (2)(1983): 265–278; Nathan, R. G., Staats, T. E., and Rosch, P. J. *The Doctors' Guide to Instant Stress Relief* (New York: G. P. Putnam's, 1987); Stroebel, C. F., Ford, M. R., Strong, P., and Szarek, B. L. "Quieting Response Training: Five-Year Evaluation of a Clinical Biofeedback Practice." (Institute for Living, Hartford, CT 06106, 1981); Stroebel, C. F., Luce, G., and Glueck, B. C. "Optimizing Compliance with Behavioral Medicine Therapies." *Current Psychiatric Therapies* (1983/1984); Pribram, K. H. *Holonomic Brain Theory* (Hillsdale, NJ: Erlbaum, 1988); Pribram. Lecture (Jun. 1987). For information on the "six-second quieting response," a method somewhat similar to the ICS, see *QR: The Quieting Reflex* by Charles F. Stroebel, M.D., Ph.D. (New York: Berkley, 1983; audiotape collection available from BMA, 200 Park Ave. So., New York, NY 10003) and *Kiddie QR* by Elizabeth Stroebel (QR Publications, 119 Forest Dr., Wethersfield, CT 06109).
84. Bandura, A., and Mahoney, M. J. "Maintenance and Transfer of Self-Reinforcement Functions." *Behaviour Research and Therapy* 12 (1974): 89–98; Denney, D. R. "Self-Control Approaches to the Treatment of Test Anxiety," in Sarason, I. G. (Ed.). *Test Anxiety: Theory, Re-*

search and Applications (Hillsdale, NJ: Erlbaum, 1980): 209–243; Goldiamond, I. "Self Reinforcement." *Journal of Applied Behavior* 9 (1976): 509–514; Stroebel et al. "Optimizing Compliance"; Stroebel. *QR.*

85. Stone, A. A. *Journal of Personality and Social Psychology* 52 (1987): 988–993; "Mood Immunity." *Psychology Today* (Nov. 1987): 14.

86. Brodish, A., et al. *Brain Research* 426 (1987): 37–46.

87. "Breathing Linked to Personality." *Psychology Today* (Jul. 1983): 109; Teich, M., and Dodeles, G. "Mind Control: How to Get It, How to Use It, How to Keep It." *Omni* (Oct. 1987): 53–60.

88. Ekman, P., Levenson, R. W., and Friesen, W. V. "Autonomic Nervous System Activity Distinguishes Among Emotions." *Science* (Sep. 16, 1983): 1208–1210; Greden, J., et al. University of Michigan. *Archives of General Psychiatry* 43 (1987): 269–274; Teich and Dodeles. "Mind Control"; Zajonc, R. B. "Emotion and Facial Efference: A Theory Reclaimed." *Science* 228 (4695) (Apr. 5, 1985): 15–21.

89. Stroebel. *QR:* 120.

90. Riskind, J. H., and Gotay, C. C. "Physical Posture: Could It Have Regulatory or Biofeedback Effects on Motivation and Emotion?" *Motivation and Emotion* 6 (3)(1982): 273–298; Weisfeld, G. E., and Beresford, J. M. "Erectness of Posture as an Indicator of Dominance or Success in Humans." *Motivation and Emotion* 6 (2)(1982): 113–131.

91. Eliot. *Is It Worth Dying For?:* 3.

92. *The Behavioral and Brain Sciences* 8 (1986): 529–566; "Brain Shows Activation Before Conscious Choice." *Brain/Mind Bulletin* (May 5, 1986): 1; Cattell, R. B. *Abilities: Their Structure, Growth and Action* (Boston: Houghton Mifflin, 1971); Pribram, K. H. Lecture at the Center for Health & Fitness Excellence, Bemidji, MN (Jun. 13–14, 1987).

93. Winter and Winter. *Building Brain:* 90.

94. Jaret, P. "Mind: Why Practice Makes Perfect." *Hippocrates* (Nov./Dec. 1987): 90–91; Salthouse, T. *Scientific American* (Feb. 1984).

95. Jaret. "Mind."

96. Jaret. "Mind"; Teich and Dodeles. "Mind Control."

97. Pribram. *Holonomic Brain Theory;* Pribram. Lecture (Jun. 1987).

98. Lamberg, L. *The American Medical Association Guide to Better Sleep* (New York: Random House, 1984).

99. Dement, W. quoted in Hopson, J. "The Unraveling of Insomnia." *Psychology Today* (Jun. 1986): 44.

100. Adam, K., and Oswald, I. "Sleep Helps Healing." *British Medical Journal* 289 (6456) (Nov. 24, 1984): 1400–1401.

101. Arnot, R. B. *CBS News* (Feb. 25, 1986).

102. Castleman, M. "How to Get a Good Night's Sleep." *Medical Self-Care* (Winter 1981): 24.

103. Lamberg. *Guide to Better Sleep;* Castleman. "A Good Night's Sleep": 124.

104. Hopson, J. "How Much Sleep Is Enough?" *Psychology Today* (Jun. 1986): 45.

105. Hopson. "How Much Sleep."

106. Ingber, D. "Is Sleep a Waste of Time? For Some, the Answer Is Yes." *Science Digest* (Apr. 1984): 84.

107. Castleman. "Good Sleep."

108. Hauri, P. "Behavioral Treatment of Insomnia." *Medical Times* 107 (6)(1986): 36–47; Regestein, Q. R. "Practical Ways to Manage Insomnia." *Medical Times* 107 (6)(1986): 19–23.

109. Hauri. "Behavioral Treatment"; Regestein. "Practical Ways"; Hopson. "How Much Sleep."

110. Hopson. "Unraveling of Insomnia"; Lamberg. *American Medical Association Guide.*

111. Shapiro, C. M., et al. "Fitness Facilitates Sleep." *European Journal of Applied Physiology* 53 (1984): 1–4; Baekland, F., Downstate Medical Center, NY, 1966 study, and Shapiro, C., and Zloty, R. B., University of Manitoba studies, both reported in Mirkin, G. *Dr. Gabe Mirkin's Fitness Clinic* (Chicago: Contemporary Books, 1986); Katch, F. I., and Katch, V. L. "To Train, Perchance to Sleep." *Muscle & Fitness* (Apr. 1986): 23, 140.

112. Kales, A., and Kales, J. D. *Evaluation and Treatment of Insomnia* (New York: Oxford University Press, 1984).

113. Lamberg, L. "White Noise on FM: Twisted Sister vs. the Sandman." *American Health* (May, 1986): 20.

114. Hauri. "Behavioral Treatment"; Regestein. "Practical Ways."

115. *Medical Journal of Australia* (Jan. 21, 1984).

116. Cailliet, R., and Gross, L. *The Rejuvenation Strategy* (New York: Doubleday, 1987): 136.

117. Dunkell, S. *Sleep Positions* (New York: Signet, 1977): 79–80.

118. Williams, G. III. "Early Morning Dangers: Why Your Body Hates to Wake Up." *American Health* (Dec. 1986): 56–59; Arnot, R. B. *CBS News* (Jan. 13, 1987).

119. Satir, V. *Making Contact* (Berkeley, CA: Celestial Arts, 1976): 1.

120. Paul, S., quoted in Gallagher, W. "The Dark Affliction of Mind and Body." *Discover* (May 1986): 76.

121. Lynch, J. J. *The Language of the Heart: The Body's Response to Human Dialogue* (New York: Basic Books, 1985).

122. Lynch. *Language:* 3–4.

123. Nichols, R. G., and Stevens, L. A. "Listening to People." *Harvard Business Review* (Sep./Oct., 1957).

124. McKay, M., Davis, M., and Fanning, P. *Messages: The Communication Book* (Richmond, CA: New Harbinger Publications, 1983): 24–28.

125. Crum, T. F. *Windstar Journal* (Spring, 1987): 30.

126. Tannen, D. *That's Not What I Meant! How Conversational Style Makes or Breaks Your Relations with Others* (New York: William Morrow, 1986): 19.

127. Tannen. *That's Not What I Meant!:* 19.

128. Miller, P. M. *The Hilton Head Executive Stamina Program* (New York: Rawson, 1986): 37; Miller, P. M.,

director of Hilton Head Health Institute. Personal communication. (Oct. 2, 1987).

129. Krueger, G. P. "Human Performance in Continuous/Sustained Operations and the Demands of Extended Work/Rest Schedules: An Annotated Bibliography." *Psychological Documents* 15 (2)(Dec. 1985): 27–28; Boothe, R. S. "Optimization of Rest Breaks: A Productivity Enhancement." *Dissertation Abstracts International* 45 (9–A)(Mar. 1985): 2927; Miller. Hilton Head: 37; Gustafson, H. W. "Efficiency of Output in Self–Paced Work, Machine-Paced Work." *Human Factors* 24 (4)(Aug. 1982): 395–410; Janaro, R. E., and Bechtold, S. E. "A Study of the Reduction of Fatigue Impact on Productivity Through Optimal Rest Break Scheduling." *Human Factors* 27 (4)(Aug. 1985): 459–466; Okogbaa, O. G. "An Empirical Model for Mental Work Output and Fatigue." *Dissertation Abstracts International* 15 (2)(Dec. 1985): 27–28; Thatcher, R. E. *Journal of Personality and Social Psychology* 52 (1987): 119–125; Zarakovski, G. M., et al. "Psychophysiological Analysis of Periodic Fluctuations in the Quality of Activity Within the Work Cycle." *Human Physiology* 8 (3)(May 1983): 208–220.

130. Emery, G. "Rapid Cognitive Therapy of Anxiety." Monograph (Los Angeles: L.A. Center for Cognitive Therapy, 1987): 39–52; Emery, G., and Campbell, J. *Rapid Relief from Emotional Distress* (New York: Fawcett, 1986); Suarez, R., Mills, R. C., and Stewart, D. *Sanity, Insanity, and Common Sense* (New York: Fawcett, 1987); Heath, C., et al. "Early Results: A Six Year Post Hoc Followup Study of the Long Term Effectiveness of Neo-Cognitive Psychotherapy." Paper presented at the Seventh Annual Conference on Psychology of Mind (Coral Gables, FL, Apr., 1988); Shuford, R., and Crystal, A. "The Efficacy of a Neo-Cognitive Approach to Positive Psychological Change." Paper presented at the Seventh Annual Conference on Psychology of Mind (Coral Gables, FL, Apr., 1988).

131. Isen, A. M. "Toward Understanding the Influence of Positive Affect on Social Behavior, Decision Making, and Problem Solving: The Role of Cognitive Organization." Paper presented at the annual meeting of the American Association for the Advancement of Science, Boston (Feb. 11–15, 1988).

132. Emery. "Rapid Therapy": 49–51.

133. Emery. "Rapid Therapy": 49–51.

134. Wurtman, J. J. *Managing Your Mind and Mood Through Food* (New York: Rawson, 1986).

135. Imai, M. *Kaizen: The Key to Japan's Competitive Success* (New York: Random House, 1986).

Step 2: Exercise Options (Chapters 11–19)

1. Kohl, H. W., and Blair, S. N. "Physical Activity, Physical Fitness, and Cardiovascular Disease Mortality in Men and Women." *American Heart Association Council on Epidemiology Newsletter* 43 (Mar., 1988): 45; Leon, A., et al. *Journal of the American Medical Association* (Nov. 6, 1987); Cooper, K. H. *The Aerobics Program for Total Well-Being* (New York: M. Evans and Company, 1982); Hage, P. "Prescribing Exercise: More Than Just a Running Program." *The Physician and Sports Medicine* 11 (1983): 123–131; Haskell, W. L., Montoye, H. J., and Orenstein, D. "Physical Activity and Exercise to Achieve Health-Related Physical Fitness Components." *Public Health Reports* 110 (1985): 202–212.

2. "Health Benefits of Exercise in an Aging Society." *Archives of Internal Medicine* 147 (1987): 353–356; Powell, K. E., et al. "Physical Activity and the Incidence of Coronary Heart Disease." *Annual Review of Public Health* 8(1987): 253–287; Proceedings of the American Heart Association's 59th Scientific Sessions, 1988.

3. Frymoyer, J. W., et al. "Epidemiologic Studies of Low Back Pain." *Spine* 5 (1980): 419–422; Kraus, H. *Backache, Stress and Tension* (New York: Fawcett, 1969).

4. Jensen, J., et al. *New England Journal of Medicine* 313 (16)(Oct. 17, 1985): 973–975; Lane, N. E., et al. "Long-Distance Running, Bone Density, and Osteoarthritis." *Journal of the American Medical Association* 255 (9)(Mar. 7, 1986): 1147–1152; Block, J. E., et al. "Does Exercise Prevent Osteoporosis?" *Journal of the American Medical Association* 257 (22)(Jun. 1987): 3115–3117.

5. Åstrand, P.-O. *Health and Fitness* (New York: Barron's, 1977): 28–30.

6. *Internal Medicine News* (Feb. 1–14, 1985); Garabrant, D. H., et al. "Job Activity and Colon Cancer Risk." *American Journal of Epidemiology* 119 (6)(1984): 1005–1014; Frisch, R. E., et al. "Lower Prevalence of Breast Cancer and Cancers of the Reproductive System Among Former College Athletes Compared to Non-Athletes." *British Journal of Cancer* 52 (6)(Dec. 1985): 885–891.

7. Harris, T. G., and Kagan, J. "The Fitness Advantage." *American Health* (Mar., 1985): 12–15; Harris, T. G., and Gurin, J. "Look Who's Getting It All Together." *American Health* (Mar., 1985): 42–47; Whitten, P. Paper presented to the Society for the Scientific Study of Sex (Nov. 7–8, 1987).

8. deVries, H. A., and Adams, G. M. "Electromyographic Comparison of Single Doses of Exercise and Meprobamate as to the Effects on Muscular Relaxation." *American Journal of Physical Medicine* 51 (1972): 130–141.

9. Sime, W. E. "Psychological Benefits of Exercise." *Advances* (Journal of the Institute for the Advancement of Health, New York) 1 (4)(Fall, 1984): 15–29 (90 references cited); Roth, D. L., and Holmes, D. S. "Influence of Aerobic Exercise Training and Relaxation Training on Physical and Psychological Health Following Stressful Life Events." *Psychosomatic Medicine* (Jul./Aug., 1987); Morgan, W. P., and Goldston, S. E. *Exercise and Mental Health* (Washington, DC: Hemisphere Publishing Co., 1987).

10. *Physical Fitness in Business and Industry* (Washington,

DC: The President's Council on Physical Fitness and Sports, 1985): 5; *Newsweek* (Apr. 1, 1985): 84–87.

11. Simon, H. B. "The Immunology of Exercise." *Journal of the American Medical Association* 252 (19)(Nov. 16, 1984); "Health Benefits." *Archives* 1987.

12. Paffenbarger, R. S., et al. *Journal of the American Medical Association* (Jul. 27, 1984); Paffenbarger, R. S., et al. *New England Journal of Medicine* (Mar. 5, 1986).

13. Packer, L. "Vitamin E, Physical Exercise, and Tissue Damage in Animals." *Medical Biology* 62 (1984): 105–109.

14. Davies, et al. "Free Radicals and Tissue Damage Produced by Exercise." *Biochemical and Biophysical Research Communications* 107 (4)(1982): 1198–1205; Dillard, et al. "Effects of Exercise, Vitamin E, and Ozone on Pulmonary Function and Lipid Peroxidation." *Journal of Applied Physiology: Respiratory, Environmental, and Exercise Physiology* 45 (6)(1978): 927–932.

15. Gyore, et al. "Human Exercise and Enzyme Induction." *Mammalian Biochemistry* 95 (1981): 445; Higuchi, et al. "Superoxide Dismutase and Catalase in Skeletal Muscle: Adaptive Response to Exercise." *Journal of Gerontology* 40 (1985): 281–286.

16. Birrer, R., quoted in "How Much Exercise Do You Really Need?" *Prevention* (Nov. 1985): 60.

17. Stamford, B., quoted in "How Much Exercise Do You Really Need?" *Prevention* (Nov., 1985): 60; Confirmed in Stamford, B. "No Pain, No Gain?" *Physician and Sports Medicine* 15 (9)(Sep. 1987): 244.

18. Cooper, K. H. *Running Without Fear: The Comprehensive New Guide to Safe Aerobic Exercise — Running, Swimming, Cycling, Skiing, and More* (New York: Bantam, 1985).

19. U.S. Department of Health and Human Services, Public Health Service, National Institutes of Health. *Exercise and Your Heart* (1981). NIH Publication No. 83-1677 (Washington, DC: U.S. Government Printing Office).

20. Hage, P. "Exercise Guidelines: Which to Believe?" *Physician and Sports Medicine* 10 (1982): 23.

21. American College of Sports Medicine. *Guidelines for Graded Exercise Testing Prescription,* 3rd edition (Philadelphia: Lea & Febiger, 1986).

22. Åstrand. *Health:* 12.

23. Cooper, K. H. *Controlling Cholesterol* (New York: Bantam, 1988): 219–243.

24. Cooper. *Cholesterol:* 231.

25. Cooper. *Running:* 160–184.

26. Dardik, I., and Waitley, D. *Quantum Fitness* (New York: Pocket Books, 1984): 91.

27. Dishman, R. K. (Ed.). *Exercise Adherence: Its Impact on Public Health* (Champaign, IL: Human Kinetics, 1988).

28. Rippe, J. M., et al. "The Health Benefits of Exercise (Part 2 of 2)." *Physician and Sports Medicine* 15 (11) (Nov., 1987).

29. Olsen, E. "Exercise, More or Less." *Hippocrates* (Jan./Feb., 1988): 65–72; Åstrand. *Health:* 12.

30. President's Council on Physical Fitness and Sports, Newsletter (May, 1986).

31. "Failing in Fitness." *Newsweek* (Apr. 1, 1985): 84–86.

32. Winter, A., and Winter, R. *Build Your Brain Power* (New York: St. Martin's, 1986): 70.

33. Hymes, A., et al. *Science of Breath* (Honesdale, PA: Himalayan Institute, 1979): 27.

34. Asimov, I. *Isaac Asimov on the Human Body and the Human Brain* (New York: Bonanza Books, 1984): 211.

35. Kannel, W. B., quoted in Malesky, G. "What It Means When You're Short of Breath." *Prevention* (Dec., 1985): 75.

36. Winter and Winter. *Building Brain:* 65.

37. Funk, E. "Avoiding Altitude Sickness." *Summit County Journal* (Brekenridge, CO: Jan. 12, 1978): 7.

38. Lynch, J. J. Study published in *Psychosomatic Medicine,* quoted in Lynch, J. *Language of the Heart* (New York: Basic Books, 1985).

39. Emery, G. "Rapid Cognitive Therapy of Anxiety." Research monograph. (L.A. Center for Cognitive Therapy, 630 S. Wilton Pl., Los Angeles, CA 90005; 1987.)

40. Clarke, J. Foreword to *Science of Breath* (Honesdale, PA: Himalayan Institute, 1979): xiii.

41. Haas, S. S. Study reported in Loehr, J. E., and McLaughlin, P. J. *Mentally Tough* (New York: M. Evans and Company, 1986): 153–154.

42. Garfield, C. *Peak Performance: Mental Training Techniques of the World's Greatest Athletes* (New York: Warner Books, 1984): 111–112.

43. Hymes et al. *Science:* 51.

44. Asimov. *Body and Brain:* 236.

45. Steincrohn, P. J. *You Live as You Breathe* (New York: David McKay Co., 1967): 134.

46. Sharkey, B. J. *Physiology of Exercise* (Champaign, IL: Human Kinetics, 1984): 336; Cailliet, R. *Understand Your Backache* (Philadelphia: F. A. Davis, 1984): 122–124; Cailliet, R., and Gross, L. *The Rejuvenation Strategy* (New York: Doubleday, 1987); Dickinson, A., and Bennet, K. "Do It Right: The Sit-up." *Shape* (Jul., 1983): 28.

47. Sharkey. *Physiology:* 336.

48. Cailliet. *Understand:* 118–121.

49. Mensendieck, E. M. *Look Better, Feel Better* (New York: Harper and Row, 1954): 48.

50. Daniels, L., and Worthingham, C. *Therapeutic Exercise for Body Alignment and Function* (Philadelphia: W. B. Saunders, 1977): 77; Yessis, M. "Kinesiology." *Muscle & Fitness* (Feb. 1985): 18–19, 142.

51. Pirie, L. *Getting Built* (New York: Warner Books, 1984): 146–148; Yessis. "Kinesiology" (Feb., 1985).

52. Lagerwerff, E. B., and Perlroth, K. A. *Mensendieck Your Posture and Your Pains* (New York: Anchor/Doubleday, 1973): 148–150; Yessis, M. "Back in Shape." *Sports Fitness* (Jun. 1986): 46, 76; Yessis, M. "The Midsection:

Your Essential Link." *Sports Fitness* (Apr. 1985): 91–93; Daniels and Worthingham. *Therapeutic:* 59.

53. Yessis, M. "Kinesiology." *Muscle & Fitness* (Nov. 1985): 21.

54. Cailliet. *Understand:* 116.

55. Sölveborn, S-A. *The Book About Stretching* (New York: Japan Publications, 1985): 19.

56. Balaskas, A., and Stirk, J. *Soft Exercise: The Complete Book of Stretching* (England: Unwin Paperbacks, 1983); Glick, J. "Muscle Strains: Prevention and Treatment." *The Physician and Sports Medicine* 8 (1980); Grahn, R., and Nordenberg, T. "Flexibility Training: Comparative Study." *GIH Report* (Stockholm, Sweden, 1979); Moore, M., and Hutton, R. "Electromyographic Investigation of Muscle Stretching Techniques." *Medicine and Science in Sports* 12 (1980); Moller, M. "Athletic Training and Flexibility." *Medical Dissertation No. 182* (Linkoping University, Sweden, 1984); Sölveborn. *Stretching;* Sady, S., et al. "Flexibility Training: Ballistic, Static or Proprioceptive Neuromuscular Facilitation." *Archives of Physical Medicine and Rehabilitation* 63 (1982).

57. Cailliet and Gross. *Rejuvenation:* 86–87.

58. Corbin, C. B., and Lindsey, R. *The Ultimate Fitness Book* (Champaign, IL: Leisure Press, 1984); Pollock, M. L., Wilmore, J. H., and Fox, S. M. *Exercise in Health and Disease* (Philadelphia: W. B. Saunders, 1984): 278.

59. Kraus, H. *Clinical Treatment of Back and Neck Pain* (New York: McGraw-Hill, 1970): 64–65; Daniels and Worthingham. *Therapeutic:* 69.

60. Sölveborn. *Stretching:* 20.

61. Daniels and Worthingham. *Therapeutic:* 58.

62. Pollock et al. *Exercise:* 278; Borysenko, J. *Minding the Body, Mending the Mind* (Reading, MA: Addison-Wesley, 1987): 77.

63. Sölveborn. *Stretching:* 20.

64. *Archives of Sexual Behavior* 14 (Feb. 1985): 13–28; Burgio, K. L., et al. "The Role of Biofeedback in Kegel Training." *American Journal of Obstetrics and Gynecology* 154 (1)(Jan. 1986): 58–64; Castleman, M. *Sexual Solutions* (New York: Simon and Schuster, 1983); Kegel, A. H. "The Physiological Treatment of Poor Tone and Function of the Genital Muscles and of Urinary Stress Incontinence." *Western Journal of Surgery, Obstetrics and Gynecology* (Nov., 1949); Kegel, A. H. "Active Exercise of the Pubococcygeus Muscle." In Meigs and Sturgis (Eds.). *Progress in Gynecology* (Orlando, FL: Grune and Stratton, 1950).

65. Burgio, et al. "Kegel Exercise."

66. *Archives of Sexual Behavior* 14 (Feb. 1985): 13–28.

67. Britton, B., and Kiesling, S. "The Little Muscle That Matters." *American Health* (Sep. 1986): 59; Rosenthal, S. *Sex over 40* (Los Angeles: J. P. Tarcher, 197).

68. Britton. "Muscle."

69. Yessis, M., and Trubo, R. *Secrets of Soviet Sports Fitness and Training* (New York: Arbor House, 1987): 74–75.

70. Nieman, D. C. *The Sports Medicine Fitness Course* (Palo Alto, CA: Bull Publishing, 1986): 441; Dardik and Waitley. *Quantum Fitness:* 114, 127; Pollock et al. *Exercise:* 292; Pirie. *Getting Built:* 82.

71. Yessis, M. "Do It Right: The Squat." *Shape* (Jul. 1985): 20.

72. Dardik and Waitley. *Quantum Fitness:* 128–129.

73. Yessis, M. "Kinesiology." *Muscle & Fitness* (Sep. 1984): 184.

74. Nieman. *Sports Medicine:* 424; Pollock et al. *Exercise:* 282; Cailliet and Gross. *Rejuvenation:* 90; Simon, H. B., and Levisohn, S. R. *The Athlete Within* (Boston: Little, Brown, 1987): 154.

75. Cailliet and Gross. *Rejuvenation:* 94–95; Pollock et al. *Exercise:* 226, 328.

76. Imrie, D., and Dimson, C. *Good Bye to Back Ache* (New York: Fawcett, 1983): 91; Cailliet and Gross. *Rejuvenation:* 118–119; Dardik and Waitley. *Quantum Fitness:* 106–107.

77. Yessis, M. "Do It Right: The Pelvic Lift." *Shape* (May 1986): 14.

78. Kraus, H. *Backache, Stress and Tension* (New York: Fawcett, 1969): 102; Kraus. *Back and Neck Pain:* 71; Cailliet and Gross. *Rejuvenation:* 118.

79. Corbin and Lindsey. *Ultimate Fitness:* 135; Kraus. *Backache:* 103; Imrie. *Back Ache:* 96–97.

80. Daniels and Worthingham. *Therapeutic:* 55, 69; Pollock et al. *Exercise:* 291–292; Corbin and Lindsey. *Ultimate Fitness:* 134; Dardik and Waitley. *Quantum Fitness:* 112; Yessis, M. "Kinesiology: Back Raises." *Muscle & Fitness* (Jan. 1985): 18–19.

81. Cooper, K. H. Personal communication. (Aug. 21, 1986).

82. Cooper, K. H. *The Aerobics Way* (New York: Bantam, 1977): 44.

83. Cooper. *Aerobics Program:* 113.

84. McArdle, W. D., Katch, F. I., and Katch, V. I. *Exercise Physiology: Energy, Nutrition, and Human Performance* (Philadelphia: Lea & Febiger, 1986).

85. Cooper. *Running:* 104.

86. American College of Sports Medicine. *Guidelines for Graded Exercise Testing and Exercise Prescription* (Philadelphia: Lea & Febiger, 1986); American College of Sports Medicine. "Position Statement: The Recommended Quantity and Quality of Exercise for Developing and Maintaining Fitness in Healthy Adults." *Medicine and Science in Sports* 10 (3)(1978): vii–x.

87. Blair, S., quoted in Cooper. *Running:* 10; Wood, P. D., et al. "Physical Activity and High-Density Lipoproteins." In Miller, N. E., and Miller, G. J. (Eds.). *Clinical and Metabolic Aspects of High-Density Lipoproteins* (Amsterdam: Elsevier, 1984): 131–165.

88. American Heart Association Committee on Exercise. *Exercise Testing and Training of Apparently Healthy Individuals: A Handbook for Physicians* (Dallas: American Heart Association): 5.

89. American College of Sports Medicine. *Guidelines.*
90. Shyne, K., and Dominquez, R. H. "To Stretch or Not to Stretch?" *The Physician and Sports Medicine* 10 (1982): 137–140; Mirkin, G. *Dr. Gabe Mirkin's Fitness Clinic* (Chicago: Contemporary Books, 1986): 16–19; Yessis and Trubo. *Soviet Sports:* 78.
91. Lawrence, R. M., and Rosenzweig, S. *Going the Distance* (Los Angeles: J. P. Tarcher, 1987): 26.
92. Shellock, F. G. "Physiological Benefits of Warm-up." *The Physician and Sports Medicine* 11 (1983): 134–139; Shellock, F. G. "Physiological, Psychological, and Injury Prevention Aspects of Warm-Up." *NSCA Journal* 8 (5)(1986): 24–27; Shellock, F. G., and Prentice, W. E. "Warming Up and Stretching for Improved Physical Performance and Prevention of Sports-Related Injuries." *Sports Medicine* 2 (1985): 267–278.
93. France, K. "Competitive vs. Non-Competitive Thinking During Exercise: Effects on Norepinephrine Levels." Paper presented at the annual meeting of the American Psychology Association, Toronto, Ontario. (Aug. 1984).
94. Brody, R. "Which Music Helps Your Muscles?" *American Health* (Jan./Feb., 1988): 80–82.
95. Ibid.
96. Nieman. *Sports Medicine:* 156.
97. Barr, A. "Water Guidelines." *American Health* (Apr. 1987): 109.
98. Lawrence and Rosenzweig. *Distance:* 135.
99. Cooper. *Running:* 114.
100. "Swimming Can Have a Positive Effect on Bone Mineral Content." *Internal Medicine News* 20 (7)(Apr. 1987): 27.
101. McArdle et al. *Exercise Physiology:* 358.
102. Longstreet, D. "Fitness Report." *American Health* (Dec. 1985): 84.
103. "Water Aerobics: A Great Workout." *Aerobics News* (Aug. 1987).
104. Taunton, J. "Running in Water." *Shape* (Apr. 1986): 60.
105. Cooper. *Running:* 125–126.
106. Cooper. *Aerobics Program:* 128.
107. Cooper. *Running:* 123.
108. Lawrence and Rosenzweig. *Distance:* 156.
109. Frederick, E. C. "Bone Jolt." *American Health* (Jul./Aug. 1982): 67.
110. "Fitness Report." *American Health* (Sep. 1987): 28.
111. Ellis, J. "Lacing Lessons." *Runner's World* (Apr. 1986): 59.
112. Schreiber, M. "More Secrets for Runners." *Sports Fitness* (May, 1986): 15.
113. Zimmerman, D. R. "Maturation and Strenuous Training in Young Female Athletes." *Physician and Sports Medicine* 15 (6)(Jun. 1987): 219–224; MacIntyre, C. "Choosing a Running Bra." *Shape* (Apr. 1986): 61.
114. Ellis, J. "The Match Game: Finding the Right Shoe for Your Biomechanics and Running Gait." *Runner's World* (Oct. 1985): 66–70.
115. Jacoby, E. "Form and Efficiency." *Runner's World* (Aug. 1985): 38–41; Yessis, M. "Sports Medicine." *Muscle & Fitness* (Dec. 1985): 13, 127, 129.
116. Selner, A., et al., quoted in *Sports Fitness* (Apr. 1986): 93.
117. Cooper. *Aerobics Program:* 129.
118. Kirch, B., et al. *Row for Your Life* (New York: Fireside Books, 1985).
119. Bassett, D. R., et al. "Energy Cost of Simulated Rowing Using a Wind-Resistance Device." *The Physician and Sports Medicine* 12 (8)(Aug. 1984): 113–118.
120. Perry, P. "Dancing on the Job." *American Health* (Oct. 1984): 46–47.
121. Priest, N. N., and Priest, J. W. "Injury Update: Are High-Impact Aerobics Safe?" *Shape* (Sep. 1987): 132; Rosenbaum, J. "Aerobics Without Injury." *Medical Self-Care* (Fall 1984): 32; Cooper. *Running:* 129.
122. Richie, D. H., Jr., et al. "Aerobic-Dance Injuries: A Retrospective Study of Instructors and Participants." *The Physician and Sports Medicine* (Feb. 1985).
123. Blair, S. *Aerobics News* (May 1987).
124. Garrick, J. G., et al. "The Epidemiology of Aerobic-Dance Injuries." *American Journal of Sports Medicine* 14 (1)(1986).
125. Ocker, G. "Aerobic-Dance Shoe Evaluation." *Shape* (Sep. 1986): 75.
126. Rosenbaum, J. *Aerobic Dance* (Durango, CO: American Aerobics Association, 1984).
127. Rosenbaum, J. Fitness Report. *Shape* (Sep. 1986): 66; Garrick. "Aerobic-Dance"; Priest. "Injury Update."
128. Johnson, S. B. "Reaching Out with Low-Impact Aerobics." *Aerobics News* (May 1987).
129. Rogers-Gould, G. "Soft Aerobics." *American Health* (Nov. 1985): 56–61.
130. Kravitz, L., and Cisar, C. J. "Worth the Weight!" *Dance-Exercise Today* 5 (9)(Nov./Dec. 1987): 21–23; Johnson. "Reaching Out."
131. Rosenbaum. *Aerobic:* 8.
132. Johnson, S. B. "Head over Heels." *Shape* (Jan. 1988): 68–69.
133. Pitreli, J., and O'Shea, P. "Rope Jumping: The Biomechanics, Techniques of and Application to Athletic Conditioning." *NSCA Journal* 8 (4)(1986): 5–11, 60–61; Davidson, D. "Jump for Joy and Fitness." *Shape* (Mar. 1983): 47–48.
134. U.S. Olympic Committee Report. Cited in Dobbins, B. "Sport Science." *Muscle & Fitness* (Mar. 1986): 14.
135. American Heart Association. "Jump Rope for Heart." Report in *Shape* (Mar. 1983): 49.
136. Larsson, B., et al. *International Journal of Sports Medicine* 6 (5)(Dec. 1984): 336–340.
137. Goldberg, L., et al. *Journal of the American Medical Association* 252 (1984): 504.

138. "Heart Rate and Lactate Levels During Weight Training Exercise in Trained and Untrained Men." *The Physician and Sports Medicine* 15 (5)(1987): 97–105; Hurley, B. F., et al. *Journal of the American Medical Association* 252 (1984): 507; "Structural Features of the Athlete Heart as Defined by Echocardiography." *Journal of the American College of Cardiology* 7 (1)(1986): 190–203; "Weight Training and Strength, Cardiorespiratory Functioning and Body Composition of Men." *British Journal of Sports Medicine* 21 (1)(1987): 40–44.

139. Hatfield, F. C. "Synergy." *Flex* (May, 1985): 64.

140. Pearl, B., and Moran, G. T. *Getting Stronger: Weight Training for Men and Women* (Bolinas, CA: Shelter Publications, 1986).

141. Pirie. *Getting Built:* 51.

142. Dishman, R. K. "The Psychology of Strength." *Sports Fitness* (Feb. 1985): 64–67, 116.

143. Yessis, M. *Soviet Sports Review* (Fall 1985).

144. Hatfield, F. C. "Machines vs. Free Weights." *Shape* (Feb. 1984): 78.

145. Cailliet and Gross. *Rejuvenation:* 42.

146. Arnold, D. "Fitness Report." *American Health* (Nov. 1985): 38.

147. Evarts, E. V. "Brain Mechanisms in Voluntary Movements." *Scientific American* (Sep. 1979): 164–179; Ehrenberg, M., and Ehrenberg, O. *Optimum Brain Power* (New York: Dodd, Mead, 1985): 223–224; Winter, A., and Winter, R. *Build Your Brain Power* (New York: St. Martin's, 1986): 47–63.

148. Sharkey. *Physiology:* 63.

149. Akselsen, A. *The Mechanics of Coordination Development* (Houston: Tri-Flex, 1976); White, J. *Jumping for Joy* (San Diego: University of California, San Diego Press, 1981): 3; Teper, L. "Coach Deluxe." *Sports Fitness* (Feb. 1986): 74; Dardik and Waitley. *Quantum Fitness:* 134.

150. Akselsen. *Rebound.*

151. White. *Jumping:* 3.

152. Liu, D. *T'ai Chi Ch'uan and I Ching* (New York: Harper and Row, 1972): 1–2, 11–14.

153. Ryan, A. Quoted in Perry, P. "Grasp the Bird's Tail: T'ai Chi, China's Centuries-old Physical Exercise of the Mind, Turns Poetry into Motion." *American Health* (Jan./Feb. 1986): 63.

154. Radcliffe, J. C., and Farentinos, R. C. *Plyometrics* (Champaign, IL: Human Kinetics Publishers, 1985): 3.

Step 3: Nutritional Wellness (Chapters 20–28)

1. Jacobson, M. F., and Brewster, L. *The Changing American Diet* (Washington, DC: Center for Science in the Public Interest, 1984): 2.

2. Jacobson, M. F. *The Complete Eater's Digest and Nutrition Scoreboard* (New York: Anchor/Doubleday, 1985): 3–5.

3. Higginson, J. In *Proceedings of the Eighth Canadian Cancer Research Conference* (Oxford: Pergamon Press, 1969): 40–75; Reddy, B., et al. "Nutrition and Its Relationship to Cancer." *Advances in Cancer Research* 32 (1980): 237–345; "How to Cut the Risk of Cancer." *FDA Consumer* (Apr. 1988): 22–29.

4. Wynder, E. L., and Gori, G. B. "Contribution of the Environment to Cancer Incidence: An Epidemiologic Exercise." *Journal of the National Cancer Institute* 58 (1977): 825–832.

5. Doll, R., and Peto, R. "The Causes of Cancer: Quantitative Estimates of Avoidable Risks of Cancer in the United States." *Journal of the National Cancer Institute* 66 (1981): 1192.

6. *Heart Facts 1986.* (American Heart Association, 7320 Greenville Ave., Dallas, TX 75231).

7. Jacobson. *Eater's Digest:* 6.

8. Liebman, B. "Are Vegetarians Healthier than the Rest of Us?" *Nutrition Action* (Jun. 1983): 8.

9. Burr, M. L., and Sweetnam, P. M. "Vegetarianism, Dietary Fiber, and Mortality." *American Journal of Clinical Nutrition* 36 (5)(Nov. 1982): 873–877; Liebman. "Vegetarians."

10. Snowdon, D. A., and Phillips, R. L. "Does a Vegetarian Diet Reduce the Occurrence of Diabetes?" *American Journal of Public Health* 75 (5)(May 1985): 507–512; "Position of the American Dietetic Association: Vegetarian Diets." *Journal of the American Dietetic Association* 88 (3)(Mar. 1988): 351; *Australian and New Zealand Journal of Medicine* (Aug. 1984); Ballentine, R. *Transition to Vegetarianism* (Honesdale, PA: Himalayan Institute, 1987); Liebman. "Vegetarians"; *British Medical Journal* 291 (Jul. 6, 1985); *Journal of the Royal Society of Medicine* 79 (Jun. 1986).

11. Dwyer, J., director, Frances Stern Nutrition Center, Tufts–New England Medical Center, quoted in *Environmental Nutrition* (May, 1987); *Environmental Nutrition* (May 1987); "A.D.A. Report: Position Paper on the Vegetarian Approach to Eating." *Journal of the American Dietetic Association* 77 (1)(1980): 61–69; *Journal of the American Dietetic Association* 88 (3)(Mar. 1988): 351.

12. Liebman. "Vegetarians."

13. *Mutagen Research* 72 (1980): 511.

14. Truesdell, D. D., et al. "Nutrients in Vegetarian Foods." *Journal of the American Dietetic Association* 84 (1984): 28–36.

15. Heinrich, H. C., et al. "Nutritional Iron Deficiency Anemia in Lacto-Ovo Vegetarians." *Klinische Wochenschrift* 57 (1979): 187–193; Dwyer, J. T., et al. "Nutritional Status of Vegetarian Children." *American Journal of Clinical Nutrition* 35 (1982): 204–216.

16. International Nutritional Anemia Consultative Group. *The Effects of Cereals and Legumes on Iron Availability* (Washington, DC: Nutrition Foundation, 1982): 8, 16–19.

17. Hallberg, L., and Rossander, L. "Improvement of Iron Nutrition in Developing Countries: Comparison of Adding Meat, Soy Protein, Ascorbic Acid, Citric Acid, and Ferrous Sulphate on Iron Absorption from a Simple Latin American Type of Meal." *American Journal of Clinical Nutrition* 39 (1984): 1469–1478.

18. International Nutritional Anemia Consultative Group. *Effects.*

19. Ballentine. *Transition:* 168.

20. Albert, M. J., et al. "Vitamin B_{12} Synthesis By Human Small Intestine Bacteria." *Nature* 283 (1980): 781–782.

21. National Academy of Sciences, National Research Council, Food and Nutrition Board: *Recommended Dietary Allowances,* 9th edition (Washington, DC, 1980): 112–120.

22. *Journal of the American Dietetic Association* 88 (3) (Mar. 1988): 351; Ballentine. *Transition:* 168–175.

23. Register, U. D., quoted in Zucker, M. *Sports Fitness* (Oct. 1985): 28.

24. Lappe, F. M., and Collins, J. *Diet for a Small Planet* (New York: Ballantine, 1982); *Food First: Beyond the Myth of Scarcity* (New York: Ballantine, 1978); and *World Hunger: Twelve Myths* (New York: Grove Press, 1986).

25. Worldwatch Institute. *State of the World 1987* (1776 Massachusetts Ave., N.W., Washington, DC 20036; 1987).

26. Brody, J. E. *Jane Brody's Good Food Book* (New York: Norton, 1985): 187.

27. Wurtman, J. J. *Managing Your Mind and Mood Through Food* (New York: Harper and Row, 1987).

28. Kostas, G., and Rojohn, K. "Nutrition Tips: Eating on the Run — The Cooper Clinic Positive Eating Program." (Aerobics Center, Dallas, TX, 1986).

29. Nandy, K. *Mechanisms of Ageing and Development* 18 (1982): 97.

30. U.S. Department of Health and Human Services report in *Prevention* (Jan. 1986): 40.

31. Brody, B. "Skip Now, Pay Later." *American Health* (Dec. 1986).

32. Pollitt, E., et al. *Journal of Psychiatric Research* 17 (2)(1982/1983).

33. Morgan, K. J., et al. "The Role of Breakfast in Nutrient Intake of 5- to 12-year-old Children." *American Journal of Clinical Nutrition* 34 (7)(Jul. 1981): 1418–1427; Service, F. J., et al. "Effects of Size, Time of Day and Sequence of Meal Ingestion on Carbohydrate Tolerance in Normal Subjects." *Diabetologia* 25 (4)(Oct. 1983): 316–321.

34. Brody. *Good Food:* 189.

35. Melnechuk, T. "Reports on Selected Scientific Conferences and Workshops." *Advances* 2 (3)(1985): 54–58.

36. "Research on Stress Hormones: Powerful Agents in Health and Disease." *Salk Institute Newsletter* (Summer 1986): 2–3.

37. Kostas, G., and Rojohn, K. "Optimal Nutrition — The Cooper Clinic Positive Eating Program." (Aerobics Center, Dallas, TX, Jan. 1985).

38. Weil, A. *Health and Healing* (Boston: Houghton Mifflin, 1983): 60.

39. Williams, R. J. *Biochemical Individuality* (Austin: University of Texas Press, 1956, 1979).

40. Kunz-Bircher, R. *The Bircher-Benner Health Guide* (Santa Barbara, CA: Woodbridge, 1980): 177.

41. Halberg, F. "Chronobiology and Nutrition." *Contemporary Nutrition* 8 (9)(1983).

42. Bircher-Benner Clinic, Zurich, Switzerland. Personal communications/interviews (1983 and 1984).

43. Pearsall, P. *Superimmunity: Master Your Emotions and Improve Your Health* (New York: McGraw-Hill, 1987): 200.

44. Migdow, J. A., and Loehr, J. E. *Take a Deep Breath* (New York: Villard, 1986): 97.

45. Hanson, P. G. *The Joy of Stress* (Kansas City, MO: Andrews, McMeel & Parker, 1986): 27.

46. Nash, J. D. *Maximize Your Body Potential* (Los Altos, CA: Bull Publishing, 1986): 130.

47. Collins, P. "Water: Do You Drink Enough?" *Mother Earth* 84 (1984).

48. McArdle, W. D., Katch, F. I., and Katch, V. L. *Exercise Physiology: Energy, Nutrition, and Human Performance* (Philadelphia: Lea & Febiger, 1986): 451; Swarth, J. *Stress and Nutrition* (San Diego: Health Media of America, 1986): 23; Brooks, G. A., and Fahey, T. D. *Exercise Physiology: Human Bioenergetics and Its Applications* (New York: Macmillan, 1985): 462.

49. Collins. "Water."

50. Colgan, M. Report in *Muscle and Fitness* (Apr. 1987): 107A.

51. Miller, P. M. *The Hilton Head Executive Stamina Program* (New York: Rawson, 1986): 26.

52. Hanson. *Stress:* 27; McArdle et al. *Exercise Physiology:* 451; Collins. "Water."

53. Goldman, B. *The "E" Factor* (New York: William Morrow, 1988): 5.

54. McArdle et al. *Exercise Physiology:* 451; Collins. "Water."

55. Collins. "Water."

56. Colgan. Report.

57. Alabaster, O. *The Power of Prevention: Reduce Your Risk of Cancer Through Diet and Nutrition* (New York: Simon and Schuster, 1985): 107.

58. Sports and Cardiovascular Nutritionists, American Dietetic Association. Report in *American Health* (May 1987): 109.

59. King, J. "Is Your Water Safe to Drink?" *Medical Self-Care* (Nov./Dec. 1985): 44–47.

60. King. "Water."

61. Brody, J. E. *Jane Brody's Nutrition Book,* revised edition (New York: Bantam, 1987): 199–200.

62. "Two-Part Report on Fluoridation." *Consumer Re-*

ports (Jul./Aug. 1978); "Fluoridation Facts" (145 scientific references). (Chicago: American Dental Association, 1980); Wulf, C. A., et al. "Abuse of the Scientific Literature in an Antifluoridation Pamphlet." (American Oral Health Institute, P.O. Box 151528, Columbus, OH 43215, 1985).
63. American Dental Association (211 E. Chicago Ave., Chicago, IL 60611; 312-440-2500).
64. King. "Water."
65. *Tufts University Diet and Nutrition Letter* 4 (2)(Apr. 1986).
66. *Medical Tribune* (Jan. 22, 1986); *Archives of Environmental Health* (Sep./Oct. 1985); Shapcott, D. in *Nutrition and Killer Diseases*. Rose, J. (Ed.) (Park Ridge, NJ: Noyes Publishing, 1982): 30; Feder, G. L. in *Aging and the Geochemical Environment* (Washington, DC: National Academy Press, 1981): 92; Marier, J. *Reviews of Cancer and Biology* 37 (1978): 115.
67. Brody. *Nutrition:* 225–226.
68. EPA Report in *Ultrasport* (Jul. 1987): 80.
69. "Water Report." *Ultrasport* (Jul. 1987): 80.
70. Young, V. *American Journal of Clinical Nutrition* (5)(1986): 770–782.
71. Ratto, T. "Protein: The Real Problem Is Getting Too Much." *Medical Self-Care* (Nov./Dec. 1986): 24–52.
72. *NHANES II: 1976–1980 Consumption Data.* Series 11, No. 231.
73. Neff, P., and Kostas, G. "Nutrition and Athletics — The Cooper Clinic Positive Eating Program." (Aerobics Center, Dallas, TX, 1986).
74. Blume, E. "Overdosing on Protein." *Nutrition Action* 14 (2)(Mar. 1987): 1–6; Morgan, B. L. G. "Protein and Your Body." *Columbia University Nutrition and Health* 8 (1)(1986): 1–6; Carroll, K. K. "Dietary Protein in Relation to Plasma Cholesterol Levels and Atherosclerosis." *Nutrition Reviews* 36 (1978): 1–5; Brenner, B. M., and Meyer, T. W. "Dietary Protein Intake and the Progressive Nature of Kidney Disease." *New England Journal of Medicine* 307 (1982): 652–654.
75. Munro, H. N., and Young, V. R. *Postgraduate Medicine* 63 (1978): 143.
76. Committee on Dietary Allowances, Food and Nutrition Board, National Academy of Sciences, 9th edition (Washington, DC, 1980): 39–51.
77. Goor, R. S., et al. *American Journal of Clinical Nutrition* 4 (1985): 299.
78. Willett, W., and MacMahon, B. "Diet and Cancer: An Overview." *New England Journal of Medicine* 310 (1984): 633–638; Alabaster. *Prevention; Journal of the National Cancer Institute* 77 (1)(1986): 33–42.
79. Brody. *Good Food:* 12.
80. Berenson, G. *American Journal of Diseases of Children* 133 (1979): 1049; *Atherosclerosis* 5 (1985): 404; Report of the American Heart Association Nutrition Committee. *Atherosclerosis* 4 (1982): 177–191; Puska, P., et al. "Con-trolled Randomized Trial of the Effect of Dietary Fat on Blood Pressure." *Lancet* (1)(1983): 1; *Journal of Hypertension* 4 (4)(1986): 407–412.
81. Williams, H. *Kidney International* 13 (1978): 410; Kromhout, D., et al. *New England Journal of Medicine* 312 (May 9, 1985): 1205.
82. *Harvard Medical School Health Letter* 13 (1)(Nov. 1987): 5; *Tufts University Diet & Nutrition Letter* 5 (3)(May 1987): 1.
83. *Tufts University Diet & Nutrition Letter* 5 (3)(May 1987): 1–2.
84. Schaefer, E. J., et al. "The Effects of Low Cholesterol, High Polyunsaturated Fat, and Low Fat Diets on Plasma Lipid and Lipoprotein Cholesterol Levels in Normal and Hypercholesterolemic Subjects." *American Journal of Clinical Nutrition* 34 (1981): 1158–1163.
85. *Tufts University Diet & Nutrition Letter* 5 (1)(Mar. 1987): 2.
86. Ibid.
87. Cooper, K. H. *Controlling Cholesterol* (New York: Bantam, 1988): 42, 44.
88. Tornberg, S. A., et al. "Risks of Cancer of the Colon and Rectum in Relation to Serum Cholesterol and Beta-Lipoprotein." *New England Journal of Medicine* 315 (26)(Dec. 25, 1986): 1629–1634; Mannes, G. A., et al. "Relation Between the Frequency of Colorectal Adenoma and the Serum Cholesterol Level." *New England Journal of Medicine* 315 (26)(Dec. 25, 1986): 1634–1638.
89. Montgomery, A. "Cholesterol Tests: How Accurate Are They?" *Nutrition Action* (May 1988): 1–7.
90. Stanford University Center for Research in Disease Prevention. "Stanford Heart Disease Prevention Program." *Prevention* (Feb. 1986): 38.
91. Hoeg, J. M., et al. "An Approach to the Management of Hyperlipoproteinemia." *Journal of the American Medical Association* 255 (4)(Jan. 24/31, 1986): 512–521; Anderson, J. W., and Chen, W. L. "Plant Fiber: Carbohydrate and Lipid Metabolism." *American Journal of Clinical Nutrition* 32 (1979): 346–363; Anderson, J. W., et al. "Hypocholesterolemic Effects of Oat-Bran or Bean Intake for Hypercholesterolemic Men." *American Journal of Clinical Nutrition* 40 (1984): 1146–1155; Kirby, R. W., et al. "Oat-Bran Intake Selectively Lowers Serum Low-Density Lipoprotein Cholesterol Concentrations of Hypercholesterolemic Men." *American Journal of Clinical Nutrition* 34 (1981): 824–828.
92. Ames, B. "Dietary Carcinogens and Anticarcinogens." *Science* 221 (1983):1256–1262; *Journal of the National Cancer Institute* 77 (33)(1986); Groto, Y. "Lipid Peroxides as a Cause of Vascular Diseases." In Yagi, K. (Ed.). *Lipid Peroxides in Biology and Medicine* (Orlando, FL: Academic Press, 1982): 295–303; Cohen, L. A. "Diet and Cancer." *Scientific American* 257 (5)(Nov. 1987): 42–48; *Cancer Research* 44 (1984): 1321.
93. Amsterdam, E. A., and Holmes, A. M. *Taking Care*

of Your Heart (New York: Facts on File, 1984): 20–22.

94. Hendler, S. S. *Complete Guide to Anti-Aging Nutrients* (New York: Simon and Schuster, 1985): 40.

95. Ballentine. *Transition:* 150.

96. Fletcher, D., and Rogers, D. *Postgraduate Medicine* 77 (5)(1985): 319–328; "Trans Fatty Acids in Processed Foods." *Environmental Nutrition* (Feb., 1988): 6–7; Kritchevsky, D. *Federation Proceedings* 41 (Sep. 1982): 2813; Smith, E. *Lancet* (Mar. 8, 1980): 534.

97. Enig, M. G., et al. "Dietary Fat and Cancer Trends — A Critique." *Federation Proceedings* 37 (1978): 2215–2220; Enig, M. G., et al. *Journal of the American Oil Chemists Society* (Oct., 1983): 1788; Kinsella, J. E., et al. "Metabolism of *trans* Fatty Acids with Emphasis on the Effects of *trans,* Trans-Octadecadienoate on Lipid Composition, Essential Fatty Acid, and Prostaglandins: An Overview." *American Journal of Clinical Nutrition* 34 (1981): 2307–2318; Thomassen, M., et al. *British Journal of Nutrition* 51 (May 1984): 315.

98. *Nutrition Week* (Sep. 17, 1987): 4.

99. Hall, R. H. *Food for Nought: Decline in Nutrition* (New York: Vintage, 1974): 247.

100. Walford, R. L. *The 120-Year Diet* (New York: Simon and Schuster, 1986): 256; Grundy, S. M. "Comparison of Monounsaturated Fatty Acids and Carbohydrates for Lowering Plasma Cholesterol." *New England Journal of Medicine* 314 (12)(Mar. 20, 1986): 745–748; Grundy, S. M., et al. "Rationale of the Diet-Heart Statement of the American Heart Association, Report of the Nutrition Committee." *Circulation* 65 (4)(1982): 841A; Mensink, R. P., and Katahn, M. B. "Effect of Monounsaturated Fatty Acids vs. Complex Carbohydrates on High-Density Lipoproteins in Healthy Men and Women." *Lancet* (Jan. 17, 1987): 122–124.

101. Mensink and Katahn. "Monounsaturated"; "More Good News for Olive Oil Lovers." *Environmental Nutrition* (Mar. 1987): 2.

102. "Will Olive Oil Lower Your Blood Pressure?" *Tufts University Diet & Nutrition Letter* 5 (7)(Sep. 1987): 1.

103. Grundy. "Comparison"; Grundy et al. "Rationale"; Mensink and Katahn. "Monounsaturated."

104. *Journal of the National Cancer Institute* 72(1984): 745; *Federation Proceedings* 43 (1984): 614; *Nutrition Action* (Jul./Aug. 1986): 5.

105. Viola, P., and Audisio, M. "Olive Oil and Health." Research compendium presented at the Third International Congress on the Biological Value of Olive Oil (Canea, Crete, Greece, Sep. 1980). Updated for distribution in 1986 (International Olive Oil Council, Bartucci-Samuel, Inc., 1 World Trade Center, Suite 7967, New York, NY 10048).

106. Blume, E. "Why Oxidized Fats Are in Your Food and Why You Wish They Weren't." *Nutrition Action* (Dec. 1987): 1–6.

107. Ballantine. *Transition:* 222–225; Brody. *Good Food:*

284; Burros, M. "Sorting Through Cooking Oils." *New York Times* (Dec. 8, 1987).

108. Wellcome Foundation. "Interferon Production." *Chemical Abstracts* 90 (1979): 157072f; Wara, E., et al. "Effect of Sodium Butyrate on Induction of Cellular and Viral DNA Synthesis in Polyoma Virus-Infected Mouse Kidney Cells." *Journal of Virology* 38 (3)(1981): 973–981; Terry, R. D., and Davies, P. "Dementia of the Alzheimer Type." *Annual Review of Neuroscience* (3)(1980): 77–9; Bradford, R. W., et al. *Butyric Acid Therapy as a New Adjunctive in the Treatment of Degenerative Diseases* (Chula Vista, CA: Bradford Research Institute, 1983); Ballentine. *Transition:* 222–225.

109. Exler, J., and Weihrauch, J. L. "Comprehensive Evaluation of Fatty Acids in Foods. VIII: Finfish." *Journal of the American Dietetic Association* 69 (3)(Sep. 1976): 243–248; Exler, J., and Weihrauch, J. L. "Comprehensive Evaluation of Fatty Acids in Foods. XII: Shellfish." *Journal of the American Dietetic Association* 71 (5)(Nov. 1977): 518–521.

110. *New England Journal of Medicine* 312 (19)(May 9, 1985): 1205–1210/1210–1217/1217–1224/1253; Nestel, P. J. "Fish Oil Attenuates the Cholesterol Induced Rise in Lipoprotein Cholesterol." *American Journal of Clinical Nutrition* 43 (5)(May, 1986): 752–757.

111. Weiner, M. A. *New England Journal of Medicine* 315 (13)(Sep. 25, 1986): 833.

112. Weiner. *New England Journal of Medicine* 315 (13)(Sep. 25, 1986): 833; Hepburn, F. N., et al. "Provisional Tables on the Content of Omega-3 Fatty Acids and Other Fat Components of Selected Foods." *Journal of the American Dietetic Association* 86 (6)(June, 1986): 788–793.

113. Simopoulous and Salem. *New England Journal of Medicine* (Sep. 25, 1986).

114. *Medical World News* (Jul. 14, 1986): 9.

115. Hendler. *Guide:* 228; *Medical World* (Jul. 14, 1986).

116. Cooper. *Cholesterol:* 259.

117. *Lipids* 22 (1987): 345.

118. Fallat, R. W., et al. "Short Term Study of Sucrose Polyester a Nonabsorbable Fat-like Material as a Dietary Agent for Lowering Plasma Cholesterol." *American Journal of Clinical Nutrition* 29 (11)(1976): 1204–1215.

119. Food Additive Petition. 7A3997 (1987).

120. *Food and Chemical Toxicology* 25 (1)(1987); Blume, E. "Finessing Fat." *Nutrition Action* (Nov. 1987): 8–9.

121. Hallfrisch, J., et al. "Modification of the United States' Diet to Effect Changes in Blood Lipids and Lipoprotein Distribution." *Atherosclerosis* 57 (2–3)(Nov. 1985): 179–188; Connor, S. L., and Connor, W. E. *The New American Diet* (New York: Simon and Schuster, 1986); Walford. *120-Year Diet:* 116; Alabaster. *Prevention:* 87–88, 107.

122. *Tufts University Diet & Nutrition Letter* 5 (1)(Mar. 1987): 2; Cooper. *Cholesterol:* 80–83.

123. World Health Organization Expert Committee on Cardiovascular Disease. *Prevention of Coronary Heart Disease.* WHO Technical Report Series, No. 678 (Geneva, 1982): 12.

124. Grundy, S. M., et al. "Rationale of the Diet-Heart Statement of the American Heart Association, Report of the Nutrition Committee." *Circulation* 65 (4)(1982): 841A.

125. Alabaster. *Prevention:* 117; Cooper. *Cholesterol:* 12, 83.

126. Story, J. *Federation Proceedings* 41 (Sep. 1982): 2797.

127. Elias, A., et al. *General Pharmacology* 15 (6)(1984): 535; Offenbacher, E., et al. *Diabetes* 29 (11)(Nov. 1980): 919.

128. Draser, B., and Irving, D. *British Journal of Cancer* 27 (1973): 167–172; Hems, G. *British Journal of Cancer* 37 (1978): 974–982; Hems, G., and Stuart, A. *British Journal of Cancer* (3)(1975): 118–123.

129. Stanford (Feb. 1986).

130. Blume, E. *Nutrition Action* (May 1987).

131. Roffers, M. "NutraSweet: The Bitter Truth." *Medical Self-Care* (Jan./Feb. 1986): 33–34. Graves, F. "How Safe Is Your Diet Soft Drink?" *Common Cause Magazine* (Jul./Aug. 1984). *Environmental Nutrition* (May 1987). "Artificial Sweeteners: Doubts Linger over Aspartame." *Environmental Nutrition* (Dec. 1987): 4–5.

132. "More Evidence on the Safety of Aspartame." *Tufts University Diet & Nutrition Letter* 5 (12)(Feb. 1988): 2.

133. Blundell, J. E., and Hill, A. J. "Paradoxical Effects of an Intense Sweetener (Aspartame) on Appetite." *Lancet* 1 (8489)(May 10, 1986): 1092–1093; *University of California, Berkeley, Wellness Letter* 2 (12)(Sep. 1986): 8; Stellman, S. D., and Garfinkel, L. "Artificial Sweetener Use and One-Year Weight Change Among Women." *Preventive Medicine* 15 (2)(Mar. 1986): 195–202.

134. Burkitt, D., in Winawer, et al. (Eds.). *Colorectal Cancer: Prevention Epidemiology and Screening* (New York: Raven Press, 1980): 13–18; Jensen, O. "Colon Cancer Epidemiology," in Atrup and Williams (Eds.). *Experimental Colon Carcinogenesis* (Boca Raton, FL: CRC Press, 1983): 3–23.

135. Alabaster. *Prevention:* 36.

136. Weininger, J., and Briggs, G. M. "Nutrition and Diabetes." *Nutrition Update* (New York: John Wiley and Sons, 1985): 59–60.

137. Anderson, J. W. "Medical Benefits of High-Fiber Intakes." *The Fiber Factor* (Quaker Oats Co., Chicago, IL, Aug. 1983); Anderson, J. W. *Plant Fiber in Foods* (Lexington, KY: HCF Diabetes Research Foundation, Inc., 1986); Kinosian, B. P., and Eisenberg, J. M. "Cutting into Cholesterol." *Journal of the American Medical Association* 259 (15)(Apr. 15, 1988); Kirby. "Oat Bran."

138. Anderson. "Medical Benefits."

139. Connor and Connor. *New American Diet:* 38; Alabaster. *Prevention:* 127.

140. Anderson. *Plant Fiber.*

141. Blackburn, H., and Prineas, R. "Diet and Hypertension." *Progress in Biochemical Pharmacology* 19 (1983): 31–79; Jacobson. *Eater's Digest.*

142. *Prevention* (Feb. 1986): 38, 114.

143. Nordin, B. E., et al. "New Approaches to the Problems of Osteoporosis." *Clinical Orthopedics* 200 (Nov. 1985): 181–197; *Prevention* (Feb. 1986): 38, 114.

144. *Prevention* (Feb. 1986): 38, 114.

145. *Internal Medicine News* (May 1–14, 1985).

146. Gussow, J. D., and Thomas, P. R. *The Nutrition Debate: Sorting Out Some Answers* (Palo Alto, CA: Bull Publishing, 1986): 261–262.

147. Ford, F. "A Grain of Truth." *New Age Journal* (Mar. 1986): 18.

148. Seymour, J., and Giradet, H. *Blueprint for a Green Planet* (New York: Prentice Hall, 1987): 40.

149. Canter, L. J. "Organic Farming Becomes Legitimate." *Science* (Jul. 1980): 254–256.

150. "Rex Oberhelman: $27,000 (Net!) from Five Organic Acres." *Mother Earth News* (Mar./Apr. 1986): 17–21.

151. National Academy of Sciences. *Regulating Pesticides in Food* (1987).

152. General Accounting Office, *Pesticides: Better Sampling and Enforcement Needed on Imported Food* (Washington, DC, 1986); General Accounting Office, *Pesticides: Need to Enhance FDA's Ability to Protect the Public from Illegal Residues* (Washington, DC, 1986).

153. *Bioscience* 28 (1978): 772; Walford. *120-Year Diet:* 252.

154. *Guess What's Coming to Dinner* (Center for Science in the Public Interest, 1501 16th St., N.W., Washington, DC 20036, 1987): 6.

155. *Washington Post* (Jul. 24, 1985).

156. Mott, L., and Snyder, K. *Pesticide Alert: A Guide to Pesticides in Fruits and Vegetables* (National Resources Defense Council, 122 E. 42nd St., New York, NY 10168, 1988).

157. Zuckerman, S. "Antibiotics: Squandering a Medical Miracle." *Nutrition Action* (Jan./Feb. 1985): 9; Chinnici, M. "Concern About Antibiotics." *Science Digest* (Feb. 1985): 16.

158. Hayes, V., et al. "Public Health Implications of the Use of Antibiotics in Animal Agriculture." *Journal of Animal Science* 62 (Suppl. 3)(1986).

159. Hayes. "Public Health."

160. *Journal of Food Protection* 48 (1985): 887; Carter Center of Emory University. *Closing the Gap* (1986).

161. *University of California, Berkeley, Wellness Letter* (Jul. 1987): 2.

162. Spika, J. S., et al. *New England Journal of Medicine* 316 (10)(Mar. 5, 1987): 565–570.

163. Ibid.

164. Natural Resources Council, data cited in *Nutrition Action* (Oct. 1987): 9.

165. *Guess:* 2; Natural Resources Council, data cited in *Nutrition Action* (Oct. 1987): 9.

166. "Toxic Chemicals in Our Meat Supply?" *Tufts University Diet and Nutrition Letter* 1 (3)(March 1983): 1.

167. Wiles, R. "Pesticide Risk to Farm Workers." *The Nation* (Oct. 5, 1985).

168. Colgan, M. *Your Personal Vitamin Profile* (New York: Quill, 1982).

169. Bashin, B. J. "The Freshness Illusion." *Harrowsmith* (Jan./Feb. 1987): 41–50.

170. Benbrook, C. M. Quoted in Bashin. "Freshness."

171. Hendler. *Guide:* 54.

172. World Health Organization, *Environmental Health Criteria 11: Mycotoxins* (1979); Tomita, I., et al. *IARC Scientific Publications* 57 (1984): 33; Blume, E. "Aflatoxin." *Nutrition Action* (Sep. 1986): 1–6.

173. *Guess:* 37.

174. Hendler. *Guide:* 54.

175. National Research Council. *Diet, Nutrition, and Cancer* (Washington, DC: National Academy Press, 1982): Chapter 13.

176. Ibid.

177. Ershoff, B. G., and Thurston, E. W. "Effects of Diet on Amaranth (FD&C Red No. 2) Toxicity in the Rat." *Journal of Nutrition* 104 (1974): 937–942; Noren, K. "Levels of Organochlorine Contaminants in Human Milk in Relation to the Dietary Habits of the Mothers." *Acta Paediatrica Scandinavica* 72 (1983): 811–816.

178. Mott and Snyder. *Pesticide Alert.*

179. Franklin, D. "The Appeal of a Peel." *Hippocrates* (Jul./Aug. 1987): 46.

180. Ibid.

181. Ibid.

182. Ames, B., Magaw, R., and Gold, L. S. "Ranking Possible Carcinogenic Hazards." *Science* (Apr. 17, 1987): 271; Harris Survey of Health Experts. "Prevention in America: The Experts Rate 65 Steps to Better Health." *Prevention* (1983). Lou Harris and Associates, Inc., #830411.

183. *Public Citizen Health Research Group Health Letter* (Mar./Apr. 1986): 7–10.

184. Blume, E., and Jacobson, M. F. "Food Irradiation: Is the Time Ripe?" *Nutrition Action* (Nov. 1986): 5.

185. *University of California, Berkeley, Wellness Letter* (Dec. 1986): 2.

186. Ibid.

187. Wolfe, S. M. *Public Citizen Health Research Group Health Letter* (Jun. 1987): 7.

188. *American Journal of Clinical Nutrition* (Feb. 1985): 130.

189. Ralston Purina Co. Final Report: Contract 53-3K06-1-29. "Animal Feeding Study for Irradiation Sterilized Chickens." (Jun. 1983).

190. *Public Citizen Health Research Group Health Letter* (Nov./Dec. 1986): 12–13; *University of California, Berkeley, Wellness Letter* (Dec. 1986): 2.

191. Rosenberg, B. "A Diner's Guide to Irradiation." *Science Digest* (Sep. 1986): 30.

192. Colgan. *Profile:* 246–247.

193. Brody. *Good Food:* 78–84.

194. Grande, F., et al. "Effect of Carbohydrates of Leguminous Seeds, Wheat and Potatoes on Serum Cholesterol Concentration in Man." *Journal of Nutrition* 86 (1965): 313–318; Jenkins, D. J. A., et al. "The Glycaemic Index of Foods Tested in Diabetic Patients: A New Basis for Carbohydrate Exchange Favouring the Use of Legumes." *Diabetology* 24 (1983): 257–264; Jenkins, D. J. A., et al. "Leguminous Seeds in the Dietary Management of Hyperlipidemia." *American Journal of Clinical Nutrition* 38 (1983): 567–573.

195. Gori, G. B. "Dietary and Nutritional Implications in the Multifactorial Etiology of Certain Prevalent Human Cancers." *Cancer* 43 (1979): 151–161.

196. Levey, G. A. "Nutrition's New Hero: Chic Beans." *American Health* (Mar., 1986): 83–92; Liebman, B. "Beans Needn't Be Bland or Embarrassing." *Nutrition Action* (Jan./Feb. 1983): 12–14.

197. Rao, D. R., et al. "Natural Inhibitors of Carcinogenesis: Fermented Milk Products," in Reddy, B. S., and Cohen, L. A. (Eds.). *Diet, Nutrition, and Cancer: A Critical Evaluation,* vol. 2 (Boca Raton, FL: CRC Press, 1986): 73; Hirayama, T. "Epidemiology of Cancer of the Stomach with Reference to Its Recent Decrease in Japan." *Cancer Research* 35 (1975): 3460–3463; Sandler, R. B., et al. "Postmenopausal Bone Density and Milk Consumption in Childhood and Adolescence." *American Journal of Clinical Nutrition* 42 (2)(Aug. 1985): 270–275.

198. Sandler, R. B., et al. "Bone Density and Milk Consumption." *American Journal of Clinical Nutrition* 42 (2)(Aug. 1985): 270–275.

199. Schaafsma, G. *The Influence of Dietary Calcium and Phosphorus on Bone Metabolism* (Ede, Netherlands, Nederlands Instituut voor Zuivelonderzoek, 1981): 25.

200. Forsythe, J. "Nutrition Report: Milk's Big Surprise." *American Health* (Dec. 1985): 100.

201. International Dairy Federation. "Cultured Dairy Foods in Human Health." (Brussels, Belgium: IDF, FIL-IDF Document 159, 1987): 22; Nair, C. R., and Mann, G. V. "A Factor in Milk Which Influences Cholesteremia in Rats." *Atherosclerosis* 26 (1977): 363–377.

202. Recker, R. R., and Heaney, R. P. "The Effect of Milk Supplements on Calcium Metabolism, Bone Metabolism and Calcium Balance." *American Journal of Clinical Nutrition* 41 (1985): 254–263.

203. Shahani, K. M., et al. *American Journal of Clinical Nutrition* 33 (1980): 2448; Shahani, K. M., et al. *Journal of Applied Nutrition* 36 (2) (1984): 125–153; Shahani, K. M., and Friend, B. A. In Skinner and Roberts (Eds.). *Food Microbiology* (London: Academic Press, 1983): 257; Deeth, H. C., and Tamine, A. Y. "Yogurt: Nutritive and Therapeutic Aspects." *Journal of Food Protein* 44 (1981):

78; *Nutrition Reviews* 42 (Nov. 1984); International Dairy. "Cultured Foods."

204. Bayless, T. M., et al. "Lactose and Milk Intolerance: Clinical Implications." *New England Journal of Medicine* 292 (22)(1975): 1156–1159.

205. Savaiano, D. A., et al. "Lactose Malabsorption from Yogurt, Pasteurized Yogurt, Sweet Acidophilus Milk, and Cultured Milk in Lactase-Deficient Individuals." *American Journal of Clinical Nutrition* 40 (1984): 1219–1223; McDonough, F., et al. *American Journal of Clinical Nutrition* 42 (Aug. 1985): 345.

206. Edington, J., et al. "Effect of Dietary Cholesterol on Plasma Cholesterol Concentration in Subjects Following Reduced Fat, High Fibre Diet." *British Medical Journal* 294 (6568)(1987): 333–337.

207. St. Louis, M. E., et al. "The Emergence of Grade A Eggs as a Major Source of Salmonella enteritidis Infections." *Journal of the American Medical Association* 259 (14)(Apr. 8, 1988): 2103–2108.

208. *New England Journal of Medicine* 312 (19)(May 9, 1985): 1205–1224, 1253.

209. Jacobson. *Eater's Digest:* 127.

210. *University of California, Berkeley, Wellness Letter* (Jan. 1988): 7.

211. U.S. Department of Agriculture. Handbook 8.

212. *Tufts University Diet and Nutrition Letter* 5 (4)(Jun. 1987).

213. Ibid.

214. *Science Digest* (Jul. 1986): 18.

215. *New England Journal of Medicine* 314 (11)(Mar. 10, 1986): 678–681, 707–709.

216. *FDA Consumer* (Feb. 1987): 19–21.

217. *Food Chemical News* (May 4, 1987): 3.

218. Haenszel, W., et al. "Large Bowel Cancer in Hawaiian Japanese." *Journal of the National Cancer Institute* 51 (1973): 1765–1779; Leveille, G. A. "Issues in Human Nutrition and Their Probable Impact on Foods of Animal Origin." *Journal of Animal Science* 41 (1975): 723–731.

219. Burch, G. E. "Pork and Hypertension." *American Heart Journal* 86 (5)(1973): 713–714.

220. Sacks, F. M., et al. "Effect of Ingestion of Meat on Plasma Cholesterol of Vegetarians." *Journal of the American Medical Association* 246 (6)(1981): 640–644.

221. Ballentine. *Transition:* 124–125.

222. Marsh, A. G., et al. "Cortical Bone Density of Adult Lacto-Ovo-Vegetarian and Omnivorous Males." *American Journal of Clinical Nutrition* 25 (1972): 555–558; Barzel, U. S., and Jowsey, J. "The Effects of Chronic Acid and Alkali Administration on Bone Turnover." *Clinical Science* 36 (1969): 517; Wachman, A., and Bernstein, D. S. "Diet and Osteoporosis." *Lancet* (1)(1968): 95.

223. Leathwood, P., and Pollet, P. "Diet-Induced Mood Changes in Normal Populations." *Journal of Psychiatric Research* 17 (1983): 147–157; Lieberman, H., et al. "The Behavioral Effects of Food Constituents: Strategies Used in Studies of Amino Acids, Protein, Carbohydrates and Caffeine." *Nutrition Reviews* (Suppl., May 1986): 61–69; Lieberman, H., et al. "Mood, Performance and Sensitivity: Changes Induced by Food Constituents." *Journal of Psychiatric Research* 17 (1984): 135–145; Spring, B. "Effects of Foods and Nutrients on the Behavior of Normal Individuals." In Wurtman, J. J., and Wurtman, R. J. (Eds.). *Nutrition and the Brain,* vol. 7 (New York: Raven Press, 1986): 1–47; Christensen, L. "Impact of Dietary Change on Emotional Distress." *Journal of Abnormal Psychology* 94 (1985): 565–579; Wurtman, J. J., and Wurtman, R. (Eds.). *Nutrition and the Brain,* vol. 7 (New York: Raven Press, 1986).

224. Wurtman, J. J. *Managing Your Mind and Mood Through Food* (New York: Harper and Row, 1987); Wurtman, J. J. Personal communication. (December 15, 1987); Spring, B., et al. "Carbohydrates, Tryptophan, and Behavior: A Methodological Review." *Psychological Bulletin* 102 (1987): 234–256; Benton. *Biological Psychiatry* 24 (1988): 95–100.

225. Wurtman, J. Quoted in "Peak Performance Brain Food." *Omni Longevity* 2 (6)(Apr. 1988): 67.

226. Spring. "Carbohydrates: Methodological Review."

227. Wurtman. *Managing Mind and Mood:* 27.

228. Hendler. *Guide:* 12.

229. Walford. *120-Year Diet:* 143.

230. Hendler, S. S., quoted in Malesky, G. "A Doctor's Guide to Anti-Aging Nutrients." *Prevention* (Aug. 1985): 30; Hendler. *Guide:* 79–80.

231. Worthington-Roberts, B., and Breskin, M. *Journal of the American Dietetic Association* 84 (7)(1984): 795–800.

232. Liebman, B. "Vitamin Supplements." *Nutrition Action* (Feb. 1986): 6.

233. Marshall, C. W. *Vitamins and Minerals: Help or Harm?* (Philadelphia: George Stickley, 1983).

234. Hendler. *Guide:* 295.

235. Ibid.

236. Fisher, H. "The Elusive Vitamin Requirement." *Prevention* (Feb. 1987): 112.

237. *Tufts University Diet & Nutrition Letter* 5 (5)(Jul. 1987): 6.

238. Fisher, H. "Nutrition in Your Life." *Prevention* (May 1987): 123–124.

239. National Research Council. *Diet, Nutrition, and Cancer* (Washington, DC: National Academy Press, 1982).

240. Alabaster. *Prevention:* 153–154.

241. Hendler. *Guide:* 117.

Step 4: Body Fat Control (Chapters 29–32)

1. Morgan, B. L. G. "Obesity." *Columbia University Nutrition and Health* 8 (5)(1987).

2. *ABC Nightline* (ABC Television, May 13, 1986); Abraham, S., and Johnson, C. L. "Prevalence of Severe Obesity in Adults in the United States." *American Journal*

of Clinical Nutrition 33 (1980): 364–370; McArdle, W. D., Katch, F. I., and Katch, V. L. *Exercise Physiology: Energy, Nutrition, and Human Performance* (Philadelphia: Lea & Febiger, 1986): 532–533.

3. Strunkard, A. J. "Obesity and the Social Environment." In Howard, A. (Ed.). *Recent Advances in Obesity Research: Proceedings of the 1st International Congress on Obesity* (Oct. 8–11, 1974; London: Royal College of Physicians, 1975): 223–225; "Dieting: The Losing Game." *Time Magazine* (Jan. 20, 1986): 54–55.

4. Hannon, B. M., and Lohman, T. G. "The Energy Cost of Overweight in the United States." *American Journal of Public Health* 68 (1978): 765; "Dieting: The Losing Game." *Time* (Jan. 20, 1986): 54–55.

5. *FDA Consumer* (Nov. 1986): 16–19; *National Institutes of Health.* "Health Implications of Obesity." NIH Consensus Development Conference Statement. 5 (9) (Washington, DC: U.S. Government Printing Office, 1985).

6. McArdle et al. *Exercise Physiology:* 532–533; *Digestive Disease Week* (May 18, 1986).

7. "Dieting-Induced Obesity: A Hidden Hazard of Weight Cycling." *Environmental Nutrition* 10 (2)(Feb. 1987): 1–6.

8. Ernsberger, P. "Yo-Yo Hypertension, the Death of Dieting." *American Health* (Feb. 1985): 29–33.

9. *FDA Consumer* (Nov. 1986): 16–19; *American Journal of Clinical Nutrition* 44 (1986): 585–595.

10. *FDA Consumer* (Nov. 1986): 16–19.

11. Sotaniemi, K. A. "Slimmer's Paralysis: Peroneal Neuropathy During Weight Reduction." *Journal of Neurology, Neurosurgery and Psychiatry* 47 (5)(May 1984): 564–566.

12. "Nutrition Report: The Trouble with Dieting — Nutritional Crashes Wreck Muscle Function." *American Health* (Feb. 1985): 72.

13. McArdle et al. *Exercise Physiology:* 544–545; *Newsweek* (May 19, 1986): 79–80; Clark, R., and Blackburn. "Danger Ahead? Fad Diets for Weight Control." *The Professional Nutritionist* (Summer 1982): 1–4; "Council on Foods and Nutrition: A Critique of Low-Carbohydrate Ketogenic Weight Reduction Regimens: A Review of Dr. Atkin's Diet Revolution." *Journal of the American Medical Association* 224 (1973): 10.

14. *Nutrition Forum* 3 (8)(Aug. 1986): 57–59; *Newsweek* (May 19, 1986): 79–80.

15. Newton, K. "Weight Management: Learning to Self-Regulate Dietary Habits." *Nutrition Report* 4 (1986): 12–16; Clark and Blackburn. "Danger Ahead?"

16. Lindner, P. "Getting Started: Don't Be Gullible!" *Shape* (Mar. 1986): 42–43.

17. Manson, J. E., et al. "Body Weight and Longevity." *Journal of the American Medical Association* 257 (3)(Jan. 16, 1987): 353–358.

18. *Nutrition Reviews* 43 (1985): 61.

19. Ratto, T. "The New Science of Weight Control." *Medical Self-Care* (Mar./Apr. 1987): 29.

20. Manson, et al. "Body Weight."

21. "Health Implications of Obesity: An NIH Consensus Development Conference Statement — Health Implications of Obesity." *Annals of Internal Medicine* 103 (1985): 981–1077; Simopoulos, A. "The Health Implications of Overweight and Obesity." *Nutrition Reviews* 43 (1985): 33–40.

22. Bray, G. A. "The Myth of Diet in the Management of Obesity." *American Journal of Clinical Nutrition* 23 (1970): 1141–1148.

23. Danforth, E. "Diet and Obesity." *American Journal of Clinical Nutrition* 41 (May 1985): 1132–1145; Liebman, B. F. "Is Dieting a Losing Game?" *Nutrition Action* (Mar. 1987): 10–11; Schwartz, R. "The Thermic Response to Carbohydrate vs. Fat Feeding in Man." *Metabolism* 34 (1985): 85–93.

24. Remington, D., Fisher, G., and Parent, E. *How to Lower Your Fat Thermostat* (Provo, UT: Vitality House, 1983): 67–68.

25. Stunkard, A. J., et al. "An Adoption Study of Human Obesity." *New England Journal of Medicine* 314 (4)(Jan. 23, 1986): 193–198; Greenwood, M., and Turkenkopf, I. *Genetic and Metabolic Aspects of Obesity,* IV (New York: Churchill Livingstone, 1983): 193–205.

26. Faust, I. "Nutrition and the Fat Cell." *International Journal of Obesity* 4 (1980): 314–321; Stunkard, A. J. *Obesity* (Philadelphia: Saunders, 1980): 1–24.

27. Rona, R. "Social and Family Factors and Obesity in Children." *Annals of Human Biology* 9 (1982): 131–145; Morris, S. "Feeding Behaviors, Food Attitudes, and Body Fatness." *Journal of the American Dietetic Association* 80 (1982): 330–333; Hertzeler, N. "Obesity-Impact on the Family." *Journal of the American Dietetic Association* 79 (1981): 525–529.

28. Harrison, D. E., et al. *Proceedings of the National Academy of Sciences, USA* 81 (1984): 1835; Bennett, W. "Dieting-Ideology vs. Physiology." *Psychology of Clinical Nutrition* 7 (1984): 321–334.

29. Remington et al. *Fat Thermostat:* 2.

30. Himms-Hagen, J. "Thermogenesis in Brown Adipose Tissue as an Energy Buffer." *New England Journal of Medicine* 311 (24)(1984): 1549–1558.

31. Bray, G. A. "Brown Tissue and Metabolic Obesity." *Nutrition Today* (Jan./Feb. 1982): 23–27; Mirkin, G. "Getting Thin: All About Fat." *Shape* (Nov. 1983): 112–122; Mirkin, G. *Getting Thin* (Boston: Little, Brown, 1983).

32. Sacks, P. "Understanding Obesity, Part II." *Nutrition Reports International* 3 (1985): 60–61; Schwartz. "Thermic Response."

33. Bray, G. A. "Brown Tissue and Metabolic Obesity." *Nutrition Today* (Jan./Feb. 1982): 23–27; Swaminathan, R. "Thermic Effect of Feeding Carbohydrate, Fat, Protein, and Mixed Meal in Lean and Obese Subjects." *American Journal of Clinical Nutrition* 38 (1983): 680–693; Bessard, T. "Energy Expenditure and Postparandial

Thermogenesis in Obese Women Before and After Weight Loss." *American Journal of Clinical Nutrition* 38 (1983): 680–693; Nair, K. "Thermic Response to Isoenergetic Protein, Carbohydrate, or Fat Meals in Obese and Lean Subjects." *Clinical Science* 65 (1983): 307–312.

34. Blackburn, G. L., quoted in Mirkin, G. *Getting Thin* (Boston: Little, Brown, 1983).

35. Griffith, W. "Food as a Regulator of Metabolism." *American Journal of Clinical Nutrition* 17 (1965): 391–398.

36. Krause, M., and Mahan, L. "Balance and Imbalance of Body Weight." In *Food, Nutrition, and Diet Therapy,* 6th edition (Philadelphia: Saunders, 1979): 553–577; Stunkard. *Obesity:* 1–24.

37. Garn, S., and Clark, D. "Trends in Fatness and Origins in Obesity." *Pediatrics* 57 (1976): 443–445.

38. Morgan. "Obesity"; Cooper, K. H. *The Aerobics News* (Dec., 1986): 2.

39. Gortmaker, S. L., et al. *American Journal of Diseases of Children* (May, 1987); Morgan. "Obesity."

40. Charney, H. C., et al. "Childhood Antecedents of Adult Obesity." *New England Journal of Medicine* 295 (1976): 6; Abraham, S., et al. "Relationship of Childhood Weight Status to Morbidity in Adults." *Public Health Report* 86(1971): 273.

41. Brooks, G. A., and Fahey, T. D. *Exercise Physiology: Human Bioenergetics and Its Applications* (New York: Macmillan, 1985): 534–535.

42. Morgan. "Obesity."

43. Berkowitz, R. I., et al. "Physical Activity and Adiposity: A Longitudinal Study from Birth to Childhood." *Journal of Pediatrics* 106 (5)(May 1985): 734–738.

44. Cooper, K. H. *The Aerobics News* (Dec., 1986): 2.

45. Berkowitz, et al. "Physical Activity and Adiposity."

46. University of California, San Francisco. News Release (Oct. 28, 1986).

47. "Dieting in Infants Can Be Dangerous." *Environmental Nutrition* (Sep., 1986): 4; *Medical World News* (May 26, 1986): 3.

48. Dahlkoetter, J. A., et al. "Obesity and the Unbalanced Energy Equation: Exercise Versus Eating Habit Change." *Journal of Consulting Clinical Psychology* 47 (1979): 898; Miller, P. M., and Sims, K. L. "Evaluation and Component Analysis of a Comprehensive Weight Control Program." *International Journal of Obesity* 5 (1981): 57; Bielinsi, R. "Energy Metabolism During Post-Exercise Recovery in Man." *American Journal of Clinical Nutrition* 42 (1985): 69–82.

49. McArdle et al. *Exercise Physiology:* 549; Brooks and Fahey. *Exercise Physiology:* 127–132.

50. Remington et al. *Fat Thermostat:* 10–11.

51. Levitsky, D. "Exercising Within Several Hours of Eating Can Burn More Kilocalories." *Journal of the American Dietetic Association* 83 (1983): 290; Welle, S. "Metabolic Responses to a Meal During Rest and Low-Intensity Exercise." *American Journal of Clinical Nutrition* 40 (1984): 990–994; Segal, K. R., and Gutin, B. "Thermic Effects of Food and Exercise in Lean and Obese Women." *Metabolism* 32 (1983): 581–589; Tremblay, A., et al. "The Effects of Exercise-Training on Energy Balance and Adipose Tissue Morphology and Metabolism." *Sports Medicine* 2 (1985): 223–233; de Vries, H. A., and Gray, D. E. "After Effects of Exercise upon Resting Metabolic Rate." *Research Quarterly* 34 (1963): 314–321.

52. "Exercising and Metabolism." *Science Digest* (Apr. 1986): 41.

53. McArdle et al. *Exercise Physiology:* 549–551; Remington et al. *Fat Thermostat:* 7.

54. Wood, P. "The No-Diet Diet." *Runner's World* (Jan. 1987): 353–359.

55. *Research Quarterly for Exercise and Sport* 55 (1985): 242–247; Clark, N. "Sit-ups Don't Melt Ab Flab." *Runner's World* (Mar. 1985): 32.

56. Pollock, M. L., et al. "Effects of Mode of Training on Cardiovascular Function and Body Composition of Adult Men." *Medicine and Science in Sports* 7 (1975): 139.

57. Johnson, S. "Cross Training to Achieve Your Fitness Goals." *The Aerobics News* (Feb. 1988): 4.

58. Gwinup, G., et al. *American Journal of Sports Medicine* (May/Jun. 1987).

59. Vash, P. D. "The Fat-Loss Payoff." *Shape* (Jan. 1987): 24, 99, 115; reconfirmed in "Good, Better, Best Weight Loss Ideas for 1988 from the American Society of Bariatric Physicians." *Prevention* (Jan. 1988): 35–41, 115–124.

60. Cooper, K. H., quoted in "The Executive's Guide to Exercise and Fat Loss." *Executive Fitness Newsletter* Supplement (Aug. 1986).

61. Roffers, M. "Sports Nutrition Myths." *Medical Self-Care* (Mar./Apr. 1986): 52.

62. Jequier, E. "Does a Thermogenic Defect Play a Role in the Pathogenesis of Human Obesity." *Clinical Physiology* 3 (1983): 1–7; "Good, Better, Best Weight Loss."

63. Danforth, E. "Diet and Obesity." *American Journal of Clinical Nutrition* 41 (May 1985): 1132–1145.

64. Wing, R. R., et al. "Mood Changes in Behavioral Weight Loss Programs." *Journal of Psychosomatic Research* 28 (3)(1984): 189–196; Liebman, B. F. "Fated to Be Fat?" *Nutrition Action* (Jan.–Feb. 1987): 5.

65. Leveille, T. "Adipose Tissue Metabolism: Influence of Eating and Diet Composition." *Federation Proceedings* 29 (1970): 1294–1301; Lukert, B. "Biology of Obesity." In Wolman, B. (Ed.). *Psychological Aspects of Obesity: A Handbook* (New York: Van Nostrand Reinhold, 1982): 1–14; Szepsi, B. "A Model of Nutritionally Induced Overweight: Weight 'Rebound' Following Caloric Restriction." In Bray, G. (Ed.). *Recent Advances in Obesity Research* (London: Newman, 1978).

66. Vash, P. D. "Outsmarting the Fat Cell." *Shape* (Mar. 1987): 72–74.

67. Mirkin. "Getting Thin": 124.

68. Stark, R. E. T. Quoted in "Good, Better, Best Weight Loss."

69. Danforth, E. "Calories: A Scientific Breakthrough." *Shape* (Mar. 1986): 47; Danforth, E. "Diet and Obesity."

70. Danforth. "Diet and Obesity"; *Proceedings of the National Academy of Sciences U.S.A.* 82 (1985): 4866.

71. "Is Fat More Fattening?" *Tufts University Diet & Nutrition Letter* 4 (12)(Feb. 1987): 1–2; *Metabolism* 31 (1982): 1234–1242.

72. Anderson, J. W. "Medical Benefits of High-Fiber Intakes." *The Fiber Factor* (Chicago: Quaker Oats Co., Aug. 1983).

73. "Myth: Artificial Sweeteners Promote Weight Loss." *University of California, Berkeley, Wellness Letter* 2 (12)(Sep. 1986).

74. Stellman, S. D., and Garfinkel, L. "Artificial Sweetener Use and One-Year Weight Change Among Women." *Preventive Medicine* 15 (2)(Mar. 1986): 195–202; MacNeil, K. "Diet Soft Drinks: Too Good to Be True?" *New York Times* (Feb. 4, 1987).

75. Blundell, J. E., and Hill, A. J. "Paradoxical Effects of an Intense Sweetener (Aspartame) on Appetite." *Lancet* 1 (8489)(May 10, 1986): 1092–1093.

76. Nash, J. D. *Maximize Your Body Potential* (Palo Alto, CA: Bull Publishing, 1986): 130.

77. Migdow, J. A., and Loehr, J. E. *Take a Deep Breath* (New York: Villard, 1986): 97.

78. Shell, E. R. "The New Science of Hunger." *American Health* (Mar. 1986): 45–49.

79. McArdle. *Exercise Physiology:* 555.

80. Tremblay, A. "The Reproducibility of a Three Day Dietary Recall." *Nutrition Research* 3 (1983): 819–830.

81. Wing, et al. "Mood Changes in Behavioral Weight Loss"; Friedman, R. "What to Tell Patients About Weight Loss Methods, Parts 1, 2, and 3." *Postgraduate Medicine* 72 (1982): 73–98; Leon, G. "The Behavior Modification Approach to Weight Control." *Contemporary Nutrition* 4 (1979): 1–2; Foreyt, J. "Limitations of Behavioral Treatment of Obesity: Review and Analysis." *Journal of Behavioral Medicine* 4 (1981): 159–171; Kirshenbaum, D. "Behavioral Treatment of Adult Obesity: Attentional Control and a Two Year Follow-up." *Behaviour Research and Therapy* 23 (1985): 675–682.

82. Mirkin. *Getting Thin:* 62–63, 84–85.

83. Nash, J. D., and Ormiston, L. *Taking Charge of Your Weight and Well Being* (Palo Alto, CA: Bull Publishing, 1978): 381–473.

84. Brownell, K. D. *The LEARN Program for Weight Control* (Department of Psychiatry, University of Pennsylvania, 133 S. 36th St., Philadelphia, PA 19104; 1985).

85. Nash, J. D. *Maximize Your Body Potential* (Palo Alto, CA: Bull Publishing, 1986): 206.

Step 5: Postural Vitality (Chapters 33–34)

1. Cailliet, R., and Gross, L. *The Rejuvenation Strategy* (Garden City, NY: Doubleday, 1987); Cailliet, R., quoted in "Good Posture: An Antidote for Aging." *Shape* (Jul. 1987): 24.

2. Åstrand, P.-O. *Health & Fitness* (New York: Barron's, 1977): 86.

3. Cailliet and Gross. *Rejuvenation:* 52.

4. Malesky, G. "Boost Your Brainpower." *Prevention* (Jan., 1985): 137–140.

5. Cailliet and Gross. *Rejuvenation:* 54.

6. Cailliet. "Good Posture."

7. Migdow, J. A., and Loehr, J. E. *Take a Deep Breath* (New York: Villard, 1986): 97.

8. Cailliet and Gross. *Rejuvenation:* 53.

9. Kraus, H. *Backache, Stress and Tension* (New York: Pocket Books, 1969): 40; Imrie, D., with Dimson, C. *Good Bye to Backache* (New York: Fawcett, 1983): 128–129.

10. Åstrand, P.-O., and Rodahl, K. *Textbook of Work Physiology: Physiological Bases of Exercise* (New York: McGraw-Hill, 1986): 112; Hanna, T. *The Body of Life* (New York: Knopf, 1980).

11. Riskind, J. H., and Gotay, C. C. "Physical Posture: Could It Have Regulatory or Biofeedback Effects on Motivation and Emotion?" *Motivation and Emotion* 6 (3)(1982): 273–298; Weisfeld, G. E., and Beresford, J. M. "Erectness of Posture as an Indicator of Dominance or Success in Humans." *Motivation and Emotion* 6 (2)(1982): 113–131; Wilson, E., and Schneider, C. "Static and Dynamic Feedback in the Treatment of Chronic Muscle Pain." Paper presented at the Biofeedback Society of America meeting (New Orleans, Apr. 16, 1985); Malesky. "Boost Brainpower."

12. Winter, A., and Winter, R. *Build Your Brain Power* (New York: St. Martin's, 1986); *The Neuropsychology of Achievement* (Sybervision Systems, Inc., Fountain Square, 6066 Civic Terrace Ave., Newark, CA 94560, 1985).

13. Heller, J., and Henkin, W. A. *Bodywise* (Los Angeles: J. P. Tarcher, 1986): 19.

14. Wilson and Schneider. "Static and Dynamic."

15. Hunt, H., quoted in Stedman, N. "Getting Straight." *Health* (Nov., 1985): 65.

16. Binder, T. *Position Technic* (Boulder, CO: Binder, 1977): 5; Barlow, W. *The Alexander Technique* (New York: Knopf, 1973): 77–78.

17. Barlow, W., quoted in *Somatics* (Spring/Summer, 1987): 11.

18. Barlow. *Alexander Technique:* 8.

19. Imrie. *Backache:* 128–129.

20. Wurm, F. "A Body to Mind." *Somatics* (Spring/Summer, 1986): 18.

21. Riskind and Gotay. "Physical Posture."

22. Ekman, P., et al. "Autonomic Nervous System Activity Distinguishes Among Emotions." *Science* (Sep. 16, 1983): 1208–1210; Greden, J., et al. *Archives of General Psychiatry* 43 (1987): 269–274; Zajonc, R. B. "Emotions and Facial Difference: A Theory Reclaimed." *Science* (Apr. 5, 1985).

23. Cooper, M. *Change Your Voice, Change Your Life* (New York: Macmillan, 1984): 5; *Wall Street Journal*

(Apr. 1, 1980); Rubin, L. S. *Voice Handbook* (Professionally Speaking, 119 W. 57th St., Suite 911, New York, NY 10019; 1986); Blumenthal, D. "Taking a Sounding." *New York Times Magazine* (Aug. 15, 1982): 51.

24. *Starling's Physiology*, 8th edition, p. 30. Cited in Wurm, F. "A Body to Mind." *Somatics* (Spring/Summer 1986): 19.

25. Sweigard, L. E. *Human Movement Potential: Its Ideokinetic Facilitation* (New York: Harper and Row, 1974): 222; Alexander, G. *Eutony* (Great Neck, NY: Felix Morrow, 1985).

26. Sweigard. *Human Movement:* 223.

27. G. Alexander. *Eutony:* 92–93.

28. Ibid.: 94.

29. Cailliet and Gross. *Rejuvenation:* 56.

30. Heller and Henkin. *Bodywise:* 92; Cailliet and Gross. *Rejuvenation:* 56.

31. Cailliet and Gross. *Rejuvenation:* 56–57.

32. Cailliet and Gross. *Rejuvenation:* 64–65.

33. Barker, S. *The Alexander Technique* (New York: Bantam, 1978): 24.

34. *Human Factors* 29 (1987): 67–71.

35. Sweigard. *Human Movement:* 272.

36. Ibid.: 176.

37. Cailliet and Gross. *Rejuvenation:* 129.

38. Travell, J. G. *Office Hours: Day and Night* (New York: World Publishing, 1968): 270, 284, 285, 301, 302. Cited in Travell, J. G., and Simons, D. G. *Myofascial Pain and Dysfunction* (Baltimore: Williams and Wilkins, 1983): 112.

39. Cailliet and Gross. *Rejuvenation:* 127.

40. "Don't Be Slack About Good Posture." *University of California, Berkeley, Wellness Letter* (Oct. 1986): 6.

41. Cailliet and Gross. *Rejuvenation:* 127.

42. Gould, N. "Back-Pocket Sciatica." *New England Journal of Medicine* 290 (1974): 633.

43. Lettvin, M. *Maggie's Back Book* (Boston: Houghton Mifflin, 1976): 131; Cailliet and Gross. *Rejuvenation:* 127.

44. *Medical Tribune* 27 (1986): 31.

Step 6: Rejuvenation and Living Environments Design (Chapters 35–42)

1. Erickson, J. M. "Vital Senses: Sources of Lifelong Learning." *Journal of Education* 167 (3)(1985).

2. Rivlin, R., and Gravelle, K. *Deciphering the Senses: The Expanding World of Human Perception* (New York: Simon and Schuster, 1984).

3. Winter, A., and Winter, R. *Build Your Brain Power* (New York: St. Martin's, 1986): 17.

4. Rosenzweig, M., Krech, D., and Diamond, M. C. "The Physiologic Imprint of Learning Investigators." Paper prepared by Luce, G. G., after interviews in Dec. 1965 and May 1966 (National Institutes of Health publication).

5. Justice, B. *Who Gets Sick? Thinking and Health* (Houston: Peak Press, 1987): 259.

6. Diamond, M. C. *How the Brain Grows in Response to Experience* (Series on the Healing Brain Cassette Recording No. T55; Los Altos, CA: Institute for the Study of Human Knowledge, 1983); *Brain/Mind Bulletin* 12 (7)(Mar. 1987): 1–5; Kiyono, S., et al. *Physiology and Behavior* 34: 431–435; Hwang, H. M., and Greenough, W. T. Paper presented at the annual meeting of the Society for Neuroscience (1986).

7. Justice. *Who Gets Sick?:* 261.

8. *Medical World News* (Jul. 22, 1985); *American Health* (May 1986): 77; Cohen, S. S. *Magic of Touch* (Harper and Row, 1987).

9. Montagu, A. *Touching: The Human Significance of the Skin*, 3rd edition (New York: Perennial Library, 1986); Ehrenberg, M., and Ehrenberg, O. *Optimum Brain Power* (New York: Dodd, Mead, 1985): 75–76.

10. Thayer, S. "Close Encounters." *Psychology Today* (Mar. 1988): 31–36.

11. Thayer, S. (Ed.). "The Psychology of Touch." *Journal of Nonverbal Behavior* 10 (Special issue, 1986).

12. Heslin, R., and Alper, T. "Touch: A Bonding Gesture." In Wiemann, J. M., and Harrison, R. P. (Eds.). *Nonverbal Interaction* (Beverly Hills, CA: Sage Publications, 1983).

13. Fisher, L. M. "What's New in Massage: Adding Massage to Office Routine." *New York Times* (Feb. 8, 1987); Brody, J. "The Ancient Art of Massage: Once a Luxury, Is Becoming a Necessity." *New York Times* (Apr. 14, 1985); "The Message About Massage." *Newsweek* (Oct. 15, 1984): 110; "Health and Fitness: Massage." *Time* (Mar. 9, 1987).

14. Winter and Winter. *Build Brain Power:* 42; Ehrenberg and Ehrenberg. *Optimum:* 75–76; Montagu. *Touching;* Cohen. *Magic of Touch.*

15. Nagler, W., quoted in Duhe, C. "The Healing Art of Massage." *UltraSport* (Aug. 1987): 42.

16. Brody. "Massage."

17. Fisher. "Massage"; Elias, M. "Office Massage Rubs Workers the Right Way." *USA Today* (Jan. 25, 1987); "Health and Fitness." *Time.*

18. *Optometric Advice on Eye Care and Eyewear* (St. Louis: American Optometric Association, 1984).

19. Henig, R. M., and Grotch, R. "Too Close for Comfort: What Makes You Nearsighted?" *American Health* (Apr. 1985).

20. United Press International (Aug. 10, 1983).

21. *University of California, Berkeley, Wellness Letter* 3 (7)(Apr. 1987): 8.

22. Taylor, C. W. "Promoting Health Strengthening and Wellness Through Environmental Variables." In Matarazzo, J. D., et al. (Eds.). *Behavioral Health: A Handbook of Health Enhancement and Disease Prevention* (New York: John Wiley, 1984): 130–148.

23. *Brain/Mind Bulletin* (Oct. 25, 1982).

24. Young, R. W. "Solar Radiation and Age-Related Macular Degeneration." *Survey of Ophthalmology* 32 (1988): 252–269.

25. Rosenthal, F. S., et al. "The Effect of Prescription Eyewear on Ocular Exposure to Ultraviolet Radiation." *American Journal of Public Health* 76 (10)(Oct. 1986): 1216–1220.

26. *Journal of Physiology* (London) 160(1962): 106–154; *Journal of Physiology* (London) 165 (1962–1963): 559–568.

27. Ehrenberg and Ehrenberg. *Optimum:* 65–66; Winter and Winter. *Build Brain Power:* 18–20.

28. Winter and Winter. *Build Brain Power:* 18–20.

29. Maslow, A. *The Farther Reaches of Human Nature* (New York: Viking, 1971).

30. Ulrich, R. S. "Natural versus Urban Scenes: Some Physiological Effects." *Environment and Behavior* 13 (5)(1981): 523–556; Ulrich, R. S. "View Through a Window May Influence Recovery from Surgery." *Science* 224 (4647)(1984): 420–421.

31. Justice. *Who Gets Sick?:* 262.

32. Kunz-Bircher, R. *The Bircher-Benner Health Guide* (Santa Barbara, CA: Woodbridge, 1980): 66; Lillyquist, M. J. *Sunlight and Health: The Positive and Negative Effects of the Sun on You* (New York: Dodd, Mead, 1985); Kime, Z. R. *Sunlight Could Save Your Life* (Penryn, CA: World Health Publications, 1980); Hollwich, F. *The Influence of Ocular Light Perception on Metabolism in Man and in Animal* (New York: Springer-Verlag, 1979); Okudaira, et al. *American Journal of Physiology* 254 (1983): R613–615.

33. Holick, M. F., quoted in *Prevention* (Mar. 1986): 122–123; Holick, M. F. *Journal of Clinical Endocrinology and Metabolism* (1987).

34. Liebmann-Smith, R. "The Man Who Patented Sunlight." *American Health* (Dec. 1985): 33–35.

35. Novick, N. L. *Saving Face* (New York: Franklin Watts, 1986): 36.

36. Lasden, M. "Sunblock Bingo." *Hippocrates* (Jul./Aug. 1987): 86.

37. *FDA Consumer* (Jun. 1987): 21–23.

38. Stern, R. S., et al. "Risk Reduction for Nonmelanoma Skin Cancer with Childhood Sunscreen Use." *Archives of Dermatology* 122 (May 1986): 537–545.

39. Stern, et al. "Risk Reduction"; "The Sunshine Kids." *University of California, Berkeley, Wellness Letter* (Jul. 1987): 6.

40. Novick. *Saving Face; FDA Consumer* (Jun. 1987).

41. Wineman, J., quoted in Meer, J. "The Light Touch." *Psychology Today* (Sep. 1985): 60–67.

42. Knowles, R., quoted in Meer, J. "The Light Touch." *Psychology Today* (Sep. 1985): 60–67.

43. Brody, J. "Surprising Health Impact Discovered for Light." *New York Times* (Nov. 13, 1984).

44. Gilbert, S. "Noise Pollution." *Science Digest* (Mar. 1985): 28.

45. Winter and Winter. *Build Brain Power:* 26.

46. Safranek, M. D. "Effect of Auditory Rhythm on Muscle Reactivity." *Physical Therapy* (Feb. 1982): 161–188.

47. "Recipe for Hearing Loss: Noise, Hypertension, and Fatty Diet." *Journal of the American Medical Association* 256 (3)(Jul. 18, 1986): 312–313.

48. Muzet and Ehrhart, cited in Vaughn, L. "Have a Happy Baby." *Prevention* (Apr. 1985): 153.

49. Halpern, S., and Savary, L. *Sound Health* (New York: Harper and Row, 1985): 31–40.

50. Westman, J. C., quoted in Halpern and Savary. *Sound Health:* 31–40.

51. "How Today's Noise Hurts Body and Mind." *Medical World News* (Jun. 13, 1969): 42–43.

52. Pierce, A., quoted in "Music Professor Teaches Fine Art of Listening." *Brain/Mind Bulletin* (Jul. 1987): 3.

53. Lapp, J., California State University, Fresno, reporting at the American Psychological Association annual meeting, 1986; Halpern and Savary. *Sound Health.*

54. Winter and Winter. *Build Brain Power:* 30.

55. Ehrenberg and Ehrenberg. *Optimum:* 78.

56. Ferguson, T., and Sobel, D. *The People's Book of Medical Tests* (New York: Summit, 1985).

57. Morse, D. R., et al. "The Effect of Stress and Meditation on Salivary Protein and Bacteria: A Review and Pilot Study." *Journal of Human Stress* 8 (4)(Dec. 1982): 31–39; Morse, D. R., et al. "Stress, Relaxation, and Saliva: Relationship to Dental Caries and Its Prevention, with a Literature Review." *Annals of Dentistry* 42 (2)(Winter 1983): 47–54; Green, L. W., et al. "Periodontal Disease as a Function of Life Events Stress." *Journal of Human Stress* 12 (1)(Spring 1986): 32–36.

58. Glass, R. T., and Lare, M. M. "Toothbrush Contamination: A Potential Health Risk." *Quintessence International* 17 (1)(Jan. 1986): 39–42; *American Health* (Aug. 1987): 26.

59. Hawkins, B., et al. *Journal of Periodontology* (Jan. 1987).

60. Wunderlich, R. C., et al. "The Therapeutic Effect of Toothbrushing on Naturally Occurring Gingivitis." *Journal of the American Dental Association* 110 (6)(Jun. 1985): 929–932.

61. Weaver, A., et al. "Mouthwash and Oral Cancer: Carcinogen or Coincidence?" *Journal of Oral Surgery* 37 (1979): 250–253; Blot, W. J., et al. "Oral Cancer and Mouthwash." *Journal of the National Cancer Institute* 70 (1983): 251–253.

62. Wynder, E. L., et al. "A Study of the Etiologic Factors in Cancer of the Mouth." *Cancer* 10 (1957): 1300–1323; Graham, S., et al. "Dentition, Diet, Tobacco, and Alcohol in the Epidemiology of Oral Cancer." *Journal of the National Cancer Institute* 59 (1977): 1611–1615.

63. Blot. "Oral Cancer."

64. Wolner, S. Z. "Mouthwash Alert." *Better Health and Living* (Dec. 1986): 14–17.

65. Wade, C. "Self-Help for Lovers: Relaxing for Romance." *American Health* (May 1985): 41–44.

66. Zilbergeld, B., quoted in Wade. "Self-Help."

67. Castleman, M. "Pillow Talk." *Medical Self-Care* (Spring 1985): 45–55.

68. Alperstein, L. P., quoted in Castleman. "Talk."

69. Castleman, M. *Sexual Solutions* (New York: Touchstone, 1983): 145.

70. Alperstein in Castleman. "Talk."

71. Castleman. *Sexual Solutions:* 162.

72. Castleman. "Talk."

73. Alperstein in Castleman. "Talk."

74. Samuels, M., and Bennett, H. Z. *Well Body, Well Earth* (San Francisco: Sierra Club Books, 1983): 194.

75. Sullivan, W. "Global Study of Changes in Earth's Livability Set." *New York Times* (Sep. 22, 1986).

76. Ferguson and Sobel. *Medical Tests;* Samuels and Bennett. *Well Earth:* 108–116.

77. Samuels and Bennett. *Well Earth:* 110.

78. Baranski, S., and Czerski, P. *Biological Effects of Microwaves* (Stroudsburg, PA: Dowden, Hutchinson, and Ross, 1976); Samuels and Bennett. *Well Earth:* 122.

79. Samuels and Bennett. *Well Earth:* 122.

80. "Researchers See More Danger in Microwave Radiation." *Business Week* (Dec. 7, 1987): 127.

81. Frey, A. Cited in Samuels and Bennett. *Well Earth:* 122.

82. Baranski. *Biological Effects.*

83. Baranski. *Biological Effects;* Shute, N. "The Other Kind of Radiation." *American Health* (Jul./Aug. 1986): 54–58.

84. *University of California, Berkeley, Wellness Letter* 3 (4)(Jan. 1987).

85. Shute. "Other Radiation."

86. Samuels and Bennett. *Well Earth:* 125.

87. Adey, W. R. "Tissue Interactions with Nonionizing Electromagnetic Fields." *Physiological Review* 61 (1981): 435–514; Singer, S. J., and Nicholson, G. L. "The Fluid Mosaic Model of the Structure of Cell Membranes." *Science* 175 (1972): 720–731; Marron, M. T., et al. "Mytotic Delay in Heterokaryons and Decreased Respiration." *Experientia* 24 (1978): 589–590; Marron, M. T., et al. "Cell Surface Effects of 60-Hz Electromagnetic Fields." *Radiation Research* 94 (1983): 217–220; Hansson, H. A. "Lamellar Bodies in Purkinje Nerve Cells Experimentally Induced by Electric Field." *Brain Research* 216 (1981): 187–191.

88. Bawin, S., and Adey, W. "Sensitivity of Calcium Binding in Cerebral Tissue to Weak Environmental Electrical Fields Oscillating at Low Frequency." *Proceedings of the National Academy of Sciences U.S.A.* 73 (1976): 1999; Wiltschko, W., and Wiltschko, R. "Magnetic Compass of European Robins." *Science* 176 (1972): 62; Larkin, R. P., and Southerland, P. J. "Migrating Birds Respond to Project Seafarers's Electromagnetic Field." *Science* 195 (1977): 777.

89. Phillips, J. L., et al. "Transferrin Binding to Two Human Carcinoma Cell Lines: Characterization and Effect of 60–Hz Electromagnetic Fields." *Cancer Research* 46 (1986): 239–244; Winters, W. D. "Biological Functions of Immunologically Reactive Human and Canine Cells Influenced by *in vitro* Exposure to 60-Hz Electric and Magnetic Fields (1986). Cited in Ahlbom, A., et al. "Panel's Final Report: Biological Effects of Power Line Fields, New York State Power Lines Project Scientific Advisory Panel Final Report." State of New York Department of Health (Jul. 1, 1987).

90. Konig, H., et al. *Biological Effects of Environmental Electromagnetism* (New York: Springer-Verlag, 1981): 218.

91. Milham, S. "Mortality from Leukemia in Workers Exposed to Electrical and Magnetic Fields." *New England Journal of Medicine* 307 (4)(Jul. 22, 1982): 249.

92. Sulzman, F. M., and Murrish, D. E. "Effects of Electromagnetic Fields on Primate Circadian Rhythms" (1986). Cited in Ahlbom et al. "Panel's Final Report."

93. Wiltschko and Wiltschko. "Magnetic Compass"; Graham, C., and Cohen, H. D. "Influence of 60-Hz Fields on Human Behavior Physiology Chemistry" (1985). Cited in Ahlbom et al. "Panel's Final Report"; Salzinger, K. "Behavioral Effects of ELF" (1987). Cited in Ahlbom et al. "Panel's Final Report"; Thomas, J. R., and Schrot, J. "Investigation of Potential Behavioral Effects of Exposure to 60-Hz Electromagnetic Fields" (1986). Cited in Ahlbom et al. "Panel's Final Report."

94. Wertheimer, N., and Leeper, E. "Electrical Wiring Configurations and Childhood Cancer." *American Journal of Epidemiology* 109 (1979): 273–284.

95. Wertheimer, N., and Leeper, E. "Adult Cancer Related to Electrical Wires Near the Home." *International Journal of Epidemiology* 11 (1982): 345–355.

96. Savitz, D. A. "Childhood Cancer and Electromagnetic Field Exposure" (1987). Cited in Ahlbom et al. "Panel's Final Report."

97. Ahlbom, et al. "Panel's Final Report": 10.

98. "EPA: Pollution Higher Indoors." *USA Today* (Sep. 11, 1986).

99. *Science News* (Sep. 28, 1985).

100. Ibid.

101. "New CPSC Study Report: Indoor Air Worse Than Outdoor." *Human Ecologist* 26 (Summer 1984): 9–10.

102. Lioy, P., quoted in Young, B. B., and Johnson, K. A. "Toxic Home Syndrome." *New Age Journal* (Apr. 1986): 48.

103. *Western Journal of Medicine* 146 (1986): 1.

104. National Center for Health Statistics report. Cited in Young and Johnson. "Toxic Home."

105. "Health Front: Lifesaving Key Chain." *Prevention* (May 1987): 12–13.

106. Lanson, G. "Is Your Dream House a Nightmare?" *American Health* (Jun. 1986): 82.

107. Brown, H. S., et al. "The Role of Skin Absorption

as a Route of Exposure for Volatile Organic Compounds in Drinking Water." *American Journal of Public Health* (May 1984).

108. Brown et al. "Skin Absorption"; Dadd, D. L. "1987 Buyer's Guide to Water Purification Devices" (Inverness, CA: Everything Natural, 1987): 5.

109. *Science News* (Sep. 28, 1985); *USA Today*. "Pollution."

110. "Formaldehyde: Assessment of Health Effects." National Academy of Sciences Commission on Toxicology (Mar. 1980): vi; Fawcett, S. "Formaldehyde: If It Smells, Watch Out!" *Medical Self-Care* (Summer 1984): 21–23.

111. *The Cancer Prevention Letter* 1 (4)(1986): 1–3; "Spider Plant Meets the Foam Monster." *Harrowsmith* (Apr./May 1986): 124.

112. Waldbott, G. L. *Health Effects of Environmental Pollutants,* 2nd edition (St. Louis: C. V. Mosby, 1978): 256.

113. Dadd, D. L. *The Nontoxic Home* (Los Angeles: J. P. Tarcher, 1986): 17.

114. Young and Johnson. "Toxic Home."

115. Waldbott. *Health Effects:* 256.

116. Shabecoff, P. "Issue of Radon Peril: New National Focus on Ecology." *New York Times* (Sep. 10, 1986); Eckholm, E. "Radon: Threat Is Real." *New York Times* (Sep. 2, 1986).

117. Lanson. "Dream House."

118. Shabecoff. "Radon Peril"; Eckholm. "Radon."

119. Dadd. *Nontoxic Home:* 17.

120. Stolwijk, J. A. J., in Feltman, J. "Do You Work in a 'Sick' Building?" *Prevention* (Apr. 1985): 52–59.

121. Robertson, A. S., et al. "Comparison of Health Problems Related to Work and Environmental Measurements in Two Office Buildings with Different Ventilation Systems." *British Medical Journal* 291 (6492)(Aug. 10, 1985): 373–375; Taylor. "Promoting Health Strengthening and Wellness."

122. "Surgeon General, Citing Risks, Urges Smoke-Free Workplace." *New York Times* (Dec. 17, 1986).

123. "Cigarette Smoking: The Bottom Line." *American Cancer Society* (Nov. 1986).

124. "Smokers Make Poor Drivers." *USA Today* (Sep. 22, 1986).

125. Abramson, L. Y. et al. "Learned Helplessness in Humans: Critique and Reformulation." *Journal of Experimental Psychology: General* 105 (1976): 3–46; Miller, S. M., and Seligman, M. E. P. "The Reformulated Model of Helplessness and Depression: Evidence and Theory." In Neufeld, R. W. J. (Ed.). *Psychological Stress and Psychopathology* (New York: McGraw-Hill, 1982): 149–179.

126. Shimer, P. "The Easiest Way to Live Longer." *Prevention* (Jan. 1986): 66–70.

127. Ibid.

128. American Automobile Association. *University of California, Berkeley, Wellness Letter* 3 (6)(Mar. 1987).

129. "Use No Restraint Buckling Up." *Prevention* (Jul. 1986): 10.

130. *University of California, Berkeley, Wellness Letter* (Apr. 1988): 7.

131. "Court Rips USA Cars' Seatbelts." *USA Today* (Dec. 12, 1986).

132. Maron, D. J., et al. "Correlates of Seat-Belt Use by Adolescents: Implications for Health Promotion." *Preventive Medicine* 15 (6)(1987): 614–623.

133. *University of California, Berkeley, Wellness Letter* (Apr. 1988): 7.

134. Shimer. "Easiest Way."

135. Lesoin, F., et al. "Has the Safety-belt Replaced the Hangman's Noose?" *Lancet* 1 (8441)(Jun. 8, 1985): 1341.

136. *University of California, Berkeley, Wellness Letter* (Oct. 1987): 7.

137. Meade, J. "Survivor Driving." *Prevention* (Jun. 1986): 64–68.

138. Horton, E. "Irrationality on the Road." *Science Digest* (Aug. 1985): 26.

139. Tsuang, M. T., quoted in Meade. "Survivor."

Step 7: Unlimited Mind and Life Unity (Chapters 43–49)

1. Hooper, J., and Teresi, D. *The Three-Pound Universe: Revolutionary Discoveries About the Brain* (New York: Macmillan, 1986): 2.

2. Winter, A., and Winter, R. *Build Your Brain Power* (New York: St. Martin's, 1986): 1.

3. Nightingale, E. "Our Changing World." Radio program. (Chicago: Nightingale-Conant Corp., 1974).

4. *Discover* (Sep. 1987): 87.

5. Rossi, E. *The Psychobiology of Mind/Body Healing* (New York: Norton, 1987).

6. Saith, T. G., Jr. Paper presented at the Society for Neuroscience meeting Atlanta, GA (Nov. 6, 1979); Frondoza, C. G., et al. "Effects of 6-Hydroxydopamine and Reserpine on the Growth of LPC-1 Plasmacytoma." Paper presented at the Annual Meeting of the Society for Neuroscience, Boston, MA (Nov. 7, 1983).

7. Black, I. B., et al. "Neurotransmitter Plasticity at the Molecular Level." *Science* 225 (4668)(1984): 1266–1270; Kandel, E. R., and Schwartz, J. H. "Molecular Biology of Learning: Modulation of Transmitter Release." *Science* 218 (4571)(1982): 433–443.

8. Merzenich, M., quoted in Hooper and Teresi. *3-Pound Universe:* 61.

9. Pollock, I., et al. "Rehabilitation of Cognitive Function in Brain-Damaged Persons." *Journal of the Medical Society of New Jersey* 81 (4)(Apr. 1984): 311–315; McCusker, E. A., et al. "Recovery from Locked-in Syndrome." *Archives of Neurology* 39 (3)(Mar. 1982): 145–147; World Health Organization. *Treatise on Neuroplasticity and Repair in the Central Nervous System* (Geneva, Switzerland, 1983).

10. Kra, S. *Aging Myths* (New York: McGraw-Hill,

1986); "Building a Better Brain." *Omni Longevity* 1 (1)(Nov. 1986): 1–2; Schaie, K. W. (Ed.). *Longitudinal Studies of Adult Psychological Development* (New York: Guildford Press, 1983); "Senility Reconsidered: Treatment Possibilities for Mental Impairment in the Elderly." Task force sponsored by the National Institute on Aging, Bethesda, MD. *Journal of the American Medical Association* (Jul. 18, 1980): 259–260; Duara, R., et al. "Cerebral Glucose Utilization as Measured with Positron Emission Tomography in 21 Resting Healthy Men Between the Ages of 21 and 83 Years." *Brain* 106 (1983): 761–775; Diamond, M. C., et al. "Differences in Occipital Cortical Synapses from Environmentally Enriched, Impoverished, and Standard Colony Rats." *Journal of Neuroscience Research* 1: 109–119; Rosenzweig, M. R. "Experience, Memory, and the Brain." *American Psychologist* (Apr. 1984).
11. Rosenzweig, M. R., and Bennett, E. "The Physiological Imprint of Aging." U.S. Department of Health Research Grant Report, National Institutes of Health (May 1966) (University of California, Lawrence Berkeley Laboratory) (Jun. 24, 1980); Goleman, D. "The Aging Mind Proves Capable of Lifelong Growth." *New York Times* (Feb. 21, 1984); Diamond, M. C., et al. "Differences."
12. Mandell, A., quoted in Hooper and Teresi. *3-Pound Universe:* 103.
13. Pert, C., quoted in Hooper and Teresi. *3-Pound Universe:* 104.
14. Pribram, K. H. *Holonomic Brain Theory: Cooperativity and Reciprocity in Processing the Configural and Cognitive Aspects of Perception* (New York: Erlbaum Associates, 1988); Pribram, K. H. Lecture, Center for Health & Fitness Excellence, Bemidji, MN (Jun. 13–14, 1987).
15. Suarez, R., Mills, R. C., and Stewart, D. *Sanity, Insanity, and Common Sense* (New York: Fawcett, 1987); Emery, G. "Rapid Cognitive Therapy of Anxiety." Research monograph (Los Angeles Center for Cognitive Therapy, 630 S. Wilton Pl., Los Angeles, CA 90005; 1987): 39–52; Emery, G., and Campbell, J. *Rapid Relief from Emotional Distress* (New York: Fawcett, 1986); Heath, C., et al. "Early Results: A Six Year Post Hoc Followup Study of the Long Term Effectiveness of Neo-Cognitive Psychotherapy." Paper presented at the Seventh Annual Conference on Psychology of Mind (Coral Gables, FL, Apr., 1988); Shuford, R., and Crystal, A. "The Efficacy of a Neo-Cognitive Approach to Positive Psychological Change." Paper presented at the Seventh Annual Conference on Psychology of Mind (Coral Gables, FL, Apr., 1988).
16. Basmajian, J. V. "Control of Individual Motor Units." *American Journal of Physical Medicine* 46 (1967): 1427–1440; Basmajian, J. V. "Electromyography Comes of Age: The Conscious Control of Individual Motor Units in Man May Be Used to Improve His Physical Performance." *Science* 176 (1972): 603–609; Lynch, J. J. *Language of the Heart: The Body's Response to Human Dialogue* (New York: Basic Books, 1985).
17. Isen, A. M. "Toward Understanding the Influence of Positive Affect on Social Behavior, Decision Making, and Problem Solving: The Role of Cognitive Organization." Paper presented at the annual meeting of the American Association for the Advancement of Science, Boston (Feb. 11–15, 1988).
18. Miller, R. C., and Berman, J. S. "The Efficacy of Cognitive Behavior Therapies: A Quantitative Review of the Research Evidence." *Psychological Bulletin* 94 (1983): 39–53; Beck, A. *Cognitive Therapy and the Emotional Disorders* (New York: International Universities Press, 1976); Beck, A., and Emery, G., with Greenberg, L. *Anxiety Disorders and Phobias* (New York: Basic Books, 1985); Burns, D. D. *Feeling Good: The New Mood Therapy* (New York: Signet, 1980); McKay, M., Davis, M., and Fanning, P. *Thoughts and Feelings: The Art of Cognitive Stress Intervention* (Richmond, CA: New Harbinger Publications, 1981).
19. Miller, S. M., and Seligman, M. E. P. "The Reformulated Model of Helplessness and Depression: Evidence and Theory." In Neufeld, R. W. J. (Ed.). *Psychological Stress and Psychopathology* (New York: McGraw-Hill, 1982): 149–179; Peterson, P., and Seligman, M. E. P. "Causal Explanations as a Risk Factor for Depression: Theory and Evidence." *Psychological Review* 91 (3)(1984): 347–374; Seligman, M. E. P. "Helplessness and Explanatory Style: Risk Factor for Depression and Disease." Paper presented at the annual meeting of the Society for Behavioral Medicine, San Francisco (Mar. 1986).
20. Seligman, M. E. P., quoted in Silver, N. "Mind Over Illness: Do Optimists Live Longer?" *American Health* (Nov., 1986): 50–53.
21. Emery. "Rapid Therapy": 49–51.
22. Ibid.
23. Sheikh, A. A. (Ed.). *Imagery: Current Theory, Research, and Application* (New York: Wiley Interscience, 1984); Marks, D. F. (Ed.). *Theories of Image Formation* (New York: Brandon House, 1986); Sheikh, A. A. (Ed.). *Imagination and Healing* (Farmingdale, NY: Baywood, 1984); Sheikh, A. A., and Sheikh, K. S. (Eds.). *Imagery in Education* (Farmingdale, NY: Baywood, 1985); Sheikh, A. A. (Ed.). *Imagery in Sports* (Farmingdale, NY: Baywood, 1988); Suinn, R. M. *Seven Steps to Peak Performance* (Lewiston, NY: Hans Huber Publishers, 1986).
24. Miller, E. E. *Power Vision: Mastering Life Through Mental Image Rehearsal.* Audiotape program and manual (Chicago: Nightingale-Conant Corp., 1987).
25. Kosslyn, S. *Visual Cognition* (Cambridge, MA: MIT Press, 1986).
26. Crum, T. F. *The Magic of Conflict* (New York: Simon and Schuster, 1987): 120.
27. Ray, M., and Myers, R. *Creativity in Business* (New York: Doubleday, 1986): 48–49.
28. Miller, E. E. *Software for the Mind* (Berkeley, CA: Celestial Arts, 1987): 49.
29. Miller. *Power Vision.*

30. Zilbergeld, B., and Lazarus, A. A. *Mind Power: Getting What You Want Through Mental Training* (Boston: Little, Brown, 1987): 19.

31. Sheikh. *Imagery:* 516; Sheikh, A. A. Lectures, Center for Health & Fitness Excellence, Bemidji, MN (Aug. 1984, Jun. 1985, Jun. 1986, and Jun. 1987).

32. *The Neuropsychology of Achievement* (Sybervision Systems, Inc., 6066 Civic Terrace Ave., Newark, CA 94560; 1985).

33. Borysenko, J. *Minding the Body, Mending the Mind* (Reading, MA: Addison-Wesley, 1987): 91–93.

34. Hahn, T. N. *The Miracle of Mindfulness* (Boston: Beacon Press, 1976): 42.

35. Hahn, T. N. *Being Peace* (Parallax Press, P.O. Box 7355, Berkeley, CA 94707, 1987): 4–5.

36. Winter and Winter. *Build Brain Power:* 17–46; 123–124.

37. Suinn. *Seven Steps to Peak Performance:* 42.

38. Elsayad, M., et al. "Intellectual Differences of Adult Men Related to Age and Physical Fitness Before and After an Exercise Program." *Journal of Gerontology* 35 (May 1980): 383–387.

39. "Building Brain." *Omni Longevity.*

40. Sime, W. E. "Psychological Benefits of Exercise." *Advances* (Journal of the Institute for the Advancement of Health, New York) 1 (4)(Fall 1984): 15–29 (90 references cited); Roth, D. L., and Holmes, D. S. "Influence of Aerobic Exercise Training and Relaxation Training on Physical and Psychological Health Following Stressful Life Events." *Psychosomatic Medicine* (Jul./Aug. 1987); Morgan, W. P., and Goldston, S. E. *Exercise and Mental Health* (Washington, DC: Hemisphere Publishing Co., 1987); *Physical Fitness in Business and Industry* (Washington, DC: The President's Council on Physical Fitness and Sports, 1985): 5.

41. Spriduso, W. W. *Journal of Gerontology* 35 (1980): 850.

42. Miller, P. M. *Hilton Head Executive Stamina Program* (New York: Rawson, 1986): 26; McArdle, W. D., Katch, F. I., and Katch, V. L. *Exercise Physiology: Energy, Nutrition, and Human Performance* (Philadelphia: Lea & Febiger, 1986): 451.

43. Goldman, B. *The "E" Factor* (New York: William Morrow, 1988): 5.

44. Wurtman, J. J. *Managing Your Mind and Mood Through Food* (New York: Harper and Row, 1987); Wurtman, R., and Wurtman, J. *Nutrition and the Brain,* vol. 7 (New York: Raven Press, 1986).

45. Goodwin, J. S., et al. "Association Between Nutritional Status and Cognitive Functioning." *Journal of the American Medical Association* 249 (21)(Jun. 3, 1983): 2917–2921.

46. *Neuropsychology* (1985); Cailliet, R., and Gross, L. *The Rejuvenation Strategy* (New York: Doubleday, 1987): 52.

47. "Stress Held Factors in IQ Scores." *New York Times* (May 31, 1983).

48. Jensen, T. S., et al. "Cerebral Atrophy in Young Torture Victims." *New England Journal of Medicine* 307 (21)(Nov. 18, 1982): 1341; McEwen, B. *Rockefeller University Research Profile* (Spring 1984).

49. *Special Report on Aging.* U.S. Department of Health, National Institutes of Health Publication No. 80-1907 (Feb. 1980).

50. Sapolsky, R. "Glucocorticoids and Hippocampal Damage." *Trends in Neurosciences* 10 (1987); McEwen. *Rockefeller University.*

51. Yesavage, J., and Lapp, D., quoted in Toal, J. "The Fear of Forgetting." *American Health* (Oct. 1986): 77–86.

52. Teich, M., and Dodeles, G. "Mind Control: How to Get It, How to Use It, How to Keep It." *Omni* (Oct. 1987): 53–60; Miller, E. E. *Software for the Mind* (Berkeley, CA: Celestial Arts, 1987); Otero, T. M. "Altering Your Inner Limits." In Sheikh, A. A. (Ed.). *Anthology of Imagery Techniques* (American Imagery Institute, P.O. Box 13453, Milwaukee, WI 53213; 1986): 289–311; Suinn. *Seven Steps;* Miller, E. E. Lectures, Center for Health & Fitness Excellence, Bemidji, MN (May 1985, May 1986, and May 1987).

Anchoring is related to holographic/holonomic theory of learning and memory: Pribram, K. H. *Holonomic Brain Theory;* Pribram, K. H. *Languages of the Brain* (New York: Brandon House, 1981). Variations of anchoring have been adapted from the "systematic desensitization" approach of Joseph Wolpe, M.D.: Wolpe, J. *Psychotherapy by Reciprocal Inhibition* (Stanford, CA: Stanford University Press, 1958); Wolpe, J. *The Practice of Behavior Therapy,* 2nd edition (New York: Pergamon Press, 1973); Wolpe, J. *Life Without Fear: Anxiety and Its Cure* (Oakland, CA: New Harbinger, 1988).

53. Teich and Dodeles. "Mind Control": 56.

54. Satir, V. *Conjoint Family Therapy* (Palo Alto, CA: Science and Behavior Books, 1966); Satir, V. *Peoplemaking* (Palo Alto, CA: Science and Behavior Books, 1972).

55. Suinn, R. M. "Visual Motor Behavior Rehearsal: The Basic Technique." *Scandinavian Journal of Behavior Therapy* 13 (3)(1984): 131–142; Suinn. *Seven Steps.*

56. Hartley, R. *Journal of Child Psychology and Psychiatry and Allied Disciplines* 27 (3)(1986); *Psychology Today* (Jan. 1987): 20.

57. McLeod, B. "Rx for Health: A Dose of Self-Confidence." *Psychology Today* (Oct. 1986): 46–50; Kazdin, A. "Covert Modeling, Imagery Assessment and Assertive Behavior." *Journal of Consulting and Clinical Psychology* 43 (5)(1975): 716–724; Kazdin, A. "Comparative Effects of Some Variations in Covert Modeling." *Journal of Behavior Therapy and Experimental Psychiatry* 5 (1974): 225–231; Thase, M. E., and Moss, M. K. "The Relative Efficacy of Covert Modeling Procedures and Guided Par-

ticipant Modeling on the Reduction of Avoidance Behavior." *Journal of Behavior Therapy and Experimental Psychiatry* 7 (1)(1976): 7–12; Kazdin, A. E. "Covert Modeling: The Therapeutic Application of Imagined Rehearsal." In Singer, J. L., and Pope, K., (Eds.). *The Power of Human Imagination* (New York: Plenum, 1978).
58. Suinn. "Visual"; Garfield, C. *Peak Performance: Mental Training Techniques of the World's Greatest Athletes* (New York: Warner, 1984); DeVore, S., and DeVore, G. R. *Sybervision: Muscle Memory Programming* (Chicago: Chicago Review Press, 1981); Loehr, J. E. "The Ideal Performance State." *Science Periodical on Research and Technology in Sport* (Canada: Government of Canada, BU-1, Jan. 1983); Lucas, J. "Anomalies of Human Physical Achievement." *Canadian Journal of History of Sport* (Dec. 1977): 231–247.
59. McLeod. "Rx Health"; McKay et al. *Thoughts and Feelings;* Cameron-Bandler, L., Gordon, D., and Lebeau, M. *The Emprint Method: A Guide to Reproducing Competence* (FuturePace, Inc., P.O. Box 1173, San Rafael, CA 94915; 1985).
60. Feltz, D., and Landers, D. "The Effects of Mental Practice on Motor Skill Learning and Performance: A Meta-Analysis." *Journal of Sports Psychology* 5 (1983): 25–57.
61. Adams, J. L. *The Care and Feeding of Ideas: A Guide to Encouraging Creativity* (Reading, MA: Addison-Wesley, 1986): 159.
62. Jaret, P. "Mind: Why Practice Makes Perfect." *Hippocrates* (Nov./Dec. 1987): 90–91.
63. Cautela, J. "Covert Modeling." Paper presented at the annual meeting of the Association for the Advancement of Behavior Therapy, Washington, DC (Sep. 1971); Kazdin (1973, 1974, 1975); Thase and Moss. "Relative Efficacy."
64. Suinn. "Visual."
65. Suinn. *Seven Steps;* Suinn. "Visual."
66. *Lancet* (Jul. 20, 1985): 134.
67. Kiecolt-Glaser, J. K., and Glaser, R. "Psychological Influences on Immunity." *Psychosomatics* 9 (1986): 621–624; Justice, B. *Who Gets Sick? Thinking and Health* (Los Angeles: J. P. Tarcher, 1987) (more than 1,200 references cited); Solomon, G. *Journal of Neuroscience Research* 18 (1988): 1–9; Hornig-Rohan, M., and Locke, S. E. (Eds.). *Psychological and Behavioral Treatments for Disorders of the Heart and Blood Vessels* (New York: Institute for the Advancement of Health, 1985) (annotated bibliography of 916 recent scientific studies); Locke, S. E. (Ed.). *Psychological and Behavioral Treatments for Disorders Associated with the Immune System* (New York: Institute for the Advancement of Health, 1986) (annotated bibliography of 1,479 recent scientific studies); Locke, S. E., and Hornig-Rohan, M. (Eds.). *Mind and Immunity: Behavioral Immunology* (New York: Institute for the Advancement of Health, 1983) (annotated bibliography of 1,453 recent scientific studies).

68. Pert, C. B., et al. "Neuropeptides and Their Receptors: A Psychosomatic Network." *Journal of Immunology* 135 (2)(1985): 820s–826s.
69. Justice. *Who Gets Sick?:* 14, 85.
70. Rubenstein, E. "Diseases Caused by Impaired Communication Among Cells." *Scientific American* 242 (3)(1980): 102–121; Pearsall, P. *Superimmunity: Master Your Emotions and Improve Your Health* (New York: McGraw-Hill, 1987): 9.
71. Borysenko, J. "Body/Mind: Getting Back in Control." *New Age Journal* (May/Jun. 1987): 17–56.
72. Franklin, J. "The Mind Fixers." *Baltimore Evening Sun* (Jul. 23–31, 1984).
73. Eccles, J. C. "How Mental Events Could Cause Neural Events Analogously to the Probability Fields of Quantum Mechanics." Paper presented at the annual meeting of the Society for Neuroscience, Dallas, TX (Oct. 1985).
74. Justice. *Who Gets Sick?:* 28–29, 38.
75. Locke, S. E. "Adaptation and Immunity: Studies in Humans." *General Hospital Psychiatry* 4 (1982): 49–58.
76. Stone, A. A. *Journal of Personality and Social Psychology* 52 (1987): 988–993.
77. Gottschalk, L. A. "Hope and Other Deterrents to Illness." *American Journal of Psychotherapy* 39 (4)(1985): 515–524; Kaplan, G. A., and Camacho, T. "Perceived Health and Mortality." *American Journal of Epidemiology* 117 (3)(1983): 292–304; Scheier, M. F., and Carver, C. S. "Optimism, Coping, and Health." *Health Psychology* 4 (3)(1985): 219–247.
78. Vaillant, G. E. "Natural History of Male Psychologic Health: Effects of Mental Health on Physical Health." *New England Journal of Medicine* 301 (1979): 1249–1254; Vaillant, G. E., quoted in Goleman, D. "Research Affirms Power of Positive Thinking." *New York Times* (Feb. 3, 1987).
79. Goleman. "Positive Thinking."
80. Case, R. B., and Heller, S. "Behavior and Survival of Type A Personalities After Acute Myocardial Infarction." *New England Journal of Medicine* 312 (12)(1985): 737–741.
81. Wechsler, R. "A New Prescription: Mind Over Malady." *Discover* (Feb. 1987): 51–61; Blalock, J. E., et al. "Peptide Hormones Shared by the Neuroendocrine and Immunologic Systems." *Journal of Immunology* 135 (1985): 858s–861s.
82. Pert, C. B. "Neuropeptides: The Emotions and Bodymind." *Noetic Sciences Review* (Spring 1987): 13–18.
83. McClelland, D. C., et al. "Stressed Power Motivation, Sympathetic Activation, Immune Function, and Illness." *Journal of Human Stress* 6 (2)(1980): 11–19.
84. Diamond, M. Quoted in "Building Brain." *Omni Longevity.*
85. Kandel, E. R., and Schwartz, J. H. "Molecular Biology of Learning: Modulation of Transmitter Release." *Science* 218 (4571)(1982): 433–443; Clark, G. "Cell Bio-

logical Analysis of Associative and Non-Associative Learning." Paper presented at the annual meeting of the American Association for the Advancement of Science, New York (May 26, 1984); News feature, University of Illinois at Urbana (May 26, 1984).

86. *Special Report on Aging.* U.S. Department of Health, National Institutes of Health Publication No. 80-1907 (Feb. 1980).

87. Coleman, P., quoted in "Building Brain." *Omni Longevity.*

88. Shaie. *Longitudinal Studies;* Rosenzweig and Bennett. "Psychological Imprint of Learning"; Winter and Winter. *Build Brain Power:* 6.

89. Toal, J. "The Seven Flavors of Intelligence." *American Health* (Jul. 1987): 63–67.

90. Diamond, M. C. "The Aging Rat Forebrain: Male-Female Left-Right: Environment and Lipofuscion." In Samuel, D., et al. (Eds.). *Aging and the Brain* (New York: Raven Press, 1983): 93–98.

91. Streufert, S., et al. "Effects of Load Stressors, Cognitive Complexity, and Type-A Coronary Prone Behavior on Visual-Motor Task Performance." *Journal of Personality and Social Psychology* 48 (3)(Mar. 1985): 728–739; Penn State study. Cited in Mazer, E. "Sharp Minds Last Forever." *Prevention* (Jul. 1985): 6.

92. Nelson, R. J., et al. "Variations in the Proportional Representations of the Hand in Somatosensory Cortex of Primates." Paper presented at the Society for Neuroscience meeting, Boston, MA (Nov. 13, 1980); Jenkins, W. M., et al. Coleman Memorial Laboratories, University of California at San Francisco. Paper presented at the Society for Neuroscience meeting, Anaheim, CA (Oct. 13, 1984).

93. "The Cerebellum: Loss of Cellular Function in the Aging Brain." *The Salk Institute Newsletter* 27 (Winter 1981): 1–4; Liebman, B. *Nutrition Action* (Nov. 1981): 9.

94. Winter and Winter. *Build Brain Power:* 17–43.

95. Cattell, R. B. *Abilities: Their Structure, Growth and Action* (Boston: Houghton Mifflin, 1971).

96. Elsayad et al. "Intellectual Differences."

97. Adams, J. L. *The Care and Feeding of Ideas: A Guide to Encouraging Creativity* (Reading, MA: Addison-Wesley, 1986): 159.

98. Sandman, C., quoted in *Psychology Today* (Nov. 1987): 20.

99. Adams. *Care:* 4–7.

100. Ray and Myers. *Creativity:* 7.

101. Gondola, J., and Tuckman, B. *Journal of Social Behavior and Personality* 1 (1)(1986).

102. Adams. *Care:* 52–53.

103. Goldberg, P. *The Intuitive Edge* (Los Angeles: J. P. Tarcher, 1984): 168–169.

104. Ray and Myers. *Creativity:* 158, 170.

105. Ruggiero, V. R. *The Art of Thinking* (New York: Harper and Row, 1984).

106. Chapman, L. S. "Spiritual Health: A Component Missing from Health Promotion." *American Journal of Health Promotion* 1 (1)(Summer 1986): 38–41.

107. Pelletier, K. R. *Longevity: Fulfilling Our Biological Potential* (New York: Delacorte, 1981); Wolf, S., et al. *Occupational Health as Human Ecology* (Springfield, IL: Thomas, 1978).

108. Bloom, A. *The Closing of the American Mind* (New York: Simon and Schuster, 1987); Bloom, A., quoted in "The Closing of the American Mind." *Publishers Weekly* (Jul. 3, 1987): 25–28.

109. Nietzsche, F., quoted in *Time* (Feb. 2, 1968): 38.

110. "Love May Speed Relief." *USA Today* (Nov. 28, 1986); Siegel, B. S. *Love, Medicine, and Miracles* (New York: Harper and Row, 1986).

111. Lynch, J. J. *Broken Heart: The Medical Consequences of Loneliness* (New York: Basic Books, 1977).

112. Allen, R. F., and Allen, J. "A Sense of Community, a Shared Vision and a Positive Culture." *American Journal of Health Promotion* 1 (3)(Winter 1987): 40–47.

113. Boyce, W. T., et al. "Permanence and Change: Psychosocial Factors." *Social Science and Medicine* 21 (11)(1985): 1279–1287.

114. Jaffe, D. T. *Healing from Within* (New York: Bantam, 1982): 130.

115. Palmore, E. B. "Physical, Mental and Social Factors in Predicting Longevity." *Gerontologist* 9 (2)(Summer 1969): 103–108; Palmore, E. B. "Predicting Longevity: A Follow-up Controlling for Age." *Gerontologist* 9 (4)(Winter 1969): 247–250.

116. Beauvoir, S. *The Coming of Age* (New York: Putnam, 1972).

117. Rimland, B. "The Altruism Paradox." *Psychological Reports* 51 (2)(Oct. 1982): 521–522.

118. Ornstein, R., and Sobel, D. *The Healing Brain* (New York: Simon and Schuster, 1987): 66.

119. Dass, R., and Gormon, P. *How Can I Help?* (New York: Knopf, 1985): 5.

120. Chapman. "Spiritual Health": 41.

Index

About the Author

Robert K. Cooper earned his Ph.D. in health education and psychology at the Union Graduate School in Cincinnati. He has also taken graduate work in psychology from the University of Michigan and in biomedical journalism from the University of Iowa and has directed university and medical school research projects.

Dr. Cooper is certified as a Health and Fitness Instructor by the American College of Sports Medicine and as a Fitness Specialist by the Institute for Aerobics Research (Kenneth H. Cooper, M.D., M.P.H., president). A health educator, performance researcher, and All-American athlete, he carries forward the University of Michigan's Honor Trophy Award for "outstanding achievement in scholarship, athletics, and leadership." He has devoted twenty years to the research and development of *Health & Fitness Excellence*.

He is a professional member of the American College of Sports Medicine, Association for the Advancement of Health Education, Association for Fitness in Business, National Wellness Association, and National Speakers Association and serves on the advisory board of the *Living Well* media series.

Dr. Cooper is the president of Advanced Excellence Systems, a corporate training and consulting firm. He presents lectures and seminars for health symposiums, business and educational organizations, and other groups worldwide.

Lectures, Seminars, Corporate Consultations, Professional Programs

Robert K. Cooper, Ph.D., is available to present a variety of programs ranging in scope from keynote addresses, lectures, and in-depth consulting to week-long seminars and workshops. Each presentation is tailored to the specific needs of corporations, professional associations, educational institutions, or the general public. For further information, contact:

Robert K. Cooper, Ph.D.
Advanced Excellence Systems
P.O. BOX 1475
BEMIDJI, MN 56601
218-854-7300

Publications and Audiotapes

To order additional copies of this book or the *Health & Fitness Excellence* audiotape series, *The Health & Fitness Excellence Cookbook,* or related publications, contact:

Advanced Excellence Systems
P.O. BOX 1085
BEMIDJI, MN 56601

To use your VISA, American Express, or MasterCard, call 218-854-7300 or, toll-free, 1-800-22-EXCEL (for orders only).